NURSING CARE PLANNING GUIDES FOR MENTAL HEALTH

NURSING CARE PLANNING GUIDES FOR MENTAL HEALTH

Edited by

JOAN W. REIGHLEY, MN, RN

Psychotherapist and Assistant Professor of Nursing
West Los Angeles College
Los Angeles, California

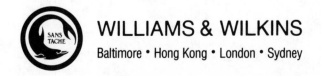

WILLIAMS & WILKINS
Baltimore • Hong Kong • London • Sydney

Editors: Rose Mary Carroll-Johnson and Mary Paquette
Associate Editor: Linda Napora
Copy Editor: Catherine Chambers
Design: JoAnne Janowiak
Cover Design: A. Marshall Licht
Production: Raymond E. Reter

Copyright © 1988
Williams & Wilkins
428 East Preston Street
Baltimore, MD 21202, USA

Printed in the United States of America

Library of Congress Cataloging in Publication Data

Nursing care planning guides for mental health/edited by Joan W. Reighley.
   p. cm.
  Bibliography: p.
  Includes index.
  1. Psychiatric nursing. 2. Nursing care plans. I. Reighley, Joan, 1936-.
  [DNLM: 1. Mental Disorders—nursing. 2. Patient Care Planning.
  WY 160 N9743]
RC440.N856 1988
610.73′68—dc19
DNLM/DLC   87-28056
for Library of Congress   CIP

ISBN 0-683-09577-3

88 89 90 91
1 2 3 4 5 6 7 8 9 10

Foreword

This book introduces what has been long overdue in psychiatric clinical nursing practice: A thorough, yet concise, portrayal of patients experiencing a variety of disturbances and behaviors with *specific* guidelines as to how to deal with them. All too often books on psychiatric nursing practice identify theory but do not offer practical information on diagnosis and intervention. So the clinician is left to "jump in where others fear to tread," without design and direction. Joan Reighley's book fills the gap between theoretical books on psychiatric and psychosocial issues and the nurse at the side of the patient.

Patients who enter a hospital or other treatment arena begin a journey on the road to relief from pain and symptoms, and an understanding of their condition. The nurse acts as a guide on this journey. The dictionary definition of guide is "to assist a person to travel through or reach a destination in an area in which he does not know the way, as by accompanying him or giving him direc-

tions." These nursing care planning guides are the accompaniment to the nurse who in turn assists the patient. Together they travel on their journey of "the plight of the human condition." The guides reflect that this journey is not a random happening but a compassionate and knowledgeable endeavor to reach a destination.

Although this book will be most useful for nurses working directly with patients, it will also be helpful to students, instructors, and administrative planning teams. It is an excellent resource to accompany more theoretical material in order to enhance understanding of the issues involved in psychiatric and psychosocial nursing.

Corrine L. Hatton, MN, RN, CS
Clinical Specialist, Mental Health
Private Practice, Los Angeles, California
Clinical Associate
Los Angeles Institute for Psychoanalytic Studies

Preface

Nursing Care Planning Guides for Mental Health is intended as a reference for planning nursing care for patients with psychosocial problems or psychiatric conditions; the expanded clinical focus includes guides on the Patient with Borderline Personality Disorder, Dependent Personality Disorder, Post-Traumatic Stress Disorder, and AIDS, as well as psychosocial problems through the lifespan: child, adolescent, adult, and aging individual. It is designed to assist the nurse or nursing student to prepare individualized care plans based on nursing process, using nursing diagnosis. Features of each guide include definition of the condition, nursing assessment, long-term goals, possible nursing diagnoses with rationale, goals for care, specific nursing interventions, and evaluation criteria to measure goal attainment. The reader is encouraged to select those aspects of care appropriate to the individual patient.

The *DSM-III-R* (*Diagnostic and Statistical Manual of Mental Disorders*, American Psychiatric Association, 1987) nomenclature have been included; this is a diagnostic classification system that is used in a variety of settings, using diagnostic categories acceptable to clinicians with a variety of professional backgrounds and theoretical orientations.

These guides should be used in conjunction with textbooks, periodicals, and other supplemental resources.

In 1981, the first edition of Nurseco's *Nursing Care Planning Guides for Psychiatric and Mental Health Care* by Margo Neal, Patricia Cohen, Phyllis Cooper, and Joan Reighley was introduced; a second edition followed in 1985. Our purpose was to assist nurses to provide the highly specialized care required in mental health settings. We are gratified to know that these books were well received and used by nurses and nursing students.

Nurses are taking increasing responsibility and accountability in providing health care in a rapidly changing and complex health care system; these guides have been written to be useful in this very important effort.

Acknowledgments

My heartfelt thanks to family and friends who have given me nourishment during this project; I also wish to thank clients, clinicians, and teachers who have shared their thoughts, feelings, and questions with me. I appreciate the professional support of Margo Neal, Rose Mary Carroll-Johnson, and the contributors to this book.

Contributors

Marjorie Buck, MN, RN
Clinical Nurse Specialist
A Child's Garden Preschool
Albuquerque, New Mexico

Marie Thonis Colucci, MN, RN
Associate Professor
Riverside City College
Riverside, California

Cindy Smith Greenberg, MS, RN, CPNP
Assistant Professor, Maternal Child Nursing
California State University, Long Beach
Long Beach, California

Wendy W. Hollis, MN, RN
Assistant Professor of Nursing
Los Angeles Harbor College
Wilmington, California

Susan Warren Horelick, MSN, RN
Staff Nurse
St. John's Lutheran Hospital
Libby, Montana

Retha Vornholt Keenan, MSN, RN
Instructor, Mental Health Nursing
Los Angeles Community College District
Los Angeles, California
El Camino Community College District
Torrance, California

Debra Jean Nash, MS, RN
Visiting Lecturer
University of California, Los Angeles
Los Angeles, California

Joan W. Reighley, MN, RN
Psychotherapist and Assistant Professor of Nursing
West Los Angeles College
Los Angeles, California

Patti Roberts, MSN Candidate, BSN, RN, CPNP
Certified Pediatric Nurse Practitioner
CIGNA Healthplans
Long Beach, California

Sarah Rothery, MS, RN
Clinical Nurse Specialist, Child Development Service
University of Massachusetts Medical Center
Worcester, Massachusetts

Ann M. Schofield, MS, RN
Lecturer in Nursing
California State University, Los Angeles
Los Angeles, California

Contents

Introduction

Nursing process is the method by which the professional nurse acts to improve the health status of patients. It is applied in the context of the patient's medical diagnosis but leads the nurse to develop strategies individual to the particular patient's needs.

There are five steps to the process
1. Assessment
2. Analysis
3. Plan
4. Implementation
5. Evaluation

The guides developed in this book detail each of these steps for commonly encountered medical conditions. By extrapolating from each section the information pertinent to the particular client and by adapting the nursing plan in light of the patient needs and the physician's orders, the reader can arrive at a plan of care designed to enhance the patient's chances of attaining maximum health.

Each part of the nursing process builds on and grows out of the preceding step. In addition, the process is cyclical and ongoing. In this context, then, specific information is presented for specific kinds of patient problems.

Assessment, the organized, systematic, and purposeful gathering of information about a patient's current or future health, is essential to permit grouping or clustering of data for analysis leading to identification of nursing concerns or nursing diagnosis. Assessment data are compiled from the patient record, through physical examination, and by interviews with the patient, family members, or other health care professionals; however, the most important source of information is the patient.

To assist the nurse in clustering data, four components of a nursing assessment have been identified. They are *pertinent history, physical findings, psychosocial concerns and developmental factors,* and *patient and family knowledge* about the condition and its treatment.

Pertinent history includes the precipitating events and/ or illnesses leading to the patient's current condition. This information may already be documented in the patient record or the nurse may have to structure the nursing interview to ensure gathering of meaningful data. Knowing the patient's history enables the nurse to better interpret other aspects of the nursing assessment, leading to more valid nursing diagnoses and appropriate selection of specific strategies likely to be effective in assisting the patient in achieving desired goals.

The nursing physical examination, routinely performed on patients at the time of admission, provides a physical overview of the patient from head to toe. In the physical findings section of each nursing care planning guide, you will find key physical assessment data especially significant for the condition under discussion. Sometimes this will be specific manifestations or abnormalities you may expect to find. In other cases it was more appropriate to list specific parameters needing assessment. Additionally, many guides include laboratory findings that aid the physician in making a diagnosis and that the nurse can expect to monitor while caring for a patient with that specific condition.

Understanding the ways in which a person has been influenced by society and by cultural heritage, and knowing the expected developmental tasks for a person of a given age are helpful in predicting patient responses and in planning specific nursing interventions to achieve desired goals. Information about previous coping strategies and existing functional support systems provides clues to identifying psychosocial nursing diagnoses. Additionally, certain patient conditions are more likely to be manifested in specific ethnic or age groups. For these reasons, the psychosocial concerns and developmental variations likely to be associated with the condition described in the nursing care planning guide are highlighted.

In current nursing practice, it is imperative that discharge planning begin at the time of admission to the health care agency. To help the nurse assess the learning needs of patients and families, important aspects of the condition and treatment plan that the patient needs to promote compliance after discharge are listed. Each nursing care planning guide includes the nursing diagnosis "Knowledge deficit." The nurse's choice to use the suggested diagnosis, to adapt it to the specific learning needs of the patient/family, or identify a more relevant diagnosis depends upon the interpretation of the assessment data obtained concerning the patient's and family's baseline knowledge.

Just as nursing diagnosis provides a framework for nursing practice, an organized nursing assessment is essential to identifying valid nursing diagnoses for a particular patient. An incomplete or incorrect database will interfere with the identification of actual or potential problems. Therefore, by systematically reviewing or obtaining information about the patient's pertinent history, physical findings, psychosocial concerns and developmental variations, and the patient's and family's knowledge of the condition and treatment, the nurse ensures that a complete database is collected. The stage is set for competent analysis leading to identification of pertinent nursing diagnoses as a framework for providing care.

A **nursing diagnosis** is a statement of a nursing problem based on a critical appraisal and analysis of the assessment data. It represents those activities the nurse performs that acknowledge her/his independent functioning. Nursing diagnosis is an ongoing process, not restricted only to the written nursing care plan.

Within the scope of individual state nurse practice law there are important aspects of both dependent and independent functions. The dependent dimensions of nursing practice describe those interventions the nurse cannot legally prescribe. For example, the nurse cannot prescribe nitroglycerin to a patient admitted with acute chest pain. The nurse requires an order from the physician prior to the administration of that medication. This represents the dependent domain of nursing. The independent dimension of nursing practice on the other hand describes those interventions the nurse can legally prescribe. An example of this is a patient in traction who complains of boredom and frustration because of confinement to bed. The nurse may in this situation prescribe diversional activities such as television or referral to volunteer services to obtain books or magazines.

The important aspect to consider when identifying nursing diagnoses is that the diagnostic statement describes an actual or potential problem that nurses, because of their education and experience, are licensed and legally responsible and accountable to treat. Therefore, nursing diagnoses are different from other patient-related problems that are the responsibility of other health care providers.

The nursing diagnosis is written as a two-part statement—the nursing diagnostic statement and the etiology/ contributing factors. For example,

Ineffective individual coping related to chronicity of disease condition, effect on usual roles and responsibilities, inadequate support system

The nursing diagnosis directs the nurse in terms of her/ his goals and interventions. Nursing diagnoses may apply to either individuals or groups. That is, not all diagnostic statements refer only to the patient. The family member or significant other may also require nursing actions in order to ensure a successful patient outcome.

Nursing diagnoses utilized in this book have been established and approved by the North American Nursing Diagnosis Association. A complete list can be found in Appendix I.

Planning is the third step in the nursing process and follows patient-specific assessment and diagnosis of nursing problems. Planning allows nursing care to be delivered in a logical, organized, goal-directed, patient-centered manner and directs the implementation and evaluation of nursing care. Planning always occurs prior to implementation of nursing actions. In emergency situations planning may occur simultaneously with implementation because of the acuity of the situation.

Planning involves
- prioritizing patient problems
- establishing patient-centered goals
- stating specific nursing actions/interventions for each problem

The changing environment of the health care setting necessitates that the nurse set priorities to allow for appropriate delivery of care to the patient in a time-efficient, cost-effective manner, thus enabling one to address the patient's biopsychosocial needs more completely. Prioritization is influenced by patient status, the degree of urgency with which the patient views the problem, the treatment plan, and potential complications. The nursing care section of each care plan has been organized in order of decreasing priority to assist the reader in this process.

When establishing goals, the nurse collaborates with the patient, when possible. Mutually agreed-upon goals foster patient compliance and motivation. The best goals reflect the prior nursing assessment and diagnosis. Included in each plan are both short- and long-term goals to promote optimal wellness. Goals need to reflect observable behaviors so that the nurse can measure progress toward the goal or lack thereof.

Implementation is the fourth step in the nursing process. It is during this step that the plan of care is put into action through ongoing assessment, actual performance of bedside nursing actions, appropriate charting of nursing care that has been given, and communication with other health team members. Nursing actions need to be individualized for each patient. They are developed to meet the established goals and should direct care to answer the questions who, where, what, when, how, and how often. The need for assessment of changing patient status is invaluable in providing current and relevant information to maintain a plan of care. As the client moves along the health-illness continuum, the nursing role increasingly focuses on patient/family education and maximizing self-care abilities. The need for quality care and equally good documentation is essential to maintain a care plan reflective of the patient's changing status.

Evaluation, the last step of the nursing process, includes observing the patient's response to the nursing actions; determining the patient's progress towards the goals, objectives, expected outcomes; and revising or modifying the written care plan accordingly.

The patient's estimation of progress towards the goal and degree of satisfaction with the outcome is an essential part of the evaluation process. In addition, family or significant others, the chart, and appropriate health team members are also consulted. Data from each source should confirm and validate the data from other sources; inconsistent findings require further investigation to determine reasons for discrepancies.

When the patient's response to the nursing actions and progress towards the goals are evaluated, a number of outcomes are possible. If the goal has been achieved and the identified need/problem has been resolved, the nurse determines the next priority. If progress is being made but the goal has not been reached, nursing interventions can be continued, discontinued, or modified. If there has been no progress toward the goal, the nurse asks the following questions:

1. Is the goal realistic for this patient and this situation? Does it need to be changed? Does the critical time need to be changed? What factors were involved in progress or lack of progress towards goal?
2. Was the nursing diagnosis accurate? Were data overlooked or are there new data to include? Have new problems emerged that need attention? Is this the patient's priority or is there some other need/problem that seems more important to the patient?
3. Are the nursing actions effective/ineffective? Are there other options to try? Consult with peers, supervisors, and current professional literature.

Revise or modify the care plan as necessary according to answers to these questions. The nursing process is dynamic and cyclic; ongoing evaluation provides valuable information to keep nursing process effective and nursing practice accountable.

The act of planning patient care by using the nursing process is an integral part of modern professional nursing care. The user of this book, be it the nursing student or the experienced nurse, will find it to be an invaluable reference not just to nursing process but to the dynamic, ever-changing arena of individualized nursing care plans.

Bibliography

Carpenito, L. (1987). *Handbook of nursing diagnosis* (2nd ed.). Philadelphia: Lippincott.

Carpenito, L. (1987). *Nursing diagnosis: Application to clinical practice* (2nd ed.). Philadelphia: Lippincott.

Gordon, M. (1986). *Nursing diagnosis: Process and application* (2nd ed.). New York: McGraw-Hill.

ADULTS

The Patient with Acquired Immune Deficiency Syndrome

Definition/Discussion

Acquired immune deficiency syndrome (AIDS) is an impairment of the body's immune system occurring in previously healthy individuals. This impairment makes these individuals vulnerable to a variety of infectious agents that might not otherwise cause disease. AIDS virus antibodies can be detected in the blood by a simple test, usually 2 weeks to 3 months after infection. Once an individual is infected, there are several possibilities. Some people remain well but even so they are able to infect others. Others may develop a disease that is less serious than AIDS, referred to as AIDS Related Complex (ARC). Other infected people may develop classic AIDS, with impairment of the immune system, opportunistic diseases, and impairment of the nervous system, and damage to the brain.

The extremely grave prognosis of AIDS, its relative newness (first identified in 1981), accelerating incidence, and the connotation of being associated with minority social groups (homosexuals and IV drug users) all combine to make AIDS a psychosocial problem as well as a medical disorder. The public is fearfully distrustful of AIDS patients, resulting in social isolation. This social isolation is distressing for all AIDS patients, but particularly for the so-called "innocent" victims of AIDS, the children who were born to high-risk women (sexual partners of high-risk males) and those who contracted AIDS after receiving contaminated blood products. There is no known cure.

Nursing Assessment

☐ PERTINENT HISTORY

Weight loss of more than 10 lb during a period of less than 2 months, unrelated to diet or increased activity; prolonged loss of appetite; unexplained, persistent, or recurrent fevers, chills, or night sweats; profound fatigue that is not transient or explained by physical activity, substance abuse, or a psychologic disorder; persistent and unexplained diarrhea or bloody stools; inclusion in a high-risk group (e.g., sexually active homosexual or bisexual men, intravenous drug users, Haitian immigrants, hemophiliacs and other frequent transfusion recipients)

☐ PHYSICAL FINDINGS

Lymphadenopathy in neck, axillae, and groin unexplained by other illness; whitish coating or spotting on the throat or tongue associated with painful swallowing; dry, persistent cough unrelated to smoking; purplish skin lesions or other new growths on top of or beneath the skin, on oral, nasal, or anal mucous membranes, or beneath the eyelids (Kaposi's sarcoma); herpetic lesions; general debility; laboratory studies indicating immunosuppression and presence of micro-organisms; myoclonus, seizures, incontinence, weakness, ataxia, tremor

☐ PSYCHOSOCIAL CONCERNS/ DEVELOPMENTAL FACTORS

Expressed or denied anxiety about uncertain etiology and grave prognosis; physical limitations imposed as disease progresses likely to interfere with ability to continue usual occupational role, possibly resulting in increased dependency in social and familial roles; effects of societal attitudes (e.g., fear, distrust, condemnation, pity, ostracism) on attainment of developmental tasks, self-esteem, social isolation, and control; symptoms of dementia (e.g., confusion, delayed verbal response, disinhibition, loss of memory, vacant stare, psychotic verbalization, hallucinations)

☐ PATIENT AND FAMILY KNOWLEDGE

Level of knowledge, readiness and willingness to learn, disease process, associated risk factors, treatments, precautions, screening tests, fears, coping strategies

Nursing Care

☐ LONG-TERM GOAL

The patient will be maintained in a state of biopsychosocial integrity with as much independence and community con-

tact as possible, adhering to treatment regimen, living within restrictions, and adjusting to actual/potential losses.

NURSING DIAGNOSIS #1

Potential for infection related to immuno-suppression

Rationale: Current investigations into the etiology of AIDS suggest it is initiated by a viral agent. The AIDS virus has been given several names: HIV (Human Immunodeficiency Virus), HTLV-III (Human T-Lymphotropic Virus Type III), LAC (Lymphadenopathy Associated Virus). The AIDS virus attacks white blood cells (t-lymphocytes) in the human blood. Because of the body's inability to fight off disease, the AIDS patient is particularly vulnerable to opportunistic infections caused by protozoa (e.g., Pneumocystis carinii, Toxoplasma gondii, and Enamoeba histolytica), viruses (e.g., cytomegalovirus [CMV], herpes simplex, and herpes zoster), bacteria (e.g., Mycobacterium tuberculosis, Klebsiella pneumonia, and Salmonella enteritidis), and fungi (e.g., Candida albicans and Cryptococcus neoformans).

☐ **GOAL**

The patient will be maintained in appropriate isolation; will be monitored for early signs of infection; staff, other patients, and visitors will be free from contagion.

☐ **IMPLEMENTATION**

- Maintain isolation as per hospital protocol; precautions include
  - gloving whenever the care giver anticipates contact with the patient's body fluids, secretions, or excretions
  - wearing a gown if the patient has copious secretions or excretions
  - wearing a mask if performing a procedure in which secretions or excretions might splatter inadvertently
- It is not necessary to use isolation techniques when entering the room to talk with the patient or to administer an oral medication.
- Arrange for a private room; do not place 2 AIDS patients in the same room since they may have different organisms involved and may acquire others through cross-contamination.
- Routinely clean patient-care surfaces with soap and water.
- Take extraordinary care to avoid self-wounds from sharp instruments contaminated with potentially infectious material (e.g., blood, excreta).
- Use disposable needles and syringes only, if feasible; if reusable syringes must be used, terminally decontaminate them before cleaning and repackaging.
- Do not bend needles after use, but promptly place in a puncture-resistant container used solely for such disposal; do not reinsert needles into their original sheaths before discarding them (a common cause of needle injury).
- Use only Luer-Lok syringes or 1-piece needle-syringe units to aspirate fluids from patients, so that collected fluid can be safely discharged through the needle.
- Maintain meticulous sterile technique; ensure used instruments are cleaned and sterilized.
- Carefully monitor vital signs and laboratory tests ordered for signs of infection.
- Administer antimicrobial therapy as ordered, carefully monitoring for side effects/toxicity.
- Caution visitors about exposing the patient to infections; teach them to observe isolation precautions, especially good handwashing, before and after entering patient's room.
- Advise pregnant women (visitors and staff) to avoid contact with the patient because of the possibility of exposure to CMV.
- Avoid unnecessary exaggeration of isolation precautions or avoiding the patient to prevent physical and emotional isolation.

☐ **EVALUATION CRITERIA/DESIRED OUTCOMES**

The Patient
- Maintains isolation precautions
- Has signs and symptoms of new infection detected early
- Is protected from cross-contamination from other patients, visitors, or staff

---

NURSING DIAGNOSES #2
a. **Impaired skin integrity** (perineal) related to immunosuppression
b. **Alteration in oral mucous membranes** related to immunosuppression

Rationale: The patient's immune deficiency increases the risk for skin and mucous membrane lesions. Common skin problems include Kaposi's sarcoma, herpetic lesions, or candidiasis.

☐ **GOAL**

The patient will experience maximum possible comfort; will maintain integrity of skin and mucous membranes.

☐ **IMPLEMENTATION**

- Provide skin care at least every 4 hours or more frequently if needed (diaphoresis and diarrhea are extremely irritating to the skin).

- Change linen frequently and give sponge baths when fever is present.
- Clean skin lesions with warm, soapy water; rinse and apply dressing and antimicrobial ointment if ordered, covering with a nonadherent pad.
- Cleanse rectal area after each bowel movement with warm, soapy water; when herpetic lesions are present, rinse and pat dry with soft cloth, not toilet paper.
- Brush teeth with soft toothbrush to treat oral candida; follow with half-strength peroxide mouthwash; offer oral care every 2-4 hours.
- Ensure position change at least every 2 hours; obtain an egg-crate or alternating pressure mattress when indicated.

☐ EVALUATION CRITERIA/DESIRED OUTCOMES

The Patient
- Expresses a feeling of comfort
- Is free from skin breakdown, oral pain or lesions

NURSING DIAGNOSES #3
a. **Ineffective airway clearance** related to viscous secretions, ineffective cough, fatigue
b. **Ineffective breathing patterns** related to severe, nonrelieved cough
c. **Impaired gas exchange** related to loss of functioning lung tissue secondary to opportunistic respiratory infection (specify causative agent if known)

Rationale: Pneumonia secondary to Pneumocystis carnii or CMV is a common complication of AIDS. If not successfully treated, respiratory failure may contribute to the cause(s) of death. A nonproductive, chronic cough may be one of the presenting symptoms that causes the person to seek medical attention initially.

☐ GOAL

The patient will maintain pulmonary function; will have a decreased risk of aspiration; will demonstrate improved gas exchange; will experience relief from symptoms of pain, weakness, and dyspnea; will demonstrate effective coughing and energy conservation.

☐ IMPLEMENTATION

- Obtain a baseline assessment of respiratory function including relevant history, respiratory rate and character, use of accessory muscles, breath sounds, skin color, general appearance, and arterial blood gases.
- Monitor use and effectiveness of ordered thera-

pies such as oxygen, mechanical ventilation, humidification, chest tubes, and pharmaceuticals.
- Reassess respiratory status every 2 hours or as necessary for signs and symptoms of respiratory insufficiency/failure (e.g., tachypnea, tachycardia, dyspnea, apprehension, irritability, or confusion).
- Administer antitussives/expectorants as ordered; note effectiveness.
- Suction at least every 2 hours; obtain specimens as ordered; carefully monitor lab results.
- Administer antimicrobials on time as ordered; observe carefully for side effects/toxicity.
- Administer antipyretic to control temperature; note effect on fever.
- Monitor blood gases; report significant changes and modify ventilatory settings as ordered.
- Provide humidification and intermittent positive pressure breathing with postural drainage as ordered; turn, cough, deep breathe, and encourage inspirometer use at least every 2 hours.
- Organize nursing care to permit periods of uninterrupted rest.
- Administer narcotic analgesics and sedatives cautiously; evaluate response.

☐ EVALUATION CRITERIA/DESIRED OUTCOMES

The Patient
- Has decreased dyspnea on exertion
- Expectorates secretions
- Expresses relief from symptoms causing discomfort
- Demonstrates improved respiratory functioning
- Has blood gas values within normal limits

NURSING DIAGNOSES #4
a. **Alteration in nutrition: less than body requirements** related to catabolic state, anorexia, difficulty swallowing
b. **Impaired swallowing** related to esophagitis

Rationale: In the presence of infection, metabolic requirements are increased. Preexisting mouth lesions or esophageal lesions may make chewing or swallowing painful, decreasing the patient's incentive to eat and further compromising the immune status.

☐ GOAL

The patient will receive adequate intake to meet metabolic requirements.

☐ IMPLEMENTATION

- Carefully record daily weights, oral intake, and calorie counts.

- Encourage full consumption of prescribed diet; give soft foods and liquids; have family and friends bring in favorite foods; provide small high-protein, high-calorie supplements between meals.
- Administer supplemental vitamins and minerals.
- Initiate referral to dietician as needed.
- If patient is unable to maintain sufficient oral intake, consult with physician about starting tube feedings. (Hyperalimentation is not advised because of the associated risk of infection.)

☐ **EVALUATION CRITERIA/DESIRED OUTCOMES**

The Patient
- Increases intake with resultant gain or stabilization of weight
- Improves skin turgor and condition of skin, hair, nails, and mucous membranes

---

NURSING DIAGNOSIS #5

Alteration in bowel elimination: diarrhea related to opportunistic bowel infection (specify agent if known), prescribed medication (specify drug), tube feeding intolerance

Rationale: Protozoan and bacterial infections of the bowel will likely present as diarrhea. Antimicrobial medications and tube feedings may be poorly tolerated by individual patients with the intolerance manifested as diarrhea.

☐ **GOAL**

The patient will experience maximum comfort and control of diarrhea.

☐ **IMPLEMENTATION**

- Encourage fluids, maintaining an oral intake of 3,000 cc/day to prevent dehydration.
- Cleanse and carefully dry rectal area after each bowel movement.
- Administer antidiarrheal agents as ordered.
- If causative factor is thought to be medication or tube feeding, consult with physician about the possibility of changing prescribed medication or tube-feeding formula.

☐ **EVALUATION CRITERIA/DESIRED OUTCOMES**

The Patient
- Has decreased number of stools/day
- Expresses a feeling of comfort
- Has a balanced intake and output

NURSING DIAGNOSES #6
a. **Grieving** related to diagnosis, loss of healthy status
b. **Ineffective individual/family coping** related to diagnosis, life-style choices
c. **Impaired social interaction** related to isolation precautions, grieving over diagnosis
d. **Social isolation** related to societal nonacceptance of disease

Rationale: The seriousness of an AIDS diagnosis challenges the coping resources of the strongest individuals and family units. For some families the time of diagnosis also necessitates adjustment to the patient's sexual orientation, thus compounding the necessary coping tasks. The physical distancing required by isolation precautions may foster social isolation if the disease process and the reasons for the required precautions are poorly understood, as is the case with AIDS.

☐ **GOAL**

The patient will deal adaptively with changes in usual social interactions; will devise new coping strategies; patient and family/friends will be able to express feelings, concerns, and fears; support systems intact prior to hospitalization will be continued.

☐ **IMPLEMENTATION**

- Assess patient and family/friends for stage of grieving; refer to *The Patient Experiencing Grief and Loss,* page 80.
- Support adaptive responses, remembering that in the initial stage any response may be adaptive except homicidal or suicidal behavior.
- Encourage realistic assessment of the situation by providing information, answering questions, and gentle truth telling.
- Recognize and support the patient's need for unique, personal adjustments to change.
- Be aware that patient's friends may withdraw out of fear of catching the disease; educate as necessary.
- Encourage family, friends, and staff to visit with the patient, avoiding unnecessary exaggeration of isolation precautions.
- Recognize the need for privacy when sexual partner is visiting, honoring wishes for confidentiality and assisting others (family, friends, and staff) to cope with patient's preference.
- Initiate referrals to mental health nurse or clinician as appropriate.

☐ **EVALUATION CRITERIA/DESIRED OUTCOMES**

The Patient
- Maintains social interaction with family, friends, and staff

- Verbalizes satisfaction with emotional support provided by staff/family/friends

---

NURSING DIAGNOSIS #7

Altered sexuality patterns related to physiologic limitations and life-style changes imposed by disease process

Rationale: *Because transmission of AIDS is believed to be through direct contact with contaminated body fluids through intimate sexual contact (as well as through sharing of contaminated needles, transfusions of blood products, and percutaneous blood exposure), intimate contact is discouraged for the patient. Since sexuality is an integral part of the patient's identity, alternate means of expression may need to be developed.*

☐ **GOAL**

The patient will explore/use alternate ways to meet sexual needs.

☐ **IMPLEMENTATION**

- Plan nursing care to permit time to encourage the patient to express feelings or concerns about sexual activity and the spread of AIDS; let the patient set the pace.
- Support the patient's partner who may feel a threat to own life because of the mode of transmission.
- Educate regarding safe sexual activity
  - abstaining from sex with partners with a known infection
  - select partners from a small group of known friends
  - avoid combination of oral and anal sex
  - use a condom during sex
- Use the word "partner" rather than "wife" or "husband" and regard the patient's partner as a "significant other" worthy of receiving information usually given to family only, if appropriate.
- Refrain from moralizing about or judging sexual choices; prevent misunderstandings about homosexuals by educating staff and holding team conferences to express feelings.
- Maintain confidentiality of homosexual patients who have not openly revealed their sexual orientation and fear the rejections of others if this information becomes known.

☐ **EVALUATION CRITERIA/DESIRED OUTCOMES**

The Patient
- Expresses satisfaction with close relationships and methods of sexual expression

---

NURSING DIAGNOSIS #8

Powerlessness related to grave prognosis

Rationale: *The patient with AIDS confronts living with a chronic disease that is poorly understood and for which there is no known cure and little hope for improvement. Powerlessness may be manifested by expressed dissatisfaction in ability to control the disease process; reluctance or refusal to participate in decision making; apathetic, aggressive, acting-out, or violent behavior; uneasiness or anxiety; or depression.*

☐ **GOAL**

The patient will be able to identify those aspects of AIDS and its treatment that can be controlled; will participate in decision making concerning treatment.

☐ **IMPLEMENTATION**

- Assess specific aspects of AIDS that are most distressing; review initial psychosocial assessment for information about usual coping patterns and identified support persons; use this information in refining planned interventions.
- Allow the patient to express fears and concerns; listen attentively without minimizing the patient's feelings; offer suggestions without directly telling the patient what to do; when possible, offer alternative solutions to patient problems and encourage the patient to make the final decision.
- Keep informed about condition, treatments, and test results.
- Provide opportunities for patient to control as many decisions as possible such as physical set-up of room and daily activities.
- Do not offer choices that do not exist; respect and follow the patient's choices when you have given the option of making a choice.
- Record preferences on care plan to ensure that others will acknowledge preferences.

☐ **EVALUATION CRITERIA/DESIRED OUTCOMES**

The Patient
- Expresses feelings of increased control over some aspects of own life
- Participates in the decision-making process regarding treatment

---

NURSING DIAGNOSIS #9

Alteration in thought processes (disorientation, forgetfulness, confusion) related to cerebral pathology

Rationale: Confusion is a state of mental disorder, derangement, and perplexion in which attention, comprehension, memory, and perceptions are disturbed or adversely affected. Evidence shows that the AIDS virus may attack the nervous system, causing damage to the brain. The damage may take years to develop and the symptoms may show up as memory loss, loss of coordination, partial paralysis, or mental disorder.

☐ GOAL

The patient will be oriented to time/place/person; will interact voluntarily with others and with environment in socially appropriate ways; will make some decisions and choices related to own care and activities.

☐ IMPLEMENTATION

- Obtain baseline mental status examination (refer to *Mental Status Exam*, page 245).
- Assess for disorientation, confusion, impaired memory, and hallucinations; describe, record, and report to physician.
- Evaluate frequently for suicidal ideation and provide suicidal precautions as needed (refer to *The Patient who is Suicidal*, page 144).
- Get patient's attention before speaking; say name, wait for eye contact, speak slowly, distinctly, and loud enough to be heard; turn off radio, television, and shut out other distractions.
- Use a voice tone that indicates sincerity, sensitivity, respect, and acceptance.
- Provide familiar and consistent care givers.
- Give patient choices when possible, but avoid sudden, unnecessary changes (e.g., in roommate, decor, routines), which may be upsetting.
- Offer information in small amounts; have patient repeat instructions to make sure they are understood.
- Answer questions repeatedly as necessary, using short, simple sentences; reinforce verbal communication with gestures; build on the sensible statements of the patient to strengthen reality-based conversation.
- Provide orientation to time/place/person every hour; use clocks, calendars, signs, pictures, night lights, and written reminders.
- Use concrete symbols (photographs, tangible creations, and products) of patient's past to strengthen and reassure patient's sense of continuity of self (now threatened with grave prognosis and brain deterioration).
- Avoid too much or too little stimulation; ask family/friends to visit 1 or 2 at a time to avoid fatigue, agitation, confusion.
- Acknowledge special events in patient's life (e.g., birthdays, anniversaries, religious days); observe

customary national holidays with quiet celebration, decorations, special refreshments, and entertainment as patient is able to tolerate.
- Refer to *The Patient with Chronic Organic Brain Syndrome*, page 158.

☐ EVALUATION CRITERIA/DESIRED OUTCOMES

The Patient
- Is oriented to time/place/person
- Interacts appropriately with others
- Participates in some decisions about ADL

NURSING DIAGNOSIS #10

Knowledge deficit regarding safe hygiene practices in the home, indications for seeking additional medical attention

Rationale: To decrease the risks of recurrent infection in the patient and transfer of AIDS to care giver(s), the patient and family need guidelines for safe care in the home and reminders of when to contact the physician.

☐ GOAL

The patient will receive safe, adequate care at home, posing a minimal risk to healthy family members.

☐ IMPLEMENTATION

- Emphasize to family and friends that AIDS is spread by intimate contact with bodily fluids and that casual, nonintimate contact is thought to be safe.
- Teach the patient/family good handwashing techniques.
- Advise disinfecting the patient's bathroom and toilet with a 1:10 solution of 5.25% bleach and water.
- Tell patient/family to wash soiled linens in a washing machine with hot water, detergent, and bleach.
- Instruct patient/family to wash eating utensils in hot soapy water.
- Demonstrate how to dispose of soiled tissues, dressings, and gloves in plastic bags, securing the closure tightly before discarding; ask for return demonstration.
- Caution patient/family to restrict visitors to those who are healthy and not susceptible to illness.
- Instruct the patient/family/significant other about the signs of AIDS and encourage them to seek medical attention should these signs become evident.
- Ensure the patient has a written list of prescribed medications with times, dosages, and possible side effects; explain measures to minimize toxic

effects and ask patient to repeat this information at another time; reinforce correct explanations and correct misinformation.
- Explain cross-infection and the signs of infection; stress the need to contact the physician immediately should these signs be noticed.
- Provide information about available community services and initial referrals as necessary; explain that relapses are possible and likely and encourage follow-up care; give the toll-free number (800/221-7044) of the National Gay Task Force crisis-line, which has up-to-date information about AIDS. (The number in New York is 212/807-6016). Public Health Service AIDS Hotline: 800/342-AIDS, 800/342-2437.

☐ EVALUATION CRITERIA/DESIRED OUTCOMES

The Patient
- Lists signs of AIDS, necessary precautions for providing home care, and indications for contacting physician
- Verbalizes plans to receive continuing care at home from family/significant others.

The Patient Manifesting Aggression

Definition/Discussion

Aggression is forceful, goal-directed behavior that may be physical, verbal, or symbolic and occurs as a defensive response to anxiety and loss of self-esteem. It may be directed toward the environment or inwardly toward the self and is pathologic when unrealistic, destructive toward the self or others, and beyond the problem-solving level.

Nursing Assessment

☐ PERTINENT HISTORY

Length, frequency, intensity of aggressive episodes; precipitating factors, life-style; alcohol or drug usage; legal difficulties; psychotic episodes

☐ PHYSICAL FINDINGS

Increased psychomotor agitation, epilepsy, endocrine or metabolic imbalance, affect intensification, abnormal vital signs

☐ PSYCHOSOCIAL CONCERNS/DEVELOPMENTAL FACTORS

School, employment, and marital history; usual coping mechanisms, reactions to stress; similarities in family members, typical or dysfunctional family dynamics

☐ PATIENT AND FAMILY KNOWLEDGE

Sources of assistance; methods of management, readiness and willingness to learn

Nursing Care

☐ LONG-TERM GOAL

The patient will develop internal controls; the patient will use assertive coping behaviors to achieve needs and desires.

NURSING DIAGNOSIS #1

Potential for violence related to physically destructive behavior

---

Rationale: If acting-out behavior escalates, the patient may lose control, resulting in physical harm to self or others.

☐ GOAL

The patient will limit or stop aggressive behaviors.

☐ IMPLEMENTATION

- Set limits on physically harmful behavior and explain why you are doing so.
- Always prepare patient both physically and verbally for what you are going to do even if you consider it a daily or usual activity.
- Watch for verbal and nonverbal signs of increasing agitation and intervene while patient is still able to respond in a reasonable manner.
- Provide nonthreatening environment.
- Keep stimuli such as radio and TV at a minimum.
- Protect other patients, visitors, etc., from physically aggressive behaviors by removing them from the area.
- Order patient to "Stop" destructive behavior; this is sometimes sufficient to prevent escalation.
- Maintain sufficient distance so that patient does not feel cornered.
- Talk to the patient calmly without becoming aggressive or defensive.
- Provide safe materials for alternative expression of physical aggression (e.g., pillows, punching bag, foam objects).
- Restrain patient physically if it becomes necessary.

☐ EVALUATION CRITERIA/DESIRED OUTCOMES

The Patient
- Has fewer periods of aggressive behaviors
- Uses substitute materials when agitated
- Displays appropriate motor activity
- Speaks in calm voice

NURSING DIAGNOSIS #2

Impaired communication: verbal related to impulsive, defensive, angry behaviors

---

Rationale: *Patients who are feeling hostile are likely to react in a nonverbal manner. Learning to describe feelings initially will prevent progression to aggressive behavior.*

☐ GOAL

The patient will verbalize aggressive feelings.

☐ IMPLEMENTATION

- Encourage verbalization to identify what is being felt (e.g., "Tell me what is happening with you.").
- Assist in verbal expression of reaction to the hospital and its attending limitations.
- Give your undivided attention; sit down and listen; use communication techniques that foster the development of a trusting relationship.
- Identify with patient factors that contribute to an increase in tension and anxiety preceding the aggressive behavior.
- Continue to accept the patient; do not avoid or retaliate; wait out verbal abuse calmly, then address the issue of using assertive techniques to respect the rights of others.

☐ EVALUATION CRITERIA/DESIRED OUTCOMES

The Patient

- Verbalizes factors precipitating increased stress and anxiety
- Describes feelings prior to exhibiting agitated behavior
- Limits verbally aggressive statements

NURSING DIAGNOSIS #3

Ineffective individual coping related to increased anxiety, fears of losing control

Rationale: *Coping with anxiety and fear is a learned behavior; aggression is a maladaptive behavior that can be replaced as the patient learns more adaptive and assertive responses.*

☐ GOAL

The patient will utilize assertive behaviors as a means of expressing independence and control.

☐ IMPLEMENTATION

- Teach the difference between assertive behavior (asking for what one wants; standing up for one's rights) and aggressive behavior (getting what one wants at the expense of others).
- Plan the nursing care and daily routine with the patient, giving as much flexibility in decision mak-

ing as possible; evaluate care on a continuing basis.
- Reinforce assertive approaches used by the patient. ("I would like . . . ," not "Do this . . . ").
- Provide opportunities for favorite activities as much as possible.
- Give honest praise for efforts to maintain independence and to use assertive techniques.
- Recognize the patient's behavior may be in response to stress or anxiety, so do not be defensive; assist patient to understand own method of coping.
- Explore alternative methods of coping and assist to identify successful present and future abilities.
- Role play alternative behaviors to prepare for future experiences.
- Assess knowledge of relaxation techniques and teach techniques appropriate to patient.
- Encourage exercise if physical condition permits; assist to plan individualized program.

☐ EVALUATION CRITERIA/DESIRED OUTCOMES

The Patient

- Demonstrates respect for the rights of others
- Participates actively in planning for own care
- Participates in milieu activities
- Utilizes relaxation techniques and exercise to decrease anxiety

---

NURSING DIAGNOSIS #4

Knowledge deficit regarding reasons for occurrence of aggressive behavior, need for continuing use of assertive techniques in management

Rationale: *People are often aggressive because they do not understand the difference between assertiveness and aggression. Teaching techniques of how to communicate needs and how to get what you want reduces the motivation for aggressive behavior.*

☐ GOAL

The patient/family will identify dynamics of aggressive behavior and the assertive techniques used in its management.

☐ IMPLEMENTATION

- Explain the reason for the patient's behavior to significant others ("It is his way of coping with frustration").
- Praise the efforts of family members in their attempts to assist the patient in coping.
- Encourage verbalization of feelings by family; ex-

plain recurrence is more likely with increased stress.

- Work with patient/family on the identification and appropriate channeling of aggressive drives into constructive areas.
- Reinforce any appropriate and useful techniques of assertive behavior that will assist in the management of aggression to both patient/family.

☐ EVALUATION CRITERIA/DESIRED OUTCOMES

The Patient/Family
- Verbalizes circumstances that trigger the aggressive response
- Describes differences between assertiveness and aggression
- Identifies and uses alternative constructive channels for aggressive drives
- Demonstrates understanding through role playing of assertive techniques

The Patient Manifesting Anger

Definition/Discussion

Anger is a strong feeling of displeasure, usually of antagonism, excited by a real or supposed injury; a learned means of avoiding anxiety that arises in response to interpersonal threat; and a normal response to loss (refer to *The Patient Experiencing Grief and Loss,* **page 80).** *Aggression* is a forceful, attacking action that may be physical, verbal, or symbolic. It is unrealistic and directed outwardly toward the environment or inwardly toward the self (refer to *The Patient Manifesting Aggression,* page 10). *Violence* is any physical behavior that is destructive to self, others, or property (refer to *The Patient who is Violent,* page 149).

Nursing Assessment

☐ **PERTINENT HISTORY**

Previous acute or chronic episodes/outbursts of angry or aggressive behavior; behavioral manifestations of anger (abusive language, frequent negative verbalizations regarding care givers and peers, refusal to conform to hospital routine, acting out, dysfunctional dependent or independent behaviors)

☐ **PHYSICAL FINDINGS**

Physical illness, trauma, organic disorder, inadequate nutrition, refusal of treatments, neglect in self-care

☐ **PSYCHOSOCIAL CONCERNS/ DEVELOPMENTAL FACTORS**

Ineffective patterns of communication, inadequate or underdeveloped socialization skills, dysfunctional family relationships, dependency, chronic or acute anxiety, feelings of inadequacy, history of emotional difficulties, hostility towards self or others, fear, depression

☐ **PATIENT AND FAMILY KNOWLEDGE**

Ability to recognize behaviors of anxiety and feelings of powerlessness, ability to assess family interactions; socialization skills and interpersonal relationships of family, readiness and willingness to learn

Nursing Care

☐ **LONG-TERM GOAL**

The patient will verbally identify causative internal and external stressors; the patient will use realistic and assertive behavior to express displeasure and anger.

NURSING DIAGNOSIS #1

Ineffective individual coping related to anxiety

Rationale: Ineffective individual coping is manifested when the individual experiences an inability to manage either internal or external stressors adequately related to inadequate resources. Anxiety is a feeling aroused by a vague nonspecific threat. The individual experiences feelings of discomfort and uneasiness, activating the autonomic nervous system. The feelings may be expressed through angry outbursts, hostility, and acting-out behavior, either overt (e.g., fighting, hitting, verbal attack) or covert (e.g., somatizing, depression, suicide).

☐ **GOAL**

The patient will eliminate the physically harmful and attacking expressions of anger; will express anger assertively rather than aggressively; will identify and use effective coping mechanisms to manage own anxiety.

☐ **IMPLEMENTATION**

- Assess level of anxiety and remove excess stimulation.
- Tell the patient you will prevent any further expression of anger that is physically harmful in nature.
- Find physical outlets for anger that are acceptable (e.g., hitting punching bag, using batakas).
- Spend time with the patient; ask what the anger is about and if patient refuses to answer, just sit with him/her while s/he is silent.

- Praise any efforts to put the anger/feelings of anxiety into words and to share the causes with you.
- Be aware that this anger is usually not meant for you personally, so do not respond defensively.
- Assist in making connections between feelings of frustration and subsequent behavior.
- Assist in reevaluation of the perceived threat and the anxiety produced.
- Have patient analyze consequences of behavior.
- Set limits on irrational or manipulative demands; state those limits clearly with consequences if limits are violated.
- Assist to develop alternative adaptive coping mechanisms for dealing with anger (e.g., discussion, one-to-one communication, physical exercise).
- Provide positive feedback when patient utilizes adaptive coping mechanisms.

☐ EVALUATION CRITERIA/DESIRED OUTCOMES

The Patient
- Verbalizes when feeling anxious or frustrated
- Describes the difference between the conversational expression of anger and physically harmful/forceful behavior
- Uses a minimum of one alternative adaptive coping mechanism when angry
- Acknowledges the limits set on manipulative or demanding behavior

---

NURSING DIAGNOSIS #2

Powerlessness related to hospitalization

Rationale: Powerlessness is a subjective state in which the individual perceives a lack of personal control over events or situations that are occurring to and about him/her. Anger may be seen as a response to feelings of powerlessness and an attempt by the individual to regain control.

☐ GOAL

The patient will discuss situations that provoke angry feelings; will verbalize both positive and negative feelings related to angry outbursts; will identify factors that contribute to a sense of powerlessness; will identify factors that s/he can control.

☐ IMPLEMENTATION

- Invite to participate in own care and discuss feelings about the hospitalization.
- Assess knowledge of hospitalization and illness.
- Assess present ability to control behavior and to make decisions.
- Determine the patient's feelings of powerlessness before beginning teaching.

- Explain all procedures, rules, and options.
- Keep informed about condition, treatments, and results.
- Provide opportunities for the patient to control decisions by offering alternatives and increase decision-making opportunities as patient progresses.
- Involve in own care on a continuing basis; ask to do specific tasks while you do others; discuss the results of this shared responsibility with the patient.
- Inform patients of scheduled tests/procedures to eliminate unpredictability of events.
- Provide specific times each shift for communication and interaction.
- Be sensitive to the factors that contribute to feelings of helplessness (e.g., strange environment, unknown outcomes, pain), and allow patient to discuss concerns and feelings.
- Direct conversation towards those aspects of the illness for which patient has the most negative feelings; use open-ended questions.
- Spend time with family explaining patient's need to have the opportunity to express both positive and negative feelings about what is happening.
- Praise the efforts of others to accept the conversational expressions by the patient of negative feelings.
- Praise staff/family efforts to support the patient and to understand the behavior without personalizing it.

☐ EVALUATION CRITERIA/DESIRED OUTCOMES

The Patient/Family
- Verbalizes behavior or demands that trigger the physically harmful aspects of patient's anger
- Shares both positive and negative feelings about an individual experience
- Participates in decision-making for self/family
- Experiences a sense of control and power

NURSING DIAGNOSIS #3

Knowledge deficit regarding use of adaptive coping mechanisms to deal with manifestations of anger

Rationale: Giving information to the patient helps decrease feelings of anxiety and powerlessness, thus reducing angry outbursts as a means of expressing these feelings. Patients who express anger in nonadaptive ways usually have not learned alternative methods of dealing with anger.

☐ GOAL

The patient/family will use adaptive coping mechanisms in dealing with angry feelings.

☐ IMPLEMENTATION

- Discuss with patient adaptive ways that patient has developed for dealing with feelings of anger, anxiety, powerlessness.
- Identify anger-producing situations with patient; use role playing to practice alternative methods of expressing anger.
- Help patient to plan ways to maintain self-care after discharge; help set personal goals.
- Discuss available community resources and support groups; supply list of such groups as needed.

☐ EVALUATION CRITERIA/DESIRED OUTCOMES

The Patient

- Identifies and expresses angry feelings in adaptive way
- States feelings and behaviors of anxiety, powerlessness that should be reported to the physician/therapist/clinic
- Knows and identifies community resources and support groups

The Patient with Anorexia Nervosa

Definition/Discussion

Anorexia nervosa is a clinical syndrome characterized by **weight loss of at least 25% of original body weight in the absence of a physical illness that would account for weight loss, extreme fear of obesity that does not diminish as weight loss progresses, body-image disturbance, emaciation, and amenorrhea.** The *DSM-III-R* classifies this problem as an eating disorder. Other eating disorders with onset in childhood and adolescence are bulimia (voracious eating from psychologic causes followed by self-induced vomiting) and pica (craving for unnatural foods such as plaster or dirt).

Occurs primarily in females (90%-95% of patients) and is on the increase in the United States and affluent countries, especially among well-educated, upper-middle-class females aged 15-25 years.

Cause is unknown but theories include

- *behavioral:* a behavior of rejecting food that is reinforced by attention; the person learns to manipulate the environment for gratification of needs
- *medical:* research presently focuses on dysfunction of the hypothalamus, increased catecholamine activity, and possible genetic predisposition
- *psychoanalytic:* maladaptive regression to oral or anal stage of development to avoid adolescent sexuality and independence
- *family interaction model:* dysfunctional family dynamics characterized by overprotection, rigidity, and lack of personal boundaries and independence; the dysfunctional family focuses on anorexia to avoid other interpersonal conflicts and conflict resolution (e.g., family avoids problems between husband and wife; problems with sexuality).

Nursing Assessment

☐ PERTINENT HISTORY

Percentage of normal body weight lost, nutritional status, amenorrhea, eating patterns: amount and type of foods ingested, eating times, history of bulimia or pica, forcing self to eat

☐ PHYSICAL FINDINGS

Weight, height, vital signs (irregular or extremely slow pulse or hypotension may indicate medical emergency), anemia, skin color (pale, brownish, or yellow-orange coloring, cyanosis of extremities)

☐ PSYCHOSOCIAL CONCERNS/ DEVELOPMENTAL FACTORS

Body-image distortion (e.g., overestimation of size of body, belief of being overweight when emaciated, denial of problem, an unrealistic ideal for own body); sexual adjustment problems or delayed psychosocial-sexual development; anxiety (may be severe and result in impulsive acts such as suicide attempts or stealing); quality of relationships with parents, friends, staff, other patients; coping mechanisms, strengths, interests

☐ PATIENT AND FAMILY KNOWLEDGE

Symptoms of acute phase and medical emergency to report to physician, prognosis, treatment plan, diet behaviors to reinforce, community resources, support groups, readiness and willingness to learn

Nursing Care

☐ LONG-TERM GOAL

The patient will regain/maintain a realistic body image and appropriate weight for height and age.

NURSING DIAGNOSIS #1

Alteration in nutrition: less than body requirements related to self-starvation

Rationale: *A reported 5%-21% of anorectics die from malnutrition, recurrent infection, or cardiac disorders resulting from electrolyte imbalance. Anorexic behavior destroys electrolyte and nutritional balance necessitating hospitalization for IV or oral feedings.*

☐ GOAL

The patient will reestablish a nutritionally adequate eating pattern; will regain/maintain fluid and electrolyte balance; will ingest adequate nutrition for growth and development.

☐ IMPLEMENTATION

- Weigh daily (or as ordered) at the same time, in hospital gown, with arms at sides, after emptying bladder to ensure accurate weight.
- Offer structured support at mealtimes; provide pleasant environment for meals, avoid discussing food or somatic complaints; focus on patient's adaptive interests, praise patient's ability to consume meal within the prescribed time period.
- Administer tube feedings, hyperalimentation, or IV feedings as ordered; approach with matter-of-fact, nonjudgmental attitude.
- Observe patient for 2 hours after eating to prevent vomiting or regurgitation.
- Provide positive reinforcements for weight gain rather than for amount of food eaten.
- Demonstrate an accepting, respectful attitude and express concern; avoid threats, pleas, and advice.
- Participate in interdisciplinary group meetings to plan goals and care; know that it is important to designate one person as primary therapist to avoid patient manipulating and possibly splitting staff.
- Hold daily staff conferences to discuss, evaluate, and provide support so that entire staff gives consistent, effective care; include patient's input, approval, and written consent of care plan via the primary therapist.
- Institute behavior modification and/or psychotherapy; outpatient psychotherapy may be used if patient agrees to participate in treatment plan and if medical emergency does not exist.

☐ EVALUATION CRITERIA/DESIRED OUTCOMES

The Patient
- Demonstrates a nutritionally adequate eating pattern
- Regains/maintains fluid and electrolyte balance
- Regains/maintains weight within normal range for height and age

---

NURSING DIAGNOSIS #2

Disturbance in self-concept: body image related to misperceptions of body size

Rationale: Self-concept is an ongoing, dynamic perception and adaptation to body image, personal identity, role performance, and self-esteem. The anorexic may have disturbances in most of these areas, the most common of which is an inability to perceive realistically body size, body functions, and

---

physical needs. The greater the body-image distortion, the greater the denial of the problem and the poorer the prognosis.

☐ GOAL

The patient will regain/maintain a realistic body image; will develop realistic attitudes and perceptions about own body size, needs, and function.

☐ IMPLEMENTATION

- Assist to express feelings and concerns about self, body size, body function, and physical needs.
- Point out verbalized misperceptions of body image (e.g., Patient: "My legs are fat." Nurse: "Your legs are beginning to look strong and healthy since you've regained your normal weight and started to walk daily. Let's talk about how the body can change and grow.").
- Teach to verbalize and visualize positive affirmations about own body (e.g., "I am healthy and energetic at my ideal weight." "I am able to choose healthy food to eat."); ask to create own statements and to practice imagining self in a positive way several times/day; review mental exercises for imagery and positive affirmations in Table 1, *Stress Management*, page 24.
- Provide support and positive feedback for accurate perceptions of body size and function as well as for demonstration of adaptive eating and health habits.
- Verbally recognize and reinforce genuine communication of feelings, concerns, and perceptions.
- Work with patient to identify abilities and strengths; offer opportunities to participate in projects or tasks that utilize existing abilities within treatment protocol.

☐ EVALUATION CRITERIA/DESIRED OUTCOMES

The Patient
- Demonstrates realistic attitudes and perception about own body size, needs, and function
- Discusses own body size, needs, and functions in realistic and positive terms

---

NURSING DIAGNOSIS #3

Ineffective individual coping related to self-care in activities of daily living (ADL)

Rationale: The anorexic patient is usually an adolescent or young adult who is still struggling with adolescent issues. Factors that may influence the anorexic Zpatient's ability to assume self-care in ADL (e.g., hygiene, diet and nutrition, exercise, rest and sleep, leisure activities) include

- conflict between longing for independence and desire for dependency
- adolescent rebellion against authority
- overwhelming feelings of inadequacy, ineffectiveness, powerlessness
- self-doubt about ability to take responsibility for self and/or ability to make decisions and problem solve.

These patients needs support and encouragement to assume self-care and take responsibility for self.

☐ GOAL

The patient will participate in treatment plan; will demonstrate effective coping with ADL.

☐ IMPLEMENTATION

- Assist to express feelings and concerns about self and treatment plan.
- Provide opportunities for choice and decision making in treatment plan and ADL such as type and time of hygiene, exercise, leisure activities, and hobbies.
- Alternate rest time with activities so that patient will not constantly exercise and expend calories that have been ingested.
- Help patient identify problem areas and assist with problem-solving techniques; refer to *Problem Solving*, page 248.
- Avoid control struggles; believe in the patient's ability to make effective decisions about ADL and to learn healthy habits.
- Set and maintain firm limits; be clear about limits and consistent with treatment plan; refer to *Behavior Modification*, page 250.
- Assist patient to identify own issues and conflicts and offer support and counseling as needed; refer to *Strategies for Counseling Adolescents*, page 252.
- Provide opportunities for staff to meet and ventilate feelings about patient's manipulative and self-destructive behavior if necessary.

☐ EVALUATION CRITERIA/DESIRED OUTCOMES

The Patient
- Participates actively in treatment plan and problem solving for ADL
- Identifies own issues and conflicts concerning self-care and participates in problem solving
- Demonstrates self-care in hygiene, exercise, diet and nutrition, sleep and rest, leisure activities

NURSING DIAGNOSIS #4

Knowledge deficit regarding coping with nutrition, ADL, anxiety, and discharge plan

Rationale: The course of anorexia nervosa varies; adherence to the treatment plan and continued emotional support can prevent acute episodes and hospitalization. Family members, in an effort to control the patient's behavior, often create more problems by their lack of knowledge about the dynamics of the illness.

☐ GOAL

The patient will discuss plan to ingest appropriate diet; will receive positive reinforcement for weight gain rather than for amount of food eaten; will make decisions for ADL; will discuss follow-up care and symptoms to report to physician.

☐ IMPLEMENTATION

- Assess level of knowledge and ability to comply with diet and treatment plan.
- Discuss schedule for follow-up care; develop a plan to put in use if patient feels anxious, depressed, or out of control.
- Assess availability of significant others; include them in discharge planning if possible.
- Teach family to give positive reinforcement for weight gain rather than amount of food eaten.
- Discuss patient plans to maintain self after discharge (e.g., caring for clothing, transportation, food shopping and meal preparation, recreation and work/school); help set personal goals and offer support in these.
- Plan for daily productive activity (e.g., occupational, vocational training); ask what patient would like to achieve, and help with this goal.
- Encourage verbalization and questions; ask patient to describe in own words medication, treatment plan, follow-up care, and symptoms to report to physician.
- Discuss community resources and support groups such as half-way houses, rehabilitation and vocational training, day-care centers.

☐ EVALUATION CRITERIA/DESIRED OUTCOMES

The Patient/Family
- Has a plan to ingest an appropriate diet
- Makes decisions for daily activities including a balance of rest and exercise, activities that utilize existing abilities, and favorite hobbies
- Has an appointment for follow-up care with physician/therapist and knows how to contact them as needed
- States symptoms of medical emergency; has telephone number of physician or clinic to call if needed

The family
- Demonstrates positive reinforcement for weight gain rather than for amount of food eaten

The Patient with an Antisocial Personality Disorder

Definition/Discussion

An antisocial personality disorder represents a cluster of personality characteristics manifested by deeply ingrained, chronically unsocialized behavior; formerly known as sociopathic or psychopathic personality. The *DSM-III-R* classification is Personality Disorder.

Nursing Assessment

☐ **PERTINENT HISTORY**

Difficulties with law, substance abuse, marital and parental performance, employment history, trigger for impulsive behaviors, recent crises, previous treatment

☐ **PHYSICAL FINDINGS**

Signs of substance use, tension, agitation, restlessness

☐ **PSYCHOSOCIAL CONCERNS/ DEVELOPMENTAL FACTORS**

Multigenerational patterns, dysfunctional family (parental rejection, lack of discipline, absent parent figure), reactions to stress, absence of anxiety, contempt for others, manipulative skills, lack of emotional attachments, cultural influences

☐ **PATIENT AND FAMILY KNOWLEDGE**

Perception of problem, degree of disruption, attitudes toward treatment, use of resources, readiness and willingness to learn

Nursing Care

☐ **LONG-TERM GOAL**

The patient will recognize and observe limits in interactions with others; the patient will accept responsibility for own actions.

NURSING DIAGNOSIS #1

Ineffective individual coping related to manipulation of others

Rationale: The antisocial patient has little trust or positive regard for others. Needs are met through manipulation, which is self-destructive and violates the rights of others.

☐ **GOAL**

The patient will recognize and observe limits in interactions with others.

☐ **IMPLEMENTATION**

• Be aware that staff commonly experience uncomfortable feelings of anger, helplessness, frustration, defensiveness, etc., when working with these patients; openly discussing and acknowledging these feelings with other staff can lead to control, thus making one less susceptible to being manipulated; refer to *The Patient Displaying Manipulation*, page 94.

• Use firm, caring approaches because of manipulative operations, patience is required; the use of authority must be rational and not punitive.

• Clearly state the expectations and limits and what the consequences will be for not adhering to the plan; implement the consequences as necessary in a matter-of-fact manner.

• Observe closely patient's behavior and interactions with staff and other patients; assess the meaning and understanding of the behavior to the patient and validate with patient and other staff; hold a staff conference to discuss, set, and inform all staff of approaches and limits for this patient.

• Be aware of other patients who could easily be used, hurt by patient and intervene as needed; work with both patients on appropriate alternatives to respond to each other; if antisocial patient refuses to cooperate, separate from rest of unit for time out; state firmly what limits will be set on behavior and that people and situations will not be used for one person's motives; make contact with patient that states specific cause and effect (e.g., "If you take Mr. H's cigarettes, you will not be allowed in the day room when he is there."); follow through on contract on all shifts; be consistent.

- Persevere in following treatment plan (indifference and resistance to treatment are common; patterns of manipulation are difficult to alter).
- Review patient requests with other staff before permission is granted or denied; do not make on-the-spot decisions if possible; remember that this patient is often an expert at pitting one staff member against another (recreating the family triangle and being the center of attention); staff must present a united front.
- Give attention when manipulative behavior is not occurring; reinforce positive behavior (often the only attention patient gets occurs after acting out or manipulative behavior; set reasonable goals with patient and reinforce positive efforts to reach them.
- Keep explanations, discussions short and simple; long, complex ones can be another aspect of manipulation.
- Know that this patient may refuse to recognize own inappropriate or manipulative behavior; it is more effective to change the subject or leave the situation than to argue or try to convince him/her.
- Be aware that patient may use tears, lies, threats to get what is wanted; limits must be followed by all staff members and may be lifted as patient shows responsibility can be managed.
- Know that patient's demands may be endless; be firm and consistent.

☐ **EVALUATION CRITERIA/DESIRED OUTCOMES**

The Patient
- States awareness of negative response by others to manipulation
- Makes fewer attempts to "split" staff
- Lessens demanding behaviors
- Conforms increasingly to limits set by environment
- Occasionally accepts trusting behaviors modeled by staff

NURSING DIAGNOSIS #2

Social isolation related to impaired interpersonal relationships

Rationale: As a result of the absence of nurturing in the developmental period, close, positive relation-

---

ships have not been experienced. This results in continued avoidance and inability to achieve permanence in personal attachments.

☐ **GOAL**

The patient will improve social skills; will initiate social contacts.

☐ **IMPLEMENTATION**

- Assess and help patient define problem areas in social relationship (e.g., blaming others, lack of concern for others).
- Encourage to discuss this problem area in group therapy and to ask others reasons for rejection (if true); structure groups to focus on interpersonal behaviors.
- Practice social skills, use role playing; give positive reinforcement for positive behavior.
- Assist to improve verbal communication skills; patterns of communication are frequently immature and underdeveloped with little experience in verbalization of feelings or recognition of the feelings of others.
- Encourage to discuss the responsibilities and rewards of interpersonal relationships; point out responses that maintain superficiality.
- Be alert for substance abuse as a means of avoiding emotional involvement.
- Stress the here and now; point out that present relationships need not be the same as unsatisfactory or unsatisfying ones from the past.
- Provide opportunities for social interactions and diversional activities when appropriate.
- Serve as a role model; be optimistic about the ability of the patient to improve relationships knowing that success may depend upon factors such as motivation to change, ego strengths and superego development, extent of commitment to life-style and support from significant others for efforts to change.

☐ **EVALUATION CRITERIA/DESIRED OUTCOMES**

The Patient
- Attends group therapy; participation is increasing gradually
- Shows decrease in solitary behaviors
- Makes fewer projective statements

NURSING DIAGNOSIS #3

Potential for violence related to impulsive, acting out behaviors

Rationale: The antisocial person has no guilt for behaviors violating the rights of others. Judgment is

also poorly developed and this may lead to callous and aggressive behaviors.

☐ GOAL

The patient will improve control of impulsive behaviors.

☐ IMPLEMENTATION

- Anticipate acting-out behavior; inform of rules and limits before escalation; do not make exceptions to rules; take whatever measures are needed to ensure safety of the patient and others (e.g., seclusion room); refer to *The Patient Who is Violent,* page 149.
- Assist to identify factors that precipitate impulsive behaviors and define what the consequences might be if the impulse is followed.
- Teach to think through actions before their execution.
- Assist to identify and verbalize awareness of impulsive feelings rather than taking immediate and unplanned action.
- Support in the realization that many impulsive acts have negative consequences and the control of these will be of value in change of life-style.
- Introduce to problem-solving techniques when able to begin alternative coping methods; refer to *Problem Solving,* page 248.
- Use behavior-modification techniques to decrease impulsive behaviors; token economies are especially effective in the adolescent population; refer to *Behavior Modification,* page 250.
- Provide alternate outlets for physical energies (e.g., foam balls, punching bag, jogging).

☐ EVALUATION CRITERIA/DESIRED OUTCOMES

The Patient

- Reduces impulsive behavior
- Shows no acting-out behavior to self or others
- Begins to verbalize prior to impulsive behaviors
- Uses approved physical activities regularly

NURSING DIAGNOSIS #4

Knowledge deficit regarding lack of socialization skills, lack of acceptance of responsibility for behavior

---

Rationale: *Socialization skills and responsibility for behavior have never been developed in the antisocial person. There is great need for learning mature, responsible, assertive behaviors as well as improved communication skills.*

☐ GOAL

The client will improve socialization skills and develop a sense of responsibility for behavior.

☐ IMPLEMENTATION

- Assess family perception of problem; involve them with the patient in relearning socially acceptable patterns of behavior.
- Teach parenting skills when applicable to prevent repeating dysfunctional behaviors in another generation.
- Encourage participation in family therapy to assist in the recognition of behaviors/reactions by family members that may unconsciously support the antisocial behavior.
- Educate regarding substance abuse and refer to community groups as ongoing sources of information and support.
- Assist to recognize the need for possible environmental changes to prevent continued antisocial behavior after discharge.
- Continue with behavior modification teaching and assertive techniques; role play frequently to increase self-confidence.
- Refer for employment counseling and training so that social responsibility may be assumed.
- Encourage to continue mental health therapy in some form after discharge.

☐ EVALUATION CRITERIA/DESIRED OUTCOMES

The Patient

- Observes some limitations voluntarily in social interactions
- Displays partial ability to maintain behavior within socially acceptable limits
- Has contacted an outpatient mental-health center
- Has made appointment with employment counselor

The Patient Experiencing Anxiety

Definition/Discussion

Anxiety is the uncomfortable feeling of tension or dread that is unconnected to a specific stimulus; it can be vague or intense. It occurs as a reaction to some unconscious threat to biologic integrity and/or self-concept. Anxiety can be assessed according to level.

- *Mild:* increased alertness and motivation and ability to cope with daily problems
- *Moderate:* decreased perception of the environment with selective inattention; decreased ability to think clearly
- *Severe:* drastically reduced perceptual field; can focus on only one detail at a time
- *Panic:* inability to integrate environment with the self; cannot function; physical activity is disorganized or the patient may be "frozen"

Nursing Assessment

☐ PERTINENT HISTORY

Recent environmental or family changes, school changes, change in life-style; family stability; employment stability; losses, absence of supportive relationships, confusion of values/beliefs; previously experienced anxiety and coping methods; financial status, health status

☐ PHYSICAL FINDINGS

Increased vital signs; muscle tension, sweating, headaches, dizziness, tremors, sweaty palms, flushing, fatigue; GI discomfort, hyperventilation, somnolence or insomnia; crying, irritability, dry mouth, capillary dilation; inability to concentrate or understand explanations

☐ PSYCHOSOCIAL CONCERNS/ DEVELOPMENTAL FACTORS

Degree of perceived disruption, patterns of dependency, coping patterns of family, socialization pattern (e.g., values, belief systems, culture)

☐ PATIENT AND FAMILY KNOWLEDGE

Identifiable cause(s)/agreement about causes and management, involvement of community agencies, level of knowledge, readiness and willingness to learn

Nursing Care

☐ LONG-TERM GOAL

The patient will recognize own anxiety and cope effectively with symptoms associated with anxiety; the patient will use anxiety as a motivation for change.

NURSING DIAGNOSIS #1

Ineffective individual coping related to perception of situation and specific symptoms associated with anxiety

Rationale: Anxiety of more than a moderate level will impair the individual's ability to cope. Narrowing of perceptual field and selective inattention result in unrealistic perceptions of the situation. Physical symptoms associated with increased anxiety may overwhelm the patient and decrease ability to function. The feeling of impending doom and "I can't cope" paralyzes the patient from making rational decisions and taking positive action.

☐ GOAL

The patient will recognize own anxiety; will cope with the anxiety and reduce it at least one level.

☐ IMPLEMENTATION

- Determine level of anxiety patient is experiencing and use interventions appropriate to that level
  - mild: does not require any intervention
  - moderate
    - spend 5-10 minutes with the patient at least 3 times daily; show interest and support
    - determine cause if possible, since anxiety may decrease if it can be explained
    - focus on the immediate problem; stay in the "here and now"
    - give careful explanations of what will occur;

22

encourage questions and verbalization of any concerns patient may have

- do not give more information than the patient can handle
- be clear and concise in communication and with explanations; repeat if needed
- attend to physical comforts and needs
- do not make demands of the patient
- do not confront patient or argue regarding unrealistic perceptions
- encourage coping mechanisms such as verbalization or physical activity ("Come walk with me.")
- allow patient to cry
- assist patient to use relaxation exercises; refer to Table 1, *Stress Management*, page 24
- do not share your own personal anxieties with the patient
- severe
  - use previously stated interventions as applicable
  - decrease environmental stimulation
  - if patient is hyperventilating, have patient take slow deep breaths and ask to focus on how body feels on expiration; breathe with patient to provide support
  - use only brief, simple communications
  - structure activities into concrete tasks that do not require concentration
  - attend to somatic complaints
  - consider use of a minor tranquilizer if ordered
  - stay with patient until anxiety is lessened
- panic
  - remain with patient; demonstrate competence
  - use physical touch judiciously; some patients are comforted by touch and some are threatened by it
  - remain calm; reassure patient that control will be maintained
  - use firm, professional manner
  - use a small room or separate area to provide privacy and security
  - direct patient's energy into motor activities; repetitive actions are helpful in concentrating attention; continue close observation
  - administer medication if ordered (imipramine [Tofranil] is often used to treat panic attacks); evaluate effectiveness

☐ EVALUATION CRITERIA/DESIRED OUTCOMES

The Patient
- Recognizes own symptoms of anxiety
- States anxiety is decreased to a tolerable level
- Channels energy into goal-directed activity
- States willingness to learn new ways to cope with anxiety
- Demonstrates adequate constructive coping

NURSING DIAGNOSIS #2

Sleep pattern disturbance related to physiologic disturbances caused by anxiety

Rationale: Physiologic disturbances caused by anxiety may be reflected in a disturbance in sleep patterns.

☐ GOAL

The patient will achieve a sleep/rest pattern appropriate to individual needs.

☐ IMPLEMENTATION

- Determine type of sleep disturbance patient is experiencing.
- Ask what the patient perceives are the reasons for the disturbed sleep pattern.
- Encourage verbalization of problems associated with anxiety.
- Provide measures appropriate to reduce insomnia, if indicated
  - quiet, secure environment
  - relaxation techniques
  - night light
  - decreased number of distractions (e.g., temperature taking during night)
  - structured bedtime routine (e.g., bath, reading, warm drink, music)
  - maximum measures for comfort of bed, clothing, etc.
  - consistent structured daytime activities that include physical exercise as tolerated
- Provide daytime stimulation and a regular schedule that discourages napping and dozing if increased somnolence is exhibited.

☐ EVALUATION CRITERIA/DESIRED OUTCOMES

The Patient
- Identifies disturbances in sleep patterns
- Utilizes measures to achieve appropriate rest and sleep without medication

---

NURSING DIAGNOSIS #3

Knowledge deficit regarding recognition and effective management of anxiety

Rationale: The individual can use anxiety as a motivating rather than a destructive force if it is recognized and successful coping mechanisms developed. Planned interactions with the patient can be increased in the duration but decreased in the number of conversations per day. It is necessary to reduce the anxiety level before beginning to teach about identifying the precipitating factors of anxiety and new coping strategies. High anxiety affects the ability to listen, take in, and remember information.

☐ GOAL

The patient will be able to identify sources of own anxiety; will employ effective measures to manage own anxiety.

☐ IMPLEMENTATION

- Be aware of the impact of anxiety on ability to learn
  - mild: learning can occur at this level
  - moderate: learning can occur but it must be directed
  - severe: inability to learn at this level
  - panic: unable to learn.
- Help patient identify those tensions and environmental factors that create a feeling of anxiety; attempt to identify precipitating factors or situations.
- Teach the signs and symptoms of anxiety and the importance of recognizing escalating anxiety before it reaches the panic stage.
- Identify with patient specific coping techniques to use in the moment to lower anxiety (e.g., deep breathing, verbalizing the feeling of anxiety to someone).
- Encourage supportive family members to be involved in prevention or management of the patient's anxiety as much as possible.
- Teach the benefits of and encourage establishment of regular physical activity to reduce stress and release anxiety.
- Praise staff and family members who are able to maintain an environment for the patient that allows an understanding of and control over the anxiety.
- Teach assertive techniques; refer to *Problem Solving*, page 248, and Table 1, *Stress Management*, page 24, to assist in keeping anxiety manageable.
- Provide information regarding community supports available for socialization, services, information, or support.

☐ EVALUATION CRITERIA/DESIRED OUTCOMES

The Patient
- Lists environmental factors that elicit anxiety
- Discusses ways of keeping responses to anxiety at a mild or moderate level and successfully cope with it
- States willingness to learn ways to cope with anxiety

The Patient/Family
- Verbalizes ways to cope with severe anxiety if it occurs

Table 1
Stress Management

Stress is a generalized, nonspecific response of the body to any demand, change, or perceived threat, whether positive or negative. *Stressors* are the circumstances or events that elicit this response and may be real or anticipated. *Distress* is damaging or unpleasant stress.

Signs of Distress
- accident proneness
- alcohol and drug abuse
- chronic fatigue
- decrease or increase of appetite
- diarrhea or constipation
- emotional instability
- emotional tension
- frequent urination
- grinding of teeth
- headache
- impulsive behavior

- inability to concentrate
- increased smoking
- insomnia
- irritability
- neck or back pain
- neurotic or psychotic
- behavior
- nightmares
- sexual problems
- stuttering
- sweating

GOAL: The patient will maintain homeostasis or optimal adaptive coping by preventing, or recognizing promptly, excessive levels of stress; the patient will utilize effective measures to manage stress by describing a plan to cope with stress in an adaptive way that includes exercise, relaxation, creative problem solving, and sharing feelings and concerns with a significant other.

Stress Reduction Techniques	Nursing Implications
Identify stressors (e.g., work, relationships, environmental, health, aging, financial, spiritual, emotional)	Have patient examine how s/he reacts to life occurrences (e.g., frustration, knot in stomach, loss of control)
	Discern between positive and negative stressors; explain that stress is unavoidable and can be useful to motivate.
Modify or eliminate stressors	Review possibilities for simple and major changes.
	Discuss alternatives, advantages and disadvantages of reducing stressors.
Develop effective coping mechanisms	
• daily exercise	Suggest methods to reduce stress through exercise (e.g., walking, running, dancing, swimming, gardening, participating in sports, body movement, exercises, yoga). Assist in developing a plan of regular activity.
	Refer to community gyms, health clubs, and YMCAs.
	Advise consultation with personal physician for contraindications to exercise program.
• develop alternative ways to relax (e.g., drawing, pottery, carpentry, writing, music, photography, reading, watching the sunset, taking a bubble bath)	Review with patient activities enjoyed and suggest s/he devote at least an hour/day to an activity. Refer to recreation departments, adult education programs, community colleges.

• relaxation techniques
  – progressive relaxation
  – autogenic training
  – guided imagery
	Guide patient through a relaxation exercise to experience its usefulness.
	Begin relaxation with deep breathing.
	Use guided imagery to induce relaxation (e.g., "Take another deep breath and let all the tension release. With each breath you become more relaxed. Now, imagine yourself in a peaceful, quiet setting [garden, beach, etc.]).
	Refer to cassettes, books, and classes on learning and practicing relaxation techniques.

• diaphragmatic breathing; periodic deep breathing	Practice diaphragmatic breathing, with patient • sit or recline in a comfortable position with legs uncrossed • place one hand on the chest and the other hand on the diaphragm, approximately 2 inches below the bottom center of the breastbone • inhale so the diaphragm expands and the hand covering the diaphragm moves out while the other hand remains almost still • as you exhale, the diaphragm relaxes and the hand covering it moves inward
• positive affirmations creating positive, active, new beliefs about oneself and immersing them into the subconscious mind by repeating them frequently)	Teach to • write out the statements and place them on mirror, steering wheel, refrigerator, desk, etc. • repeat the statements several times daily • be specific, positive, and brief (e.g., "I am relaxed," not "I am not tense.") • use the present tense "I am," not "I will." (e.g., "I am learning to express my feelings. I am expressing anger in a positive way. I am loveable.")
• balance work and recreation	Teach importance of • seeking work that one enjoys and is capable of doing or learning • taking relaxation breaks • taking regularly scheduled vacations • taking a "mental health" day away from work in lieu of a sick day

Stress Reduction Techniques	Nursing Implications
• improve self-care	Discuss personal habits that contribute to distress • self-medication • poor nutrition • neglecting early warning signs of tension • nonassertiveness • drinking, smoking Demonstrate positive ways to express and become more aware of feelings. Teach creative problem solving; brainstorm alternatives and other possibilities. Discuss importance of setting priorities, taking one thing at a time.

Table 2
Minor Tranquilizers

Drug Type, Actions, Examples	Side and Toxic Effects	Nursing Implications
Propanediols • Skeletal muscle relaxant, antianxiety *meprobamate (Equanil, Miltown)*	Drowsiness, lethargy, slurred speech, ataxia, paradoxical excitement, physical and psychologic dependence, compulsive use	• Warn patient to avoid operating dangerous machinery. • Teach patient dangers of combining with alcohol, narcotics, or other sedatives.
Benzodiazepines • CNS depressant, antianxiety, anticonvulsant, skeletal muscle relaxant *alprazolam (Xanax)* *chlordiazepoxide (Librium, in Librax)* *clorazepate dipotassium (Tranxene)* *clorazepate monopotassium (Azene)* *clonazepam (Klonopin)* *diazepam (Valium)* *lorazepam (Ativan)* *oxazepam (Serax)* *halazepam (Paxipam)* *prazepam (Verstran, Centrax)*	Sedation, dizziness, fatigue, ataxia, drowsiness. Less frequently: confusion, depression, headache, nausea, incontinence, lowered BP, paradoxical excitement or sleep disorders. Serious but rare: jaundice, skin rashes, respiratory depression, bone-marrow depression. Withdrawal symptoms: nausea and vomiting, anxiety, irritability, seizures.	• Check vital signs daily. • Observe and record behavioral responses. • Same as above re operation of machinery. • Observe for postural hypotension; if present, teach patient to sit up slowly, pause, and make a gradual change to being upright. • Observe skin color, condition; withhold drug, report to physician. • Observe and closely monitor gradual withdrawal of medication. • Supervise carefully patient intake of exact dosage; prevent hoarding.
Diphenylmethane Derivative • Mildly sedative, tranquilizer, antiemetic, antispasmodic *hydroxyzine (Atarax, Vistaril)*	Drowsiness, dry mouth, involuntary motor activity (tremors), convulsions. Can cause birth defects. Reports of tissue irritation with injections.	• Warn female patients not to take tranquilizers during pregnancy if possible. • Same as above for other tranquilizers.

The Patient Experiencing a Body-Image Disturbance

Definition/Discussion

Body image is a person's image or concept of his/her own body. It is formed from internal development as well as from environmental experiences including input from others, societal views, cultural practices, and previous experience with persons whose bodies have changed.

A body-image disturbance reflects the inability of an individual to perceive and/or adapt to an alteration in structure, function, or appearance of a part of or the entire body.

Nursing Assessment

☐ PERTINENT HISTORY

Surgeries, illness, trauma causing change in body form; rapidity of change; permanent or temporary refusal to participate in care; denial of change(s), willingness to discuss change in body or limitation of function

☐ PHYSICAL FINDINGS

Loss of body part and/or its function; neurologic, metabolic, or toxic disorders; progressively deforming disorders; acute dismemberment; disability or handicap; visibility of change; withdrawal, apathy, crying, agitation

☐ PSYCHOSOCIAL CONCERNS/ DEVELOPMENTAL FACTORS

Previous experience with someone with altered physical appearance, cultural practices, coping patterns, personality style, dependency patterns; depression, shame

☐ PATIENT AND FAMILY KNOWLEDGE

Possibility of rehabilitation or repair, degree of change in life-style and functional significance, value placed on alteration, perception of what change means, available community agencies, level of knowledge, readiness and willingness to learn

Nursing Care

☐ LONG-TERM GOAL

The patient will acknowledge and integrate body change(s) into adaptive and realistic management of own life.

NURSING DIAGNOSIS #1

Disturbance in self-concept: body image related to altered body structure or function

Rationale: *A real or perceived change in body image results in a need to modify one's self-concept. Certain areas of the body have greater value and meaning to an individual; threats to these areas cause more disruption and require more adjustment.*

☐ GOAL

The patient will acknowledge and begin to accept body change(s).

☐ IMPLEMENTATION

- Provide openings to enable patient to express feelings by validating your observations and feelings (e.g., "You look down in the dumps. How are things going for you today?" or "You seem upset/ sad. Are you?"); be a good listener and accept what patient verbalizes; remember not to take anger or hostility personally (this may be the only way possible for the patient to handle these feelings).
- Focus on the patient's feelings and deal with the presenting behavior (e.g., do not challenge patient's denial that a body change has actually occurred).
- Determine what the body-image change means to the patient and what effect the patient thinks it will have on life; if you think these perceptions are unrealistic, do not challenge them but continue to provide opportunities for patient to share these perceptions and feelings with you.

- Include in nursing care plan patient's own perception of meaning of body change, the objectives, and nursing actions; share plan with all care givers, including family.
- Be accepting of patient's body changes; if patient is repulsed or ashamed of physical changes, s/he will be watching the faces of others for negative signs; assist the family to accept changes also and to avoid reinforcement of the patient's negative feelings.
- Provide basic needs for patient; very dependent behaviors may be exhibited at this time.
- Let the patient know that the feelings and concerns that are being experienced are normal and that you are there to listen as well as to help cope with the changes.

☐ EVALUATION CRITERIA/DESIRED OUTCOMES

The Patient
- States that a change in the body has occurred
- Begins verbalization of feelings regarding the change
- Exhibits fewer negative reactions to staff and environment
- Shows occasional interest in self-care

NURSING DIAGNOSIS #2

Grieving related to loss or alteration in body form, function

Rationale: *Resolution of a loss through successful management of the grief process will allow the patient to progress effectively toward adjustment to changes in body structure and function. Individual responses to grief are determined by ego strengths, perception and meaning of loss, previous experiences, and present support systems. The nurse's personal feelings toward loss must be recognized before the nurse can accept those of others.*

☐ GOAL

The patient will acknowledge and express feelings of grief related to change(s) in body form or function.

☐ IMPLEMENTATION

- Recognize individual responses to grief: sadness, guilt, anger, depression, helplessness, denial, shock and disbelief; refer to *The Patient Experiencing Grief and Loss*, page 80.
- Listen to family members' feelings and concerns; give them emotional support so they will increase their ability to support patient.
- Be empathic and understanding; educate family/patient regarding normal grief reactions to permit more realistic expectations.

- Encourage verbalization of feelings toward the loss of the body part or function, the pleasures provided, and the needs it fulfilled in the past in order to promote grieving and to lessen denial.
- Allow patient to cry.
- Be alert for signs of depression (e.g., isolation or withdrawal, inability to grieve, fatigue, anorexia).
- Do not encourage fantasizing or false hopes regarding reversal of change in body form or function.
- Know that resolution of loss is accomplished a little at a time; be realistic about time required to achieve resolution.

☐ EVALUATION CRITERIA/DESIRED OUTCOMES

The Patient
- Verbalizes sadness and feelings of loss; identifies this as part of the normal grieving process
- States what the change in body part or function means
- Is able to cry
- Begins to share feelings of loss with family or friend
- Begins to regard the future in a positive way

NURSING DIAGNOSIS #3

Ineffective individual coping related to adaptation to alteration in body part or function

Rationale: *When changes in one's body occur, new coping mechanisms and changes in life-style may be required for successful adjustment.*

☐ GOAL

The patient will accept the alteration in body image and successfully adapt to required changes in life-style.

☐ IMPLEMENTATION

- Give positive reinforcement for efforts to adapt; patient behavior will indicate when acceptance of body alterations has begun (e.g., may ask questions; will start to look at the incision, dressings; will discuss limitations).
- Accept, but do not support, expressions of denial.
- If a prosthesis will be used, assist patient in choice by providing information and arranging for a visit by a member of an ostomy club, Reach to Recovery, or other appropriate group; let patient determine time of visit, but try to arrange it as soon as possible.
- Involve in self-care activities; begin slowly and add new activities one at a time; reinforce any efforts to participate.
- Listen and support realistic perceptions of the ex-

tent of the loss since there is frequently a lag between initial alteration and realistic perception.
- Tell family how they can help by listening, supporting reality, allowing expressions of anger, denial, and not challenging patient's statements, permitting patient to cry, and giving positive reinforcement for all efforts to cope/adapt; praise the family for participation in efforts to assist.
- Hold a team conference, including family if you wish, and share information on grief and loss, and crisis intervention; discuss what parts of these concepts apply at this time; revise the care plan as necessary.
- Refer for employment counseling if change in occupation is required.

- Refer for continued contact with community support group, home health nurse, and appropriate community agencies.

☐ EVALUATION CRITERIA/DESIRED OUTCOMES

The Patient
- Accepts continued support and positive input from family
- Utilizes community resources such as Reach to Recovery, ostomy club to provide ongoing support, reassurance, and assistance in recovery
- Resumes activities and role-related responsibilities with adaptation to limitations or changes

The Patient with a Borderline Personality Disorder

Definition/Discussion

The person with a borderline personality disorder characteristically displays a marked instability in several areas and leads a life that is consistently chaotic. There is a lack of close relationships (a result of alternately clinging and distancing behaviors), an inability to control anger and impulsivity that may result in substance abuse or suicidal behaviors, shifts in mood that can rapidly change from euphoria to manifestations of anxiety and depression, uncertainty regarding gender identity and self-image, and chronic feelings of emptiness and boredom. Psychosis may occur but is usually transient and follows increased stress or crises and characteristically does not include delusions and hallucinations.

The roots of this disorder lie in the failure to resolve the developmental process of separation and individuation, which is usually completed prior to the age of 3. At this time, the child establishes him/herself as an autonomous individual and learns that parents are composites of both positive and negative characteristics. The inability to integrate this concept creates the perspective that others are either "all good" or "all bad." This results in the overutilization of the ego defense mechanism of splitting in which self, others, and situations are judged in this way and no middle ground exists. In this way the perceptions of reality are impaired.

Because the hospitalized borderline patient idealizes some staff members and devalues others, a real challenge exists to present a united front. The attempts to manipulate staff are not done consciously, however, and all staff must consistently adhere to the nursing care plan to be successful.

Nursing Assessment

☐ PERTINENT HISTORY

Patterns of unstable relationships, recent crises or stressors, substance abuse, problems with impulse control, legal difficulties, suicide attempts, anxiety or panic attacks, transient psychotic episodes

☐ PHYSICAL FINDINGS

Depression, crying, anxiety, irritability, clinging, anger, agitation, apathy

☐ PSYCHOSOCIAL CONCERNS/ DEVELOPMENTAL FACTORS

Social and employment history, usual coping mechanisms, problems with sexual relatedness, life-style, indefinite career goals, unstable home life, mood swings, inability to tolerate solitude or frustration, erratic school progress, boredom, patterns of manipulation

☐ PATIENT AND FAMILY KNOWLEDGE

Perception of degree of disruption, awareness of pattern of functioning, community resources, readiness and willingness to learn

Nursing Care

☐ LONG-TERM GOAL

The patient will achieve control of impulsive behaviors; the patient will learn to integrate realistic perceptions and acceptance of self and others.

NURSING DIAGNOSIS #1

Potential for violence related to inability to control anger, impulsive behavior

Rationale: *The anger felt by the borderline patient is a result of inability to develop and achieve autonomy. Frustration with the problems of adult life results in the projection of violence onto the present situation or inward to the self.*

GOAL

The patient will not exhibit self-mutilating or suicidal behaviors; will manage anger and impulsive behaviors in safe, socially acceptable ways.

IMPLEMENTATION

- Assess environment for potential for harm to self or others; refer to *The Patient who is Suicidal*, page 144; provide safety at all times.
- State explicitly the unacceptability of destructive behaviors to self, others, or property; refer to *The Patient who is Violent*, page 149; use restraints or seclusion when necessary, explaining reasons and then carrying out to minimize escalation.
- Monitor for use of chemicals; be alert for signs of drug or alcohol consumption; provide adequate supervision during all activities; negotiate a contract for expectations of acceptable behavior.
- Monitor for self-abusive behaviors (e.g., excessive alcohol or food consumption, drug abuse, accidents); discuss possible referrals for long-term follow up.
- Assist patient to identify factors that precipitate acting-out behavior and encourage verbalization of what is being felt rather than acting on it; work with patient to find alternative acceptable behaviors; know that established patterns of behavior are difficult to change and require long-term, patient, and persistent communication.
- Substitute physical activities when possible (e.g., punching bag, jogging); refer to *The Patient Manifesting Anger*, page 13.
- Explain limit setting in nonpunitive manner with clear statements of expectations; ensure that all personnel on all shifts perceive the necessity of consistent reinforcement; adjust limits according to progress in handling responsibility for self.
- Be alert for testing behavior; withdraw attention when acting out occurs unless it is destructive; if self-mutilation occurs, give treatment, then focus on feelings of patient.
- Give positive feedback when any control of acting-out behavior is achieved; assist in developing skill in communicating verbally what is being felt.

EVALUATION CRITERIA/DESIRED OUTCOMES

The Patient
- Displays fewer acting-out and impulsive behaviors
- Identifies stress-producing situations
- Verbalizes feelings of anger in appropriate ways
- Does not ingest chemicals
- Identifies and demonstrates alternative constructive behaviors to control impulsivity

---

NURSING DIAGNOSIS #2

Ineffective individual coping related to inability to express feelings and use coping skills constructively

---

Rationale: The lack of development of a strong and integrated ego results in poorly developed coping skills, chronic boredom, and denial of feelings.

GOAL

The patient will identify feelings; will develop problem-solving and sublimating skills.

IMPLEMENTATION

- Assist to develop problem-solving skills; refer to *Problem Solving*, page 248.
- Encourage verbalization of underlying feelings to redirect energy from conflict to constructive channels.
- Teach recognition of distancing and dependency behaviors; assist to define consequences of these behaviors and alternatives that can be developed; provide constructive feedback.
- Encourage participation in psychodrama if possible to provide opportunity for expression of painful emotions.
- Promote identification and expansion of previous interests, hobbies, and talents to decrease the hopelessness of chronic boredom; assist to identify activities that alleviate boredom and promote development of constructive autonomy; encourage creativity in adjunctive therapies.
- Assist in identifying strengths and successes so that appropriate self-esteem is developed rather than continued feelings of grandiosity, entitlement, or devaluation; refer to *The Patient Experiencing a Threat to Self-Esteem*, page 127.
- Determine what coping mechanisms have been used successfully in the past and encourage their continued use; make a written list to emphasize positive aspects of life.
- Use role playing to rehearse new behaviors and develop expertise in usage.
- Teach assertive techniques as ways of coping.
- Provide increased structure in activities during establishment of new coping skills.

EVALUATION CRITERIA/DESIRED OUTCOMES

The Patient
- Identifies feelings of boredom and strategies to counteract them
- Verbalizes strengths and weaknesses realistically
- Actively pursues 1 hobby
- Demonstrates understanding of the use of assertive techniques and problem-solving skills

---

NURSING DIAGNOSIS #3

Social isolation related to instability of social and interpersonal relationships

---

Rationale: The inconsistency of the patient's behavior produces frustration and uncertainty in others. The patient's fear of abandonment produces clinging behavior which in turn leads to distancing when needs are not met and disappointment occurs. Manipulation and the perception of others as either "all good" (idealization) or "all bad" (devaluation) alienates others, leaving the patient with feelings of loneliness and emptiness.

☐ GOAL

The patient will establish social contacts; will begin to identify positive and negative aspects of self and others.

☐ IMPLEMENTATION

- Assist patient to identify expectations of self and others; determine how realistic these expectations are and how they can be changed if unrealistic.
- Examine with patient how his/her behaviors affect the behavior of others; help establish patterns in relationships (e.g., absence of relationships, dual relationships to avoid closeness, superficiality, idealization, devaluing).
- Point out self-defeating patterns of behavior that alienate others; refer to *The Patient Displaying Manipulation*, page 94; assist to identify how this behavior results in loneliness and emptiness.
- Discuss which persons are being idealized or devalued; point out obvious contradictions.
- Assist to develop awareness of assigning value to people; ask patient how these perceptions of others relate to self (e.g., "I wonder if you ever felt this way about yourself") when excessive use of projection is displayed.
- Establish a trusting relationship by modeling consistency in behavior; use staff conferences to decrease conflicts among personnel and attempts by patient to split staff; remain nondefensive and examine own feelings about patient.
- Encourage group therapy, especially social skills groups; role play and rehearse new ways of relating to others; give feedback to emphasize appropriate patterns of relatedness; identify goals in relationships and discuss how they can be achieved.
- Help patient to establish positive contacts by beginning with 1 contact/day and increase as tolerated; assist to learn supportive behavior of others and give positive feedback for progress displayed; discuss concept of ambivalence and acceptance of others.
- Discuss available social support systems and contacts for developing and maintaining constructive relationships.

☐ EVALUATION CRITERIA/DESIRED OUTCOMES

The Patient
- Identifies behaviors that cause difficulties in relationships
- Describes situations that increase useage of splitting people into good/bad
- Identifies both positive and negative characteristics of self and others
- Accepts ambivalence in self and others
- Establishes 1 positive peer relationship

NURSING DIAGNOSIS #4

Disturbance in self-concept: personal identity related to weak ego formation, inability to master autonomy

Rationale: The failure to master separation produces an identity disturbance and difficulty determining reality. The patient may be confused regarding gender, identity, long-term goals, values, and beliefs.

☐ GOAL

The patient will identify differences between self and others; will clarify long-term goals and values.

☐ IMPLEMENTATION

- Assist to identify self-perception and discuss if perception is realistic; interpret to patient how others may perceive him/her and discuss differences (realistic feedback will decrease use of projection).
- Encourage verbalization of personal feelings, uncertainties, and thoughts that are of concern to patient; remain nonjudgmental and continue to exhibit positive regard for the patient.
- Support attempts to attain self-knowledge and deepen self-understanding; give information when indicated regarding careers, choices, education, etc.
- Request patient's opinions and contributions on appropriate topics; assist in development of identity and values.
- Encourage participation in group therapy to provide access to ideas and values of others.
- Encourage establishment of a regular exercise routine to strengthen body image and give patient an increased sense of reality, strengths, and weaknesses.
- Support efforts to determine long-term goals and interests.
- Encourage tolerance of differences between self and others.
- Suggest patient maintain written daily journal of

feelings and activities to help clarify thoughts, values, and beliefs.

☐ EVALUATION CRITERIA/DESIRED OUTCOMES

The Patient
- States realistic perception of self
- Accepts differences in values and beliefs of others
- Exercises regularly
- Makes journal entries daily
- Identifies 1 realistic long-term goal

NURSING DIAGNOSIS #5

Anxiety related to fear of abandonment

Rationale: The lack of the development of autonomy and individuation results in the persistent fear of abandonment. This produces anxiety, depression, irritability, and feelings of alienation and emptiness that can be intensified during periods of stress.

☐ GOAL

The patient will manage anxiety appropriately; will display stable affective behavior.

☐ IMPLEMENTATION

- Assist to identify factors that precipitate or intensify anxiety.
- Discuss concept of separation versus abandonment; work with patient to identify ways to gradually increase tolerance for periods of solitude.
- Discuss management of anxiety relative to the level displayed; refer to *The Patient Experiencing Anxiety*, page 22.
- Monitor for panic attacks (may precede self-mutilation or suicide attempts).
- Teach relaxation techniques; refer to Table 1, *Stress Management*, page 24.
- Role play management of anxiety-producing situations until discomfort is decreased.
- Monitor for signs of depression; refer to *The Patient Experiencing Depression*, page 57.
- Teach that old anxieties may not be relevant to current situations; assist to deal with regressive feelings prior to discharge; consider use of transitional objects such as a journal or telephone calls to help cope with separation anxiety.
- Give positive feedback for responsibility taken in the appropriate management of anxiety and self-defeating affective behaviors.
- Consider referral to a group that promotes self-monitoring of chronic anxiety (e.g., Recovery, Inc.) for community support.

☐ EVALUATION CRITERIA/DESIRED OUTCOMES

The Patient
- Describes anxiety-producing behaviors or situations
- Demonstrates understanding of stress management techniques
- Displays fewer expressions of inappropriate affect
- Maintains journal to use for assistance in transition to community

---

NURSING DIAGNOSIS #6

Knowledge deficit regarding family dynamics contributing to lack of development of autonomy and necessity of rehabilitative therapy

Rationale: Since the roots of the borderline personality are found in failure to develop in the separation-individuation phase prior to the age of 3, knowledge of appropriate parenting may allow for developmental progression. Once pathology has developed, treatment may be long term, and many resources may need to be utilized.

☐ GOAL

The patient/family will discuss and participate in ongoing treatment and rehabilitation of borderline individual.

☐ IMPLEMENTATION

- Determine patterns of family coping; refer to family therapy for prevention and treatment if at all possible.
- Educate parents about fostering independence in children prior to age 3 and the possible need for intensive psychotherapy and long-term treatment in the borderline adolescent.
- Teach drug regimen to patient/family when indicated.
- Inform patient/family of community services and agencies providing psychotherapy on an individual or group basis; make appropriate referrals prior to discharge.
- Provide referral for vocational education programs when indicated for retraining.
- Provide information regarding self-help groups (e.g., Alcoholics Anonymous, Narcotics Anonymous, Gamblers Anonymous, Overeaters Anonymous) for appropriate individuals.
- Assist in identifying high-risk situations that may result in need for crisis intervention; provide local telephone numbers for agencies providing these services (e.g., Suicide Prevention Center).
- Identify individuals and groups to provide support and assistance to patient/family and information as to use, availability, and cost.

☐ EVALUATION CRITERIA/DESIRED OUTCOMES

The Patient/Family
- Identifies dynamics that may contribute to borderline pathology
- Has a list of community support groups available
- Describes drug regimen correctly
- Acknowledges need for family therapy
- Demonstrates knowledge of postdischarge follow up

The Patient with Bulimia

Definition/Discussion

Bulimia is a clinical syndrome characterized by a morbid fear of becoming overweight combined with voluntary restriction of food intake followed by "binge" overeating, self-induced vomiting, and overuse of laxatives to rid the body of food. The *DSM-III-R* classifies this problem as an eating disorder. Other eating disorders with onset in childhood and adolescence are anorexia nervosa and pica (craving for unnatural foods such as plaster or dirt).

Nursing Assessment

☐ PERTINENT HISTORY

Ongoing problem with weight control, restrictive dieting, out-of-control binge/purge episodes (often related to difficulty handling specific emotions such as anger, depression, loneliness, boredom, and interpersonal conflicts with parents or friends); pattern of secret overeating of high-calorie, easily digested food until physically uncomfortable; history of inducing vomiting or purging with laxatives; history of poor impulse control

☐ PHYSICAL FINDINGS

Change in vital signs, anemia, dehydration, electrolyte imbalance, obesity, hypertension

☐ PSYCHOSOCIAL CONCERNS/ DEVELOPMENTAL FACTORS

Body-image distortion (e.g., overestimation of size of body, belief of being overweight when within normal weight limit, an unrealistic ideal for own body), unrealistic expectations about body needs for food and exercise, feelings of guilt, depression, and self-disgust after binge

☐ PATIENT AND FAMILY KNOWLEDGE

Knowledge distortion about body functions and needs; symptoms to report to physician, realistic expections for self (including body needs for food and exercise), treatment plan, diet behaviors to reinforce, community resources and support groups, readiness and willingness to learn

Nursing Care

☐ LONG-TERM GOAL

The patient will accept and adjust to a comprehensive program of weight management; the patient will regain/maintain a realistic body image.

NURSING DIAGNOSIS #1

Alteration in nutrition: less than body requirements related to binging/purging

Rationale: Out-of-control binging and purging episodes cause rapid changes in weight and may contribute to electrolyte imbalance, cardiac dysrhythmias, hypertension, and secondary complications of obesity. Prognosis is good with weight-treatment plan and use of a follow-up support group. There is an increased risk of complications and death if bulimia associated with anorexia nervosa or if patient does not comply with treatment.

☐ GOAL

The patient will participate in a weight-treatment plan that includes a healthy diet and exercise appropriate to own life-style; will decrease or be free from binging and purging episodes; will be free from electrolyte imbalance, cardiac dysrhythmias, complications associated with obesity.

☐ IMPLEMENTATION

- Refer to *Strategies for Counseling Adolescents*, page 252.
- Assess patient/family attitudes toward food.
- Consult with physician, dietician, patient/family to develop an individualized, suitable weight-treatment plan.
- Encourage questions and invite participation in meal planning and cooking adaptations.
- Assist to express feelings and concerns about self and weight-treatment plan; be accepting and nonjudgmental about history of out-of-control eating

and purging episodes, and focus instead on patient's perceptions of the difficulties of dealing with weight management and coping with stress of daily life.
- Offer hope that patient can learn to manage daily life and weight problem; refrain from lecturing, shaming, or giving unwanted advice.
- Be clear and consistent about treatment plan and set firm limits on appropriate behavior; refer to *Behavior Modification*, page 250.
- Provide support and positive reinforcement for demonstration of adaptive eating.
- Know that motivation for change has to come from within patient; help patient identify problem behaviors and set goals; refer to *Problem Solving*, page 248.
- Help to locate an appropriate mutual-support peer group or group therapy program for ongoing support.

☐ **EVALUATION CRITERIA/DESIRED OUTCOMES**

The Patient
- Participates in weight-treatment plan, including diet and exercise
- Decreases or remains free from binging and purging episodes
- Regains/maintains fluid and electrolyte balance
- Ingests adequate nutrition to maintain weight within normal range for height and body
- Verbalizes importance of ongoing support group to maintain weight-treatment plan

---

NURSING DIAGNOSIS #2

Disturbance in self-concept related to distorted perceptions of body size, body image

Rationale: Self-concept is an ongoing perception and adaptation to body image, personal identity, role performance, and self-esteem. The bulemic may have disturbances in most of these areas; the most common disturbance is an ability to perceive body size, body functions, and physical needs realistically.

☐ **GOAL**

The patient will regain/maintain a realistic body image; will develop realistic attitudes and perceptions about own body size, needs, and functions.

☐ **IMPLEMENTATION**
- Assist patient to express feelings and concerns about self, body size/function, and physical needs.
- Consistently point out misperceptions and teach as needed; provide support and positive feedback

for accurate perceptions of size and body function.
- Work with patient to identify abilities and strengths; offer opportunities to participate in projects or tasks that utilize existing abilities.
- Use appropriate strategies to increase patient's self-esteem; refer to *The Patient Experiencing a Threat to Self-Esteem*, page 127.
- Teach to verbalize positive affirmations about body (e.g., "I am healthy and energetic at my ideal weight." "I am flexible and at ease." "I am learning to listen to my body."); have patient create own statements and practice imagining self in a positive way several times a day.

☐ **EVALUATION CRITERIA/DESIRED OUTCOMES**

The Patient
- Discusses own body size, needs, and functions in realistic and positive terms
- Demonstrates realistic attitudes and perceptions about own body size, needs, functions

---

NURSING DIAGNOSIS #3
a. **Ineffective individual coping** related to anxiety, intense feelings, inability to control eating habits
b. **Knowledge deficit** regarding coping with anxiety, intense feelings, inability to control eating habits, treatment plan

Rationale: Out-of-control binge/purge behaviors are an ineffective way to cope with anxiety, intense feelings, and the stress of everyday life. This patient may also have a history of poor impulse control, especially when anxious. The patient with bulimia is often struggling with adolescent issues of identity, independence versus dependency, self-doubt about ability to take responsibility for self/inability to make decisions and problem solve. The patient can learn adaptive coping mechanisms and self-control.

☐ **GOAL**

The patient will develop a plan and practice strategies to cope effectively with anxiety, intense feelings, activities of daily living (ADL), and the stress of everyday life; will be free from out-of-control binge/purge behaviors.

☐ **IMPLEMENTATION**
- Explore patterns of behavior with patient, especially noting pattern of events that occur before binge/purge episodes.
- Assist to find adaptive ways to cope with anxiety, feelings/stressors (e.g., to identify, name, and express feelings in effective ways (such as assertion

techniques, communication skills, "I" statements [" *I'm* feeling upset about what just happened. *I'd* like to sit down and talk about it. Are you willing to sit down and talk with me now?"]).

- Help patient to explore alternate ways to express feelings
  - to express anger try handball, racketball, hitting a punching bag or bed, shouting, singing, confronting with words, tearing up telephone books, throwing sponges or bean bags
  - to express guilt explore situations and persons with whom the patient experiences guilt: "I feel guilty when I . . .;" then have the patient try to replace the word "guilt" with "resentment"; explore feelings about this
- Know that most situations that involve guilt also involve feelings of anger and resentment; work with patient on expressing these feelings.
- Provide opportunities for choice and decision making in treatment plan and ADL (e.g., in hygiene, exercise, leisure activities).
- Avoid control struggles, reassure patient that healthy habits of ADL and independent problem solving can be learned.
- Identify hobbies and pastimes that patient enjoys; assist to include these on a daily basis.
- Teach to reward self for healthy eating habits, utilizing enjoyable pastimes and hobbies.
- Identify specific examples of times when patient feels especially anxious or needy (e.g., lonely, bored, dissatisfied with life, needing love, appreciation, companionship); explore these situations, the intense feelings that accompany them, and the lack of impulse control (e.g., overeating, binge/purge syndrome); work with patient to develop alternative ways to nurture self at these times

(e.g., taking a warm bubble bath, calling friend and arranging to go for walk and talk, getting a massage, going to gym to swim or work out, involving self with enjoyable hobby or pastime).

- Plan for daily outlets for productive activity (e.g., occupational, industrial therapy); ask what patient would like to achieve and help with this goal.
- Encourage verbalization and questions; ask patient to describe in own words medication, treatment plan, follow-up care, and symptoms to report to physician.
- Discuss community resources (e.g., support groups, rehabilitation and vocational training, day-care centers).
- Offer opportunities to practice adaptive coping by utilizing problem situations to role play and practice communication skills, assertion techniques, use of relaxation techniques, positive affirmations, and guided imagery (refer to Table 1, *Stress Management*, page 24).
- Provide support and positive reinforcement for demonstration of adaptive coping with ADL, stress, or intense feelings

☐ EVALUATION CRITERIA/DESIRED OUTCOMES

The Patient
- Demonstrates ability to cope effectively with anxiety and intense feelings
- Discusses plan to cope effectively with stress of everyday life
- Is free from out-of-control binge/purge behaviors
- Demonstrates self-control in eating habits
- Discusses follow-up plan, symptoms to report to physician, and community resources

The Patient Experiencing Chronic Illness

Definition/Discussion

Chronic illness is considered to be any impairment or deviation from normal health that has some of the following characteristics: **permanent, nonreversible, or residual impairment; insidious onset; need for a long period of supervision of care.** The role in chronic illness consists of behaviors related to the limitations that are defined by society as appropriate. Chronic illness involves a lifelong period of treatment, usually with remissions and exacerbation of symptoms; this role is not seen as attractive or desired, and the patient is often separated from the well population during periods of exacerbation. Impairment requires special training for rehabilitation.

Nursing Assessment

☐ **PERTINENT HISTORY**

Length of chronic illness to date and role behaviors developed thus far, remissions and exacerbations, hospitalizations and treatment

☐ **PHYSICAL FINDINGS**

Physical limitations, disfigurement, deformities caused by pathophysiology; projected course of pathophysiology and if permanent or progressive; projected level of rehabilitation; pain and other noxious stimuli; apathy, withdrawal, depression; restlessness, anxiety

☐ **PSYCHOSOCIAL CONCERNS/ DEVELOPMENTAL FACTORS**

Developmental stage and tasks; powerlessness; progression and current responses in grief process, support systems, stigmatization, guilt, motivation to retain roles and tasks; financial base/support

☐ **PATIENT AND FAMILY KNOWLEDGE**

Medical and rehabilitation plan, projected course of convalescence and level of independence, self-help groups, psychotherapists/clinic to aid acceptance of role of chronically ill; necessary equipment/aids; readiness and willingness to learn

Nursing Care

☐ **LONG-TERM GOAL**

The patient will adapt to limitations imposed by chronic illness; the patient will care for self and be as independent as possible; the patient will retain as many previous tasks and roles as are possible.

NURSING DIAGNOSIS #1

Grieving related to change in body image, roles in chronic illness

Rationale: *Numerous losses occur with the onset of chronic illness (e.g., loss of function, health, self-image, self-esteem, performance). Grief is a natural response to loss and is present in a person adjusting to a chronic illness.*

☐ **GOAL**

The patient will work through the stages of the grief process.

☐ **IMPLEMENTATION**

- Assess for behaviors of shock and disbelief, denial, and other behaviors of loss; listen and give emotional support, accepting the patient's need to cope with the situation at own pace; accept patient's denial at this time but do not support it; refer to *The Patient Manifesting Denial,* page 52.
- Protect patient from injury caused by denying or ignoring limitations; strive to prevent complications and deformities; refer to *The Patient Manifesting Noncompliance,* page 97.
- Assess patient/family for knowledge of chronic disease process, treatment plan, treatments, medications and for feelings and concerns; give positive reinforcement for knowledge and cooperation.
- Offer brief explanations if requested; wait until initial grief and mourning period is over to begin teaching.

- Be aware of adaptive and maladaptive behaviors associated with loss; assess patient's behaviors and support adaptive ones; refer to *The Patient Experiencing Grief and Loss*, page 80.
- Assist through feelings of anger by encouraging verbalization; know that the expression of anger toward the environment occurs because of inability to control losses; assist family to accept this; refer to *The Patient Experiencing Powerlessness*, page 115.
- Allow patient/family to cry; be empathic; spend time with them and continue to show positive regard and respect; encourage communication between family members and patient; use touch appropriately.
- Reassure that grieving responses to loss are universal, that stages overlap, that time is needed to achieve the restitution phase.
- Be alert for signs of dysfunctional grieving in both patient and family; assist in progressing through stages (e.g., role play to express feelings); praise them when progress is made.
- Determine successful coping methods used in previous losses and support their use.
- Help patient/family to identify changes which are imminent due to alterations in role and financial resources; assist to find satisfactory alternatives to previous methods of coping; refer to *Problem Solving*, page 248.

☐ EVALUATION CRITERIA/DESIRED OUTCOMES

The Patient
- Expresses feelings and concerns about loss (body part, function, independence, role)
- Begins to state meaning of loss and is realistic about limitations
- Discusses plans for present realistically

NURSING DIAGNOSIS #2

Self-care deficit related to limitations of chronic disease or disability

Rationale: Self-care tasks and roles change with a chronic illness. The patient will need to learn new methods for meeting basic needs because of the additional requirements of coping with treatments, medications, and rehabilitation. Usual self-care may be drastically altered by the limitations of the illness.

☐ GOAL

The patient begins to recognize and cope with limitations and becomes committed to rehabilitation program

☐ IMPLEMENTATION

- Emphasize patient's assets and strengths; give positive reinforcement with praise and attention as patient begins to show progress and commitment to treatment plan and rehabilitative program; refer to *The Patient Experiencing the Sick Role*, page 134.
- Set short-term goals in order to increase patient's ability to be independent in activities of daily living (ADL); encourage independence in therapeutic exercises and range of motion as ordered by physician and physical therapist.
- Teach safe practices in self-care, making modifications in activity commensurate with abilities; involve family in adjustments.
- Encourage patient to participate in planning own care and to do as much self-care as limitations of chronic disease or disability will allow; be aware that patient may become very dependent on first hearing diagnosis.
- Help to minimize fatigue by keeping stressors at a minimum; know that inability to care for his/herself increases anxiety and frustration; refer to *The Patient Experiencing Anxiety*, page 22.
- Teach that participation in ADL and exercise program is essential to restore motivation and optimism as well as to retain muscle tone and ROM.
- Be creative with the patient and the health care team to assist the patient to use self-help devices when there is difficulty performing an activity; self-help devices may include adaptive equipment for mobility, personal care aids, communication, writing and typewriting aids.
- Assess for readiness to learn about disease process, treatment plan, medication, and prognosis; teach patient/family as indicated; refer *Guidelines for Teaching Patients and Families*, page 229.
- Be prepared to give emotional support, comfort measures, and treatment of acute symptoms during exacerbations; patient may fear further disability, pain, increased dependence, and death; refer to *The Patient Experiencing Fear*, page 78.

☐ EVALUATION CRITERIA/DESIRED OUTCOMES

The Patient
- Begins to participate in ADL and exercise program
- Discusses disease process, treatment plan, medications, and adjustments to limitations in self-care
- Assumes roles in realistic fashion
- Discusses concerns, fears, and problems anticipated
- Begins to plan for the future

NURSING DIAGNOSIS #3

Disturbance in self-concept: body image, self-esteem related to chronic illness

---

Rationale: One of the major changes brought about by chronic illness may be the loss or alteration of a body part which results in a lowered self-esteem. This can lead to depression and hopelessness in the patient.

☐ GOAL

The patient will develop constructive adjustment to altered body image and maintain adequate self-esteem.

☐ IMPLEMENTATION

- Encourage verbalization of feelings regarding alteration of appearance and promote gradual acceptance of changes; if indicated, assist patient to touch area that is changed so that acceptance of changes in body can begin.
- Assist patient to improve appearance and body image; provide cleanliness, make-up, hair grooming, own clothing, etc.; praise when efforts are made to accomplish this with increasing independence.
- Teach use of rehabilitative and cosmetic services if indicated.
- Monitor for symptoms of depression; refer to *The Patient Experiencing Depression,* page 57.
- Assist patient to identify own strengths and limitations; assist in modifying activities to experience successes in ADL.
- Assist patient to retain roles and tasks to extent possible within existing limitations.
- Assist to identify activities and interests which are positive and able to be mastered; know that this gives patient some continuity and hope for the future.
- Teach patient to reward self for accomplishments; involve family whenever possible.
- Recognize that patients with chronic illnesses or disabilities are still sexual beings; assist patient to deal with sexual concerns by teaching, counseling, or referral to a specialist in counseling the handicapped.
- Assist patient to find one positive aspect of every day, to define something hopeful for each day, and to take one day at a time.

☐ EVALUATION CRITERIA/DESIRED OUTCOMES

The Patient
- Identifies current strengths and limitations
- States one activity that has been mastered
- Identifies one positive aspect of self every day

NURSING DIAGNOSIS #4
Ineffective individual coping related to multiple stressors imposed by chronic illness

---

Rationale: The existence of a chronic illness may produce extreme stress in an individual. The inability to meet basic needs and the changes in life-style necessitated by physical/mental limitations may decrease the ability to cope adequately. The patient is in a state of conflict imposed by limitations and threat to life-style and may need to temporarily regress and depend on others.

☐ GOAL

The patient will develop coping strengths adequate for altered role.

☐ IMPLEMENTATION

- Assess abilities to cope with stress of chronic illness; identify previous successful coping patterns.
- Monitor dependent and regressive behavior; offer hope and assistance towards independent self-care; give feedback to patient on behaviors that are unnecessarily dependent.
- Encourage verbalization about changes s/he feels should be made; assist to identify new or alternate ways of coping; involve family whenever possible.
- Provide information and teaching in stress management (e.g., relaxation techniques, setting realistic goals, making decisions, assertive communication); refer to Table 1, *Stress Management,* page 24.
- Assist patient to become comfortable with these skills and encourage and support both patient and family whenever possible.

☐ EVALUATION CRITERIA/DESIRED OUTCOMES

The Patient
- Discusses feelings and concerns regarding stressors imposed by chronic illness
- Identifies one effective method of coping with stress of chronic illness
- Demonstrates use of assertive communication
- Develops realistic goals and expectations

NURSING DIAGNOSIS #5
Social isolation related to limitations in outside contacts and activities imposed by chronic illness

Rationale: The decrease in ability to be mobile, the social stigma of illness, and the alteration of physical/mental state may contribute to the lack of social interaction of the chronic illness patient. Once contact is decreased significantly with others, it may be difficult to resume, adding to the withdrawal and/or depression of the patient and the burden on the family.

☐ GOAL

The patient will maintain social ties; will participate in family life; will decrease feelings of social isolation.

☐ IMPLEMENTATION

- Assess state of loneliness and/or withdrawal of patient and family; explore feelings of "being different" or "looking different"; provide accurate information regarding these negative results of chronic illness and encourage ventilation of feelings.
- Foster healthy development of acceptance of necessary changes in life-style; determine what this means to the patient/family, and which outside contacts can be preserved and which cannot.
- Assess hobbies and pastimes that can decrease monotony; involve others whenever possible.
- Explore feelings about curiosity of others if body changes are visible; role play with patient/family how to respond in a manner that preserves self-esteem.
- Encourage communication between family and patient to determine how each feels about restriction; know that the care giver may experience increased isolation due to the increased burdens and responsibilities and this results in decreased life satisfaction for both.
- Encourage patient/family to discuss stresses felt in maintaining social ties; discuss ways of alternating care givers and changing surroundings of patient.
- Explore use of community contacts and support groups that can be of assistance in patient care and socialization (e.g., senior citizen or day-care groups).
- Involve as many family, friends, and appropriate outside agencies as possible to maximize the quality of life of the patient/family; for some, the addition of a pet to the household will decrease loneliness and promote a sense of companionship.

☐ EVALUATION CRITERIA/DESIRED OUTCOMES

The Patient
- Discusses ways of increasing supportive relationships
- Accepts assistance from friends and family
- Experiences decreased feelings of social isolation
- States one hobby which will be resumed or developed

NURSING DIAGNOSIS #6

Knowledge deficit regarding home maintenance management

Rationale: Patient needs to anticipate returning home and coping with limitations. Environmental changes are often required, as well as purchase of equipment and supplies. An altered daily routine

---

needs to be planned for and implemented so the patient will not be overwhelmed by the changes.

☐ GOAL

The patient will identify home management needs; will plan for dealing with the problems before discharge.

☐ IMPLEMENTATION

- Begin planning for discharge on the day of admission; reassess the patient's functional potential so that discharge plans can be made by health care team; know that chronic illnesses have remissions and exacerbations; teach patient/family to prepare for changes required with increased symptoms.
- Assist patient/family to acquire needed skills or assistance for going home.
- Give increased support when discharge is near; many patients experience some separation anxiety and have concerns about leaving hospital.
- Assess attitudes and concerns of family members; family therapy may be indicated for rejection and avoidance.
- Send ADL assessment home or to extended care facility so that visiting nurse or staff will be able to reinforce independent progress in ADL.
- Advise patient/family of Rehabilitation Services Administration, which provides diagnosis, treatment, counseling, training, and placement services to help towards vocational objectives.
- Inform patient of voluntary and self-help groups in community.
- Teach about needed equipment/aids and where to buy or rent.
- Tell patient/family about the Directory of National Information Sources on Handicapping Conditions and Related Services (contains abstracts and addresses of organizations offering services, information, and resources to handicapped individuals); obtain a copy from Superintendent of Documents, Government Printing Office, Washington, DC 20420.
- Educate person/family when additional assistance is indicated and under what conditions to notify physician and visiting nurse.

☐ EVALUATION CRITERIA/DESIRED OUTCOMES

The Patient
- Can describe in own words chronic disease process and medical treatment plan, including action and side effects of medication, exercise program, diet, etc.
- Can identify symptoms or side effects of medications to be reported to physician right away.
- Can describe rehabilitation program and adapt to limitations of chronic illness

- Can discuss appropriate support services and how to contact (e.g., social worker, rehabilitation services, self-help groups)

The Patient Experiencing Confusion

Definition/Discussion

Confusion is a quality or state of being perplexed. It is the inability to comprehend and/or integrate words or events and may be of a temporary or permanent nature. Refer to *The Patient with Alzheimer's Disease*, page 155, and *The Patient with Chronic Organic Brain Syndrome*, page 158, for discussion of irreversible confusion.

Nursing Assessment

☐ PERTINENT HISTORY

Characteristics and duration of confusion; polypharmacy, recent trauma, stresses or changes in environment or life-style; past and present coping mechanisms and support systems; recent losses; personality changes; changes in orientation and judgment; lability; seizures; exposure to toxic substances

☐ PHYSICAL FINDINGS

Sensory-perceptual deficits; abnormal vital signs, hydration; nutritional status; presence of infectious disease; metabolic, neurologic, cardiac, or respiratory system disturbance; drug/alcohol use, abuse, or withdrawal; dysmnesia (poor memory), agitation; apathy; poor hygiene

☐ PSYCHOSOCIAL CONCERNS/ DEVELOPMENTAL FACTORS

Personality style, history of deviant behaviors, social support systems, history of compulsive/paranoid behaviors; previous coping with crisis or similar situations

☐ PATIENT AND FAMILY KNOWLEDGE

Community agencies, severity of problem, degree of disruption, ways to cope

Nursing Care

☐ LONG-TERM GOAL

The patient will regain/maintain reality orientation to the extent possible.

NURSING DIAGNOSIS #1

Alteration in thought processes related to metabolic disturbances, neurologic trauma or dysfunction

Rationale: *The confused patient has dysfunction in perception, comprehension, attention, and memory, which causes problems in interpersonal relationships and communication (sending and receiving), and disorientation.*

☐ GOAL

The patient will recover from confusion; will regain as much contact with reality as possible.

☐ IMPLEMENTATION

- Always address the patient by name and state who you are (the patient may hear and understand you even if no acknowledgment is made).
- Be consistent in informing the patient what you are going to do; do not assume confusion is so great that understanding is not possible.
- Be patient in the need for continuing explanations; use clear, concise communication whenever possible.
- Involve the patient in decision making and activity whenever possible.
- Be honest, do not just go along with patient's "reality" and do not encourage a denial of the confusion; be sensitive to patient's needs.
- Avoid letting the patient ramble, bring the conversation back to reality at every opportunity.
- Use clear concise statements and questions; speak slowly and allow plenty of time for answers; do not rush patient.
- Have patient keep familiar objects (e.g., clock, own sleepwear, pictures of family and friends).
- Identify and assist in providing diversional activities appropriate for level of ability.
- Support and praise efforts to maintain conversation and reality-oriented behavior; encourage staff/family to praise patient for these efforts.

- Recognize cultural differences that may account for behaviors of patient/family.
- Reduce the amount of sensory overload/deprivation the patient is experiencing
  - overload: turn down lights or reduce noise level; schedule nursing care activities to allow for periods of uninterrupted quiet
  - deprivation: have a staff member or another alert patient spend time with patient, especially at mealtimes; put the patient with others or encourage familiar and positive visitors; whenever near, touch the patient, say hello, bring patient out of room into areas where additional sensory stimuli are available.
- Use the same staff as much as possible to provide continuity of care.

☐ EVALUATION CRITERIA/DESIRED OUTCOMES

The Patient
- Is increasingly oriented to person, place, and time
- Responds with increased alertness when asked for preferences in self-care
- Follows simple directions
- Recognizes family visitors

NURSING DIAGNOSIS #2

Potential for injury related to confusion, loss of memory, misperception

Rationale: The alteration of perception that results in impaired reality orientation may cause other people or the environment to appear threatening (e.g., patient may pull out IVs, trip over things, fall down). Dysmnesia may also produce unsafe situations (e.g., patient may forget to eat, take medications, do self-care, use safety devices, or may forget own limitations and loss of function).

☐ GOAL

The patient will accept necessary safety measures; will be free from accidents or injury related to confused state.

☐ IMPLEMENTATION

- Be alert to potential for injury; use mittens or restraints only if absolutely necessary.
- Orient frequently to environment; if intrusive procedures are necessary, assist to feel and see tubes, bottles, etc.; this will decrease fear and misperceptions.
- Assess for precipitating factors for the "sundown syndrome" (i.e., a patient is oriented and alert in daylight and becomes increasingly more confused at nightfall and in dark rooms); attempt to adjust

cause (e.g., isolation, darkness, drugs, noises, or fatigue).
- Provide a night light to assist in maintaining orientation.
- Use sedatives and pain medications judiciously; assess for increased confusion as a possible side effect.
- Protect patient and others from impulsive, labile, or negative behaviors; it is not always possible for the patient to control emotional response even when aware of actions.
- Watch for manifestation of illusions (misinterpretations of reality); listen and determine the basis; do not support the illusion but consistently and calmly reinforce reality to prevent anxiety.
- Support realistic expectations of abilities; praise for accomplishments whenever possible.
- Teach necessity for and methods of maintaining safe environment.
- Organize and maintain a regular routine.
- Make changes slowly so patient can maintain a feeling of security.

☐ EVALUATION CRITERIA/DESIRED OUTCOMES

The Patient
- Displays few misinterpretations of reality
- Is free from accidents and injury
- Accepts safety measures
- Sleeps better with night light
- Follows regular routine of activities

NURSING DIAGNOSIS #3

Social isolation related to confusion, withdrawal

Rationale: The inability to perceive or comprehend reality may cause the patient to withdraw from family and social interactions.

☐ GOAL

The patient will regain/maintain family and social contacts.

☐ IMPLEMENTATION

- Assess for proper working of hearing aids, and for eyeglasses that provide adequate vision for client (inability to hear or see well may cause withdrawal).
- Offer socialization opportunities (e.g., seat patient in hallway, bring to day room and encourage observation or participation in activities).
- Accompany to occupational or recreational therapy and support in any efforts to join activities.
- Offer socialization at mealtime (e.g., provide meals in dining area rather than in room, arrange

for patient to sit with family member or alert patient).
- Encourage family to visit as often as possible even though they may feel they are not recognized or their presence is not noticed.
- Have family members or friends share "old times"; reminiscing is valuable in maintaining self-esteem.
- Praise any efforts at being with others and involved with the environment.
- Use touch judiciously in combination with verbal communication, knowing that a combination of stimulation from 2 senses is more effective than from 1 alone.
- Provide a mirror and encourage use to maintain a sense of body.

- Enlist the support of all disciplines so the care plan will reflect consistent efforts to decrease isolation.
- Refer to a resocialization group if available and involve family members whenever possible.

☐ EVALUATION CRITERIA/DESIRED OUTCOMES

The Patient
- Socializes at mealtime
- Participates in hobbies, occupational therapy, or recreational therapy
- Uses glasses, hearing aid as needed
- Decreases withdrawal behaviors
- Increases verbal communication with peers

The Patient with a Conversion Disorder

Definition/Discussion

A conversion disorder is an unconscious process in which underlying psychologic conflict and anxiety are converted into symbolic physical symptoms that have no organic basis. Symptoms are temporary and symbolic in nature, such as paralysis in the arms and hands in a typist or pianist; they occur with increased stresses related to mastery of the developmental tasks of adolescent and adult life; cognitive functioning remains intact. The *DSM-III-R* classification is Somataform Disorder. Prior to 1979, this was considered to be hysterical neurosis, conversion type.

Careful assessment and testing must be done to rule out any organic basis for symptoms resembling those of neurologic lesions, endocrine disorders, or malingering (to feign an illness).

Nursing Assessment

☐ **PERTINENT HISTORY**

Onset of physical symptoms, recent history of increased stress or loss, present state of health, current medications

☐ **PHYSICAL FINDINGS**

Symptoms of physical disorder: sensory disturbances (e.g., blindness, deafness, numbness); motor disturbances of the voluntary nervous system (e.g., paralysis, tics, tremors, or convulsions); vital signs

☐ **PSYCHOSOCIAL CONCERNS/ DEVELOPMENTAL FACTORS**

Affect, patient's perception of disorder, *"la belle indifférence,"* forgetfulness, lack of concentration, distractability, lack of ability to sustain intellectual effort; adaptive/maladaptive coping mechanisms; strengths, weaknesses, stressors, relationships with significant other, family, friends; ability to carry out own activities of daily living (ADL)

☐ **PATIENT AND FAMILY KNOWLEDGE**

Symptoms of acute phase and prognosis, treatment, coping methods for anxiety and conflict, community resources and support groups, readiness and willingness to learn

Nursing Care

☐ **LONG-TERM GOAL**

The patient will verbalize relief from physical symptoms; the patient will cope more effectively with anxiety and conflict; the patient will increase ability to tolerate intense feelings, to cope with dependency needs, and to participate in independent self-care.

NURSING DIAGNOSIS #1

Self-care deficit (specify level) related to conversion symptoms

Rationale: Conversion symptoms (e.g., blindness, deafness, numbness, paralysis) may limit ability to perform self-care. In addition, the patient may tend to forget, have poor concentration, and regress to dependency on others for care.

☐ **GOAL**

The patient will verbalize relief of physical symptoms; will perform ADL independently.

☐ **IMPLEMENTATION**

- Approach in accepting and calm manner.
- Allow patient to discuss feelings and concerns.
- Do not confront patient with symptoms or lack of organic basis; listen to patient's perceptions and offer hope that patient will be able to be more independent and have fewer physical symptoms.
- Involve patient in decision making in ADL; offer choices when appropriate and let patient do as much independent decision making and self-care in hygiene, grooming, daily tasks, and pastimes as symptoms allow; assist with hygiene and ADL as needed until patient is able to do for self.
- Assist patient to focus on independent self-care activities and healthy interests such as friends,

hobbies, exercise; do not focus on physical symptoms.
- Engage in alternative activities with patient; give verbal praise and attention to patient when engaged in independent self-care activities.

☐ EVALUATION CRITERIA/DESIRED OUTCOMES

The Patient
- Experiences relief from physical symptoms
- Decreases focus on physical symptoms
- Performs ADL independently

NURSING DIAGNOSIS #2

Ineffective individual coping related to anxiety, conflict, and dependency needs

Rationale: The ego defense mechanism used is repression of conflict and anxiety; repressed feelings are converted into physical symptom(s) and the patient experiences psychologic relief and complacency; the characteristic lack of affect and lack of concern about the physical symptoms is called "la belle indifférence." Secondary gains usually include relief from unpleasant or feared responsibilities associated with developmental tasks, relief of dependency/independency conflicts, and increased attention and sympathy from family, friends, staff.

☐ GOAL

The patient will identify and express feelings; will discuss own needs and preferences; will demonstrate methods to effectively cope with conflict and anxiety.

☐ IMPLEMENTATION

- Observe verbal and nonverbal expressions of feelings; share your observations in nonjudgmental ways such as, "This is what I notice and I'm wondering what you're feeling right now?" or "You don't look upset right now, but if this (specify) happened to me I'd be hurt and angry. What are your thoughts and feelings about this?"
- Explore patient's feelings and concerns and assist to identify and name feelings; note ambivalence and conflict areas and allow patient to focus on these, verbally acknowledging that the patient is dealing with intense feelings and conflicting needs.
- Listen attentively when patient discusses or expresses feelings.
- Explore new ways to help patient express feelings, e.g., utilize role playing, assertive techniques, imagery (refer to Table 1, *Stress Management*, page 24), poetry, music, dance, sports.
- Allow to express needs and desires; identify one

nurse with whom the patient can consistently work and come to for help.
- Ignore manipulative behavior as much as possible and respond to direct expressions of feelings and needs; praise assertive, nonmanipulative, independent behavior.
- Acknowledge adaptive coping mechanisms and strengths, and explore ways to utilize these strengths to cope more effectively with intense feelings, anxiety, and conflict; refer to *Problem Solving,* page 248, *Behavior Modification,* page 250, and *The Patient Displaying Manipulation,* page 94.

☐ EVALUATION CRITERIA/DESIRED OUTCOMES

The Patient
- Identifies and explores feelings
- Demonstrates ability to express feelings effectively

NURSING DIAGNOSIS #3

Knowledge deficit regarding dynamics of disorder, treatment, ability to cope with anxiety, conflict, and stress, community resources and support groups

Rationale: The course of conversion disorders varies; after the conversion symptom is decreased or absent, the patient needs to continue to learn to cope with anxiety and stress, or regression into conversion symptoms may recur. Inadequate preparation for discharge or inadequate continuing follow-up care puts the patient at risk.

☐ GOAL

The patient/family will discuss treatment plan and follow-up care, including medication schedule and side effects to watch for; will plan to maintain independent ADL and to cope with stressors and anxiety.

☐ IMPLEMENTATION

- Assess level of knowledge and ability to comply with medication and treatment plan.
- Discuss a follow-up care schedule, and develop a plan to use in case patient feels anxious or overwhelmed with feelings.
- Assess availability of family; include them in discharge planning if possible.
- Encourage verbalization and questions; ask patient to describe in own words: medication, treatment plan, follow-up care, and symptoms to report to MD.
- Discuss community resources such as support groups, rehabilitation and vocational training, day-care centers.

☐ EVALUATION CRITERIA/DESIRED OUTCOMES

The Patient

- Has appointment for follow-up care with MD, clinic, or day care center, and can state how to contact them for appointment as needed
- Has plan to maintain independent ADL and to cope with stressors

The Patient Requiring Crisis Intervention

Definition/Discussion

Crisis intervention refers to those approaches used to restore a patient to a state of emotional equilibrium, from one of disequilibrium (the crisis state), that is equal to or better than the functioning at the precrisis level.

Nursing Assessment

☐ **PERTINENT HISTORY**

Recent illness or loss; stresses of the past year; transitions; trauma, catastrophic illness or accident; marriage, job, family stability; decreased ability to carry out activities of daily living (ADL); current threatening event

☐ **PHYSICAL FINDINGS**

Altered vital signs, anxiety (severe to panic), decreased concentration, somatic complaints, agitation, tension, neglect in self-care

☐ **PSYCHOSOCIAL CONCERNS/ DEVELOPMENTAL FACTORS**

Normal coping methods, supportive nuclear or dysfunctional family history, ego strengths, dependency patterns, apathy, distorted perceptions, regression to lower levels of functioning

☐ **PATIENT AND FAMILY KNOWLEDGE**

Previous experiences; perception of the problem, severity of disruption; internal and outside support or agencies; ability to decrease anxiety; socialization, interpersonal, and communication skills

Nursing Care

☐ **LONG-TERM GOAL**

The patient will achieve adaptive resolution of the crisis; the patient will return to usual job/roles with a realistic perception of what has occurred and with adequate coping mechanisms.

NURSING DIAGNOSIS #1

Ineffective individual coping related to perceived inability to deal with problem, distorted perception of the problem

Rationale: Usual coping mechanisms may not be able to prevent increased stress when a threatening event occurs. The individual may have a distorted perception of the problem and may feel unable to deal with it. The inability to manage the stress situation results in disequilibrium.

☐ **GOAL**

The patient will state perception of stressful situation and develop coping mechanisms effective in the crisis state.

☐ **IMPLEMENTATION**

- Ask to identify feelings regarding the stressful event and what patient perceives the problem to be; remember perception is what is important and patient's may differ from yours.
- Allow to respond at length and in detail to your questions; do not challenge any statements; try to determine exactly what is most threatening; listen and encourage patient to keep talking.
- Determine the real/anticipated patient loss/losses involved; assess behavior in light of the grief and mourning process; see *The Patient Experiencing Grief and Loss,* page 80.
- Determine the usual ways patient copes with a problem and how successful these methods are.
- Encourage verbalization about supportive individuals or agencies and whether or not they would be of value in the present situation.
- Ask what you could do to make patient feel better right now; if at all possible, provide it.
- Provide basic needs; patient may be very dependent in ADL; allow this dependency to occur for the immediate time.
- Help patient to gradually increase independence

in ADL: involve in self-care, slowly at first, then gradually add more activities.
- Provide opportunities for patient to make decisions about daily care (to give some control over own life); praise patient for making decisions, for coping with current stress, for helping self to feel better.
- Ask for patient's ideas on what can be done next to improve the situation; incorporate your ideas with patient's to give a sense of control.
- When behavior indicates that patient is beginning to adapt or cope (e.g., begins to ask questions, focus on reality), support and reinforce reality; share with patient how you see it; ask patient to clarify or validate your perceptions.
- Incorporate into the nursing care plan suggestions for new methods of coping with the crisis state; enlist the cooperation of staff in assisting the patient with these.

☐ **EVALUATION CRITERIA/DESIRED OUTCOMES**

The Patient
- Appraises situation realistically
- Verbalizes feelings regarding the threatening event
- Identifies usual methods of coping with problems
- States need for new ways to handle the disequilibrium
- Identifies at least two effective strategies

NURSING DIAGNOSIS #2

Anxiety related to feelings of being overwhelmed by threatening event

Rationale: Situations perceived as threatening produce increased anxiety that can result in inability to manage situation, which leads to feeling overwhelmed.

☐ **GOAL**

The patient will identify causes of threat; will achieve skill in managing the anxiety.

☐ **IMPLEMENTATION**
- Refer to *The Patient Experiencing Anxiety*, page 22.
- Ask what the patient is feeling at this time (e.g., scared, anxious, panicky) and what occurred to cause these feelings (e.g., new diagnosis, new roommate, new equipment).
- Encourage verbalization of all feelings of anxiety and discern those that are the most threatening; listen actively and with empathy.
- Make any environmental changes that are possible to decrease the impact of the threat (e.g., change room, allow family to stay for additional support).

- Share information regarding tests, procedures, etc.; tell what to expect and how orders are carried out.
- Enlist the help of other personnel in planning for care that will decrease anxiety; share your perceptions and information with them.
- Teach simple relaxation techniques (e.g., deep breathing) to use whenever needed to keep anxiety from increasing.
- When leaving room, tell patient when you will be back; return at the appointed time.

☐ **EVALUATION CRITERIA/DESIRED OUTCOMES**

The Patient
- Verbalizes causes of threat and describes threatening event
- Can make realistic requests to keep anxiety manageable
- Uses relaxation techniques
- Requests staff assistance appropriately

NURSING DIAGNOSIS #3

Grieving related to an actual or perceived loss

Rationale: An individual's grief is affected by many factors, including personality, previous losses, intimacy of relationship, and personal resources. Unresolved grief is a pathologic response of prolonged denial of the loss or a profound psychotic response that leads to problems in coping. Dysfunctional grieving is evidenced by loss of self-esteem, depression, excessively strong dependency needs, and ambivalent feelings for the lost person or object. Such unresolved grief leaves the individual susceptible to further psychologic trauma that can in turn lead to crisis, depression, and suicide.

☐ **GOAL**

The patient will describe loss and the meaning of the loss; will express and share grief with family; will resolve the loss in an adaptive manner.

☐ **IMPLEMENTATION**
- Review *The Patient Experiencing Grief and Loss*, page 80.
- Assess for any contributing/causative factors that may delay the grief work.
- Listen to patient, encourage expression of feelings (e.g., fear, despair, anger, sadness).
- Develop a relationship of trust through one-to-one interactions.
- Give support and reassurance by accepting patient's feelings and experiences.
- Explore what it is that makes patient feel hopeless, worthless, that life is not worth living.

- Provide support for the patient/family members by discussing feelings and coping mechanisms.
- Encourage patient/family to share grief and provide support for each other.
- Discuss new coping mechanisms; encourage to practice them.
- Involve patient in the decision making process.

☐ EVALUATION CRITERIA/DESIRED OUTCOMES

The Patient
- Expresses feelings
- Shares feelings and concerns with family members
- Participates in decision making for the future

NURSING DIAGNOSIS #4

Alteration in family process related to situational or pathophysiologic stressor

Rationale: When the normally supportive and adaptively functioning family experiences a stressor, the family's previously effective functioning ability may be challenged. Common factors that contribute to an alteration in family process include illness of a family member, trauma, loss of a family member or valued object, gain of a new family member, disaster, economic crisis, change in family roles, conflict, psychiatric illness, and social deviance. When the patient's/family's usual problem-solving methods are inadequate to resolve the situation, a crisis may occur. The patient/family in response to crisis will either return to precrisis functioning, develop a higher level of functioning, or develop an ineffective (lower) form of functioning.

☐ GOAL

The patient/family will return to the precrisis level of functioning; will verbalize feelings to nurse and to each other on a regular basis; will participate in care of family members; will maintain a functional system of mutual support for each other.

☐ IMPLEMENTATION

- Assess patient/family patterns of interaction and coping.
- Help patient/family members identify feelings of stress, past and current methods of coping, strengths and weaknesses.
- Encourage to share thoughts and feelings with each other, to interact and communicate daily.
- Encourage verbalization of guilt, anger, hostility, blame, and to recognize own feelings in patient/family members.
- Help patient/family to make realistic appraisal of the situation.
- Urge to list choices, available resources.

- Assist to reorganize roles as needed at home and to set priorities to maintain family integrity and to reduce stress.

☐ EVALUATION CRITERIA/DESIRED OUTCOMES

The Patient/Family
- Share feelings and concerns
- Participate in care appropriately
- Set priorities and implement adaptive coping strategies
- Reorganize home roles as needed
- Avoid crisis or return to precrisis level of functioning

NURSING DIAGNOSIS #5

Knowledge deficit regarding utilization of support systems, problem-solving techniques needed to avert a crisis state

Rationale: A crisis will not develop if situational supports are sufficient, perception of the problem is realistic, and effective coping solutions are available.

☐ GOAL

The patient will identify available support; will develop alternative coping to solve current problem.

☐ IMPLEMENTATION

- Continue to give as much information as needed about hospitalization, treatment therapy, etc.; ask for feedback to ensure understanding.
- Teach to brainstorm alternate solutions to current problem, to look at the pros and cons of each one; do not tell patient what to do, but ask if one of the solutions could possibly work.
- Check the effectiveness of patient's new coping options by asking what actions patient would take if confronted with a situation similar to the one just experienced; reinforce positive adaptation and coping and teach as necessary.
- Refer to outside support or agency to correct family or individual dysfunction once crisis is resolved.

☐ EVALUATION CRITERIA/DESIRED OUTCOMES

The Patient/Family
- Has a realistic expectation of what occurred
- Has adequate situational supports in the form of family, friends, job
- States at least 3 options available to use to cope with stress
- Has name of a community resource to go to if another threatening situation occurs

The Patient Manifesting Denial

Definition/Discussion

Denial is the manifestation of a person's inability to consciously acknowledge some anxiety-provoking aspect of self or of external reality. It is an unconscious defense mechanism used to allay anxiety.

Nursing Assessment

☐ **PERTINENT HISTORY**

Usual methods of coping, causes for behavior, compliance with treatment plan

☐ **PHYSICAL FINDINGS**

Symptoms of physical neglect (e.g., colostomy bag not changed, no mouth care), disheveled appearance, not eating, ignoring basic needs

☐ **PSYCHOSOCIAL CONCERNS/ DEVELOPMENTAL FACTORS**

Apathy, exaggerated cheerfulness, usual methods of communication; disbelief of diagnosis, symptoms, progress, information given; information changed in such a way that it can be termed distorted; refusal to discuss hospitalization, trauma, or diagnosis; refusal of medication, food, all treatments; refusal to follow recommendations that do not produce any increase in discomfort and may actually increase comfort

☐ **PATIENT AND FAMILY KNOWLEDGE**

Past experiences with illness, trauma, and changes in life-style; perception of situation; degree of disruption

Nursing Care

☐ **LONG-TERM GOAL**

The patient will interact with the environment in a way that maintains integrity and control and is not harmful to self.

NURSING DIAGNOSIS #1

Potential for injury related to denial of reality, need for treatment

Rationale: The mechanism of denial allows reality to be redefined so that it is no longer threatening; this may result in refusal to acknowledge physical limitations or the need for treatment.

☐ **GOAL**

The patient will eliminate the physically harmful aspects of the denial.

☐ **IMPLEMENTATION**

- Relieve anxiety through the establishment of a trusting relationship.
- Spend time listening to patient verbalize about areas of own life other than the focus of denial.
- Identify and support use of other coping mechanisms (e.g., talking, crying).
- Attempt to identify the most threatening aspects of reality by observing what the patient reacts to most intensely (e.g., patient is on a 1,000-calorie diet and has the family bring in fattening foods).
- Do not support the denial but give adequate care and converse with patient frequently; do not avoid patient; be alert for indications patient is willing to verbalize about the focus of denial.
- Allow time to adjust; do not give additional information until able to tolerate or denial may be increased.
- Attempt to introduce realities slowly by beginning with the least threatening part of the reality (e.g., if patient refuses to begin looking at or caring for colostomy, begin by discussing diet and then gradually move the conversation into discussing diet for colostomy patients).
- Assess motivation for behavior, then identify and assist to meet needs in nondestructive manner.

52

EVALUATION CRITERIA/DESIRED OUTCOMES

The Patient
- Accepts the need for treatment and the plan for care
- Uses necessary precautionary measures
- Consents to changes in activities of daily living (ADL)

NURSING DIAGNOSIS #2

Anxiety related to actual or perceived threat to the status quo

Rationale: Changes brought about by trauma, illness, or life-style alterations may cause anxiety that may increase as denial lessens.

GOAL

The patient will recognize and manage anxiety in an adaptive manner.

IMPLEMENTATION

- Assess level of anxiety and assist in reduction to manageable proportions; refer to *The Patient Experiencing Anxiety*, page 22.
- Teach simple relaxation techniques.
- Provide empathy; show you are concerned and interested.
- Encourage verbalization of fears, worries; give attention to the patient's questions.
- Use clear, concise communication techniques.
- Keep environment serene (e.g., lower lights and noise level, limit numbers of people).
- Focus on positive aspects of life and inherent strengths.
- Provide diversions to occupy time and provide sources of pleasure.

EVALUATION CRITERIA/DESIRED OUTCOMES

The Patient
- Acknowledges anxiety and verbalizes related feelings

- Utilizes relaxation techniques
- Shows decreased physiologic/psychologic discomfort
- Identifies and uses diversionary activities

NURSING DIAGNOSIS #3

Knowledge deficit regarding denial in response to changes in life-style, altered management of ADL

Rationale: The acceptance of life changes can be a slow and difficult process. Continued teaching will assist in decreasing the denial and achieving successful adjustment.

GOAL

The patient/family will express an understanding of and willingness to maintain healthy practices.

IMPLEMENTATION

- Continue to involve the patient in own care when planning time, place, and kind of care.
- Praise and encourage any interest shown in knowing more about the change/illness.
- Praise efforts in caring for self, beginning recognition of reality.
- Spend time with family to explain to them what is happening and what they can do to assist and support patient's positive efforts to cope.
- Help other staff/family realize the importance of refraining from chastising the patient/family when they are using denial to cope.
- Inform, when indicated, of self-help groups for continuing support for patient/family.

EVALUATION CRITERIA/DESIRED OUTCOMES

The Patient/Family
- Discusses the positive and negative aspects of the change/illness
- Follows those aspects of daily regimen that maintain life at optimum level
- Accepts responsibility for possible effects of noncompliance with recommended regimen

The Patient with a Dependent Personality Disorder

Definition/Discussion

The person with a dependent personality disorder has a current and long-term pattern of functioning in which s/he passively allows others to be responsible for major areas of life because of a lack of self-confidence, low self-esteem, and an inability to function independently. This individual avoids self-reliance, puts other persons' needs first, and has problems identifying own needs. There is frequent belittling of self and problems with depression and hopelessness. Because of an underlying fear of abandonment, anxiety is produced, which results in clinging, needy, and demanding behavior. These characteristics result from lack of fulfillment of dependency needs early in life.

Nursing Assessment

☐ **PERTINENT HISTORY**

Usual coping mechanisms, length and extent of dependency; exacerbation by environment, substance abuse, recent stress, depression, chronic illness as a child or adolescent, anxiety or panic attacks

☐ **PHYSICAL FINDINGS**

Apathy, withdrawal, crying, clinging, irritability, anger, tension, agitation, demanding, refusal to participate in care, tremulousness, sweating, vertigo, shortness of breath, dyspnea

☐ **PSYCHOSOCIAL CONCERNS/ DEVELOPMENTAL FACTORS**

Social and employment history, life-style, ability to manage stress or crisis, absence of parent in early life, chaotic home environment, childhood fears, nightmares, inability to tolerate solitude or frustration

☐ **PATIENT AND FAMILY KNOWLEDGE**

Perception of degree of disruption, previous similar situations and experiences, involvement of outside agencies, awareness of pattern of functioning, acceptance of passivity by self and family

Nursing Care

☐ **LONG-TERM GOAL**

The patient will accept responsibility for major life decisions and will demonstrate increased self-reliance, self-esteem, and ability to function more independently.

NURSING DIAGNOSIS #1

Ineffective individual coping related to subordinating own needs to the needs and decisions of others

Rationale: The development of a long-term pattern of passive dependence and excessive or unnecessary reliance on others results in an individual's inability to assume responsibility for the management of his/her own life. Feelings of depression associated with inability or failure to function independently interfere with the individual's progress towards effective coping.

☐ **GOAL**

The patient will decrease dependent behaviors; will progress toward self-responsibility in daily functioning.

☐ **IMPLEMENTATION**

- Assess level of functioning on a continuing basis; display confidence in patient's abilities after careful explanation; set limits on the amount and type of dependent behavior that will be tolerated by the staff; be consistent in maintaining limits.
- Ask for patient's perceptions of dependent and independent functioning; explore how needs are

met by passive dependence as well as independent action.

- Give feedback on what you observe; assist patient to identify problem areas and situations in which patient wishes to take more independent action.
- Listen to patient's description of own needs, ideas, and feelings; convey to him/her you consider his/her opinions valuable and worthwhile.
- Actively involve patient in plan of care whenever possible; assist to identify realistic and attainable goals acceptable to both patient and treatment team.
- Role play assertive techniques so that increased control over decisions can be achieved.
- Assist to develop coping strategies that are effective; teach patient problem-solving techniques; refer to *Problem Solving*, page 248.
- Use behavior modification when indicated; recognize and reinforce attention to own needs and decisions that are appropriate and ignore passive, dependent behaviors; refer to *Behavior Modification*, page 250.
- Praise any independent behavior and/or increase in autonomy; be honest and do not flatter; do not take on patient's responsibilities or make decisions for patient or allow other staff to do so.
- Explain carefully to family patient's need to be more independent; tell them they can be helpful by urging patient to make own decisions; offer praise when this occurs.
- Watch for signs of depression and institute appropriate interventions; refer to *The Patient Experiencing Depression*, page 57.
- Use interdisciplinary team planning to support independence in all areas of functioning.

☐ EVALUATION CRITERIA/DESIRED OUTCOMES

The Patient
- Demonstrates increased autonomy in daily life
- States own wishes and feelings more frequently
- Verbally communicates realistic requests
- Uses assertive communication
- Participates increasingly in ADL
- Cooperates with interdisciplinary team members

NURSING DIAGNOSIS #2

Anxiety related to fear of abandonment and perceived inability to meet own needs

Rationale: The patient believes that s/he is unable to function independently to meet own needs. The patient's fear that s/he will be isolated and not be assisted if a perceived need arises creates an increased anxiety level. This may be accompanied by demanding behavior and feelings of powerlessness and frustration.

☐ GOAL

The patient will recognize and achieve reduction of anxiety.

☐ IMPLEMENTATION

- Assess level of anxiety; assist patient to manage anxiety; refer to *The Patient Experiencing Anxiety*, page 22.
- Use clear, concise communication; answer questions honestly.
- Assist to identify feelings of helplessness caused by illness or hospitalization; refer to *The Patient Experiencing Powerlessness*, page 115.
- Discuss demanding behavior with patient; mutually define expectations and set limits on unrealistic demands.
- Anticipate patient's needs before level of anxiety increases; give attention at times other than when a request is made.
- Be consistent in care; return at stated times; sit and listen to patient so attention can be given to his/her needs, wants, and feelings.
- Work with family so they can recognize and cope with their own anxiety and tolerate/support the patient's efforts toward independence.
- Encourage discussion of feelings of anger or frustration; listen actively and with empathy; give explanations and information when indicated.
- Do not withdraw from clinging behavior; recognize own feelings and reactions so that cycle of increased avoidance associated with increased patient demands is not perpetuated.
- Provide therapeutic, serene environment.
- Teach simple relaxation techniques (e.g., deep breathing).
- Assist patient to develop interest in diversionary activities to reduce tension.

☐ EVALUATION CRITERIA/DESIRED OUTCOMES

The Patient
- Recognizes and verbalizes feelings of anxiety
- Uses relaxation techniques
- Demonstrates fewer demanding or clinging behaviors
- Participates in diversionary activities

NURSING DIAGNOSIS #3

Disturbance in self-concept: self-esteem related to lack of appreciation for own value, lack of confidence in ability to accomplish what is desired

Rationale: Continued dependency results in poor role performance with a lack of self-confidence in ability to function and lack of appreciation for own abilities and value. This may be reinforced by fam-

ily or the environment. New patterns of relating to others and the environment are needed to achieve more positive perceptions of oneself and one's abilities.

☐ GOAL

The patient will exhibit increased self-esteem and confidence in ability to accomplish specific tasks and functions.

☐ IMPLEMENTATION

- Assist patient to identify strengths and areas of positive accomplishments; point out that each individual is responsible for own behavior.
- Structure activities so that success is possible; begin with simple decisions and reinforce positive efforts.
- Be realistic in expectations; a life-long pattern of behavior does not change readily.

- Communicate positive regard to patient; draw attention to self-denegrating remarks (e.g., "I'm so stupid."); tell patient you see capabilities and possibilities for growth if efforts are made in this direction.
- Be consistent and attentive to increase patient's trust in the ability of others to meet his/her needs; since patient feels unwanted/unloved, it is difficult to perceive that others could care about him/her.
- Encourage verbalization of own desires so increased self-reliance can be achieved; refer to *The Patient Experiencing a Threat to Self-Esteem*, page 127.

☐ EVALUATION CRITERIA/DESIRED OUTCOMES

The Patient
- Verbalizes strengths and positive abilities
- Makes decisions for self
- States fewer self-deprecatory remarks
- Defers less to others

The Patient Experiencing Depression

Definition/Discussion

Depression is an alteration in mood, usually related to a loss, characterized by sadness, pessimism, despondence, hopelessness, and emptiness. It can also be related to internalization of anger or aggressive feelings. Levels of depression include mild, moderate, severe. For discussion of severe depression (major depressive episode), refer to *The Patient Experiencing Depression: Severe*, page 60. The *DSM-III-R* categorization is Affective Disorder. Mild depression is referred to as a reactive depression (precipitated by environmental events such as loss). Moderate depression is classified as a dysthymic disorder or depressive neurosis (chronic depression and loss of pleasure or interest in most of usual activities).

Nursing Assessment

☐ PERTINENT HISTORY

Recent or unresolved loss; crises; suicidal ideation; cultural or social isolation; changes in location, status, employment, home, body, school, health, abilities, finances; alcohol or substance abuse; anhedonia, withdrawal; sleep disturbances; onset of depression

☐ PHYSICAL FINDINGS

Psychomotor retardation, crying, anorexia or overeating, apathy, decreased concentration, anxiety, fatigue, sad expression, poor eye contact, change in body weight

☐ PSYCHOSOCIAL CONCERNS/ DEVELOPMENTAL FACTORS

Personality, normal coping patterns, self-esteem, introjection of anger, feelings of failure, familial pattern of depression or dependency, importance of real or perceived loss, degree of disruption perceived; adolescents: acting-out, problem behaviors; elderly: sensory-perceptual changes

☐ PATIENT AND FAMILY KNOWLEDGE

Dynamics of depression, community resources, treatment plan, readiness and willingness to learn

Nursing Care

☐ LONG-TERM GOAL

The patient will be able to acknowledge and resolve the loss; the patient will resume management of own life and plan for the future.

NURSING DIAGNOSIS #1

Ineffective individual coping related to feelings of depression associated with loss, failure

Rationale: *Feelings of depression associated with loss or failure prevent the individual from effective role performance and coping with activities of daily living (ADL).*

☐ GOAL

The patient will express feelings; will develop skills to effectively manage readjustment.

☐ IMPLEMENTATION

- Make frequent, intermittent contact with the patient, both verbal and nonverbal.
- Give attention consistently, even when the patient is unwilling/unable to converse with you; this approach will establish you as an interested, caring person; be aware that depressed patients usually feel alone and worthless; a belief that someone is interested in and cares about them is the most helpful intervention.
- Involve in self-care and activities of daily living (ADL); start with one activity and gradually add others; prevent withdrawal by encouraging social interactions; recognize patient's efforts.
- Explore how patient feels about listening to others' feelings (often people who have problems tolerating their own feelings tend to feel overwhelmed with those of others').
- Use open-ended questions to elicit expression of feelings, (e.g., "You look sad today. What is it

that makes you feel this way?"); acknowledge and reinforce any expression of feelings.

- Do not tell patient the feeling of depression is not as bad as it is perceived to be; this approach only serves to reinforce the feeling that no one understands.
- Ensure that staff knows not to chastize the patient when feelings of sadness are evident; allow the patient to cry.
- Praise for any involvement in self-care or other activities; encourage staff/family to praise patient for these efforts; structure schedule to provide adequate and enjoyable activities.
- Help patient do things for self and explain that activity usually helps people to feel better.
- Assist staff in their efforts to draw out the patient; direct them to pay as much attention as possible.
- Monitor physical needs and encourage patient to maintain good hygiene and grooming.
- Provide sufficient nourishment; allow favorite foods and choice of diet when possible.
- Assess sleep and activity pattern; provide adequate rest and a regular bedtime routine that promotes sleep without medications; limit daytime sleeping; encourage morning activities as patient will usually feel best then.
- Encourage participation in regular exercise program if possible.
- Help patient focus on meaning of loss, somatic symptoms, depressed feeling tone (e.g., "You've had a hard time lately and you're learning to deal with your feelings." "You've lost functioning and you're going through grief and mourning.")
- Reinforce reality and realistic expectations.
- Identify problem areas and work out alternatives with patient; take care to consider individual preferences and needs.
- Assess areas in which patient is making own decisions and give positive reinforcement to self-enhancing ones; assist with decision making when profoundly depressed; as depression lifts, expect patient to make own decisions with support.

☐ EVALUATION CRITERIA

The Patient
- Identifies events/loss that led to feeling depressed
- Demonstrates increasing self-direction in self-care and activities
- Has stable physical condition
- Participates actively in unit activities
- Participates in regular exercise

NURSING DIAGNOSIS #2

Disturbance in self-concept: self-esteem related to lack of appreciation for own value and abilities

---

Rationale: The characteristic present in all depressions is lowered self-esteem. Attention to improving self-esteem will assist in lifting depression.

☐ GOAL

The patient will experience an increase in self-esteem.

☐ IMPLEMENTATION

- Approach the patient in accepting, respectful way; keep promises and agreements to demonstrate caring.
- Recognize patient's prior abilities and display a positive attitude toward recovery; do not reassure but ask patient to describe feelings.
- Offer alternative statements to ruminative or self-deprecatory remarks but do not argue with the patient.
- Determine interests and activities that were enjoyed previously and try to incorporate these into the care plan.
- Ask patient to describe positive thoughts and write them down; suggest that when negative thoughts occur, producing feelings of helplessness, that the patient state "I will stop thinking about that."
- Begin with small tasks and activities where success will be possible and give honest praise for accomplishments; increase requirements as patient improves; provide recognition consistently.
- Encourage verbal interaction and communication with staff and other patients to prevent isolation; role play situations of potential concern to the patient.
- Encourage increasing decision making in as many areas as possible; ask for participation in planning for own care.
- Support any evidence of motivation or initiative and praise efforts and progress.
- Assist in reevaluation of goals and expectations and recognize efforts being made to adjust; continue to focus on positive aspects and strengths.
- Encourage attendance and participation in group therapy, occupational therapy, and recreational activities.
- Convey an attitude of confidence in the abilities of the patient.

☐ EVALUATION CRITERIA

The Patient
- Identifies successful aspects of life
- Demonstrates adequate communication skills; makes few self-deprecatory remarks
- Participates in therapies and plan for care

NURSING DIAGNOSIS #3

Knowledge deficit regarding behaviors of depression, responses to loss, treatment plan, need for support system

Rationale: *Often new supports and adjustments in life-style are necessary to cope with changes that precipitated the depression. Patients can learn new coping strategies and problem solving.*

☐ GOAL

The patient will adapt to changes, utilize support systems, and plan constructively for the future.

☐ IMPLEMENTATION

- Assist to understand behaviors that usually occur with depression and how the resolution of a loss may be accomplished; refer to *The Patient Experiencing Grief and Loss* , page 80.
- Encourage development of techniques to help in management of life changes and alterations of mood; refer to Table 1, *Stress Management*, page 24.
- Teach assertive techniques and their appropriate application.
- Instruct regarding prescribed medication: actions, side effects, compliance, how to obtain refills.
- Educate regarding symptoms of recurring depression so early assistance can be obtained.
- Encourage evaluation of environmental situation and assist with changes if indicated; involve the social worker in areas indicated.
- Encourage continuation of social contacts and discuss the importance of their maintenance.
- Inform patient/family regarding self-help or informational groups for outpatient assistance (e.g., Reach-to-Recovery, spouse groups.)
- Tell about local mental health center, crisis and suicide prevention centers.
- Inform regarding benefits of continuing individual, family, or group therapy; ensure understanding of indicated referrals; arrange for follow-up appointment prior to discharge.

☐ EVALUATION CRITERIA/DESIRED OUTCOMES

The Patient

- Understands need to monitor follow-up care
- States understanding of causes of depression
- Has plans for alterations in life-style
- Describes correct use of medications
- States optimism and a constructive plan for the future

The Patient Experiencing Depression: Severe

Definition/Discussion

Severe depression is a clinical entity classified in the *DSM-III-R* as an affective disorder in which an alteration in mood is the dominant factor.

Although intensity of the depression varies greatly, the prominent and persistent features are extreme sadness and loss of interest and/or pleasure in all or most of the activities of daily living. The patient may say "I just don't care about anything anymore," or may not be aware of significant changes that family members notice. Feelings of lowered self-esteem, helplessness, hopelessness, powerlessness, and guilt are frequent, and suicidal ideation may be present. Psychosis may be present as the patient manifests a distorted view of reality.

Some depressions are considered to be self-limiting, but patients may benefit greatly from a combination of psychotherapy, medication, and adjunctive therapies. Electroconvulsive therapy (ECT) is done only with the permission of the patient and when psychotherapy and use of medication fail to lift the depression.

Depression may occur at any age, and the prevalence is greater in women by a 2:1 ratio. It is the most frequently occurring psychiatric illness, accounting for more psychiatric hospitalizations than any other diagnosis.

Although there is no one totally accepted theory for the causes of depression, some of the most frequently proposed are
- *Biologic*: low levels of norepinephrine and serotonin are present in the blood of depressed persons. This can be reversed by the tricyclic antidepressants and monoamine oxidase inhibitors. There is a possibility that a genetic influence may occur in some types of depression due to the increased risk that is present in first-generation relatives of diagnosed depressives.
- *Cognitive*: symptoms of depression may occur because of the negative perception that the patient has of him/herself, the world, and the future. This narrow perspective produces pessimism and hopelessness.
- *Psychologic*: an intrapsychic theory in which the feelings from an early loss are reactivated by a perceived real or symbolic loss of anything valued, such as love, status, or self-esteem. This

perception causes feelings of dependency, powerlessness, helplessness, and guilt.
- *Sociocultural*: the environment and society contribute to the development of the individual. Feelings of low self-esteem and powerlessness may result from lack of positive reinforcement, excessive stress, discriminatory status, or familial dysfunction.

Nursing Assessment

☐ **PERTINENT HISTORY**

Recent or past losses, real or perceived crises situations; suicide attempts (frequency, outcome); social network, friends; changes in environment, employment, home, abilities, finances, health status; cultural isolation; alcohol or substance abuse, past or present; delusion, hallucinations, illusions; previous depression (extent, treatment, outcome); anhedonia, hopelessness, guilt, hostility, anger, aggression, poor self-esteem

☐ **PHYSICAL FINDINGS**

Confusion, agitation, flat affect, somatizing, restlessness, apathy, withdrawal, passivity, insomnia, amenorrhea, impotence, weight gain or loss, poor hygiene, constipation, urinary retention, poor posture, inability to concentrate, fatigue, tears, anxiety, anorexia/overeating, headache, psychomotor retardation, irritability, morning-evening mood variations, impaired sleep pattern

☐ **PSYCHOSOCIAL CONCERNS/ DEVELOPMENTAL FACTORS**

Patterns of failure, frustration; mood swings, temper outbursts, poor mechanisms to cope with stress; familial depression or suicide; poor communication patterns; family dynamics; usual life-style, mood, coping mechanisms, expectations of family, self; identifiable, perceived losses
Adolescent: alienation from peers; loss of relationship; parental rejection; isolation; poor school, job performance; acting out behaviors; dependency, ambivalence, melancholia, emptiness/heaviness

Elderly: Loss of spouse, home, friends, health; social isolation; poverty; retirement

☐ PATIENT AND FAMILY KNOWLEDGE

Degree of disruption; involvement of outside agencies (amount, acceptance); previous experiences, outcome; acceptance of involvement/rejection of treatment; readiness and willingness to learn

Nursing Care _____

☐ LONG-TERM GOAL

The patient will deal with painful feelings by learning to share, express, and resolve them; the patient will resume effective management of own life, carry out activities of daily living, and resume job or usual roles.

NURSING DIAGNOSIS #1

Ineffective individual coping related to feelings of ambivalence, anxiety, helplessness, and hopelessness associated with depression

Rationale: The depressed patient feels unworthy and unlovable and has neither the volition or energy to cope effectively with the management of life's tasks. This results in self-deprecating and non-productive behaviors that further the pattern of failure, lack of pleasure, dependency, and withdrawal.

☐ GOAL

The patient will identify feelings of ambivalence, anxiety, helplessness, and hopelessness and develop new, effective techniques for their management.

☐ IMPLEMENTATION

- Built rapport and relationship by spending time with patient at least twice daily; start with 5-10 minutes, and increase time as you and patient can tolerate it; encourage patient to identify and share feelings with you, accepting what is said; use silence (just the presence of a caring person is helpful when learning to cope with painful feelings); avoid reassurance.
- Focus on patient's feelings; allow ventilation in ways that seem comfortable to him/her; share with patient that the only way to get through the feelings is to stay with them and experience them.
- Explore how patient feels about listening to others' feelings (often people who have problems tolerating their feelings tend to feel overwhelmed by others); practice sharing feelings of being overwhelmed and setting limits on listening to problems; if other patients are willing and available, practice reciprocal sharing of feelings, with discussion of how to set limits and keep relationship.
- Communicate clear, concise directions when pa-

tient demonstrates ambivalence; assess areas where patient makes own decisions and give positive reinforcement to self-enhancing ones; as depression lifts expect patient to make more decisions; give appropriate support; recognize the need for acceptance by the patient and be patient when indecisive behaviors occur.

- Assess for overt or covert anxiety; in the depressed, anxiety is frequently expressed with agitated, restless, purposeless motor behaviors; accompany the patient during pacing or walking; do not require that patient "sit still" as this will increase the anxiety; provide exercise and recreation to keep anxiety level manageable; refer to *The Patient Experiencing Anxiety*, page 22; consider the use of medication if indicated.
- Deter helpless behaviors by assisting the patient only when necessary (the dependency may fill a need the patient either does not want to recognize or is unwilling to modify); encourage to verbalize what is possible to be changed, to write down small successes, and to look for positive directions rather than to be overwhelmed by difficulties perceived; set limits on irrational demands and be consistent.
- Assess for feelings of powerlessness in everyday situations and encourage to verbalize regarding alternatives that can be derived from patient's own strengths and experiences.
- Retain and share hope with patient (e.g., "I know you're feeling low now; you're getting treatment and these feelings will lift.").
- Assist them to look to the future, to identify what can be enjoyed; in the elderly, remind them of what is left that is positive and encourage life review.
- Encourage verbalization of feelings of hopelessness as those most deeply felt are frequently not discussed, especially in the adolescent; explore how these perceptions can be altered and replaced with future oriented possibilities.

☐ EVALUATION CRITERIA/DESIRED OUTCOMES

The Patient
- Makes some small daily decisions regarding care without assistance
- Verbalizes feelings more readily
- Displays some insight regarding coping with negative feelings and developing more effective ways to handle them
- States one positive aspect to be anticipated in the future

NURSING DIAGNOSIS #2

Self-care deficit: feeding, bathing/hygiene, dressing/grooming, toileting related to depression

---

Rationale: The depressed person may be unable to perform self-care activities in a manner consistent with body requirements. The absence of appetite, lack of activity, and slowed metabolism of the severely depressed can result in malnutrition, urinary retention, and constipation. The patient may experience fatigue and a feeling of heaviness accompanied by excessive or lack of restful sleep. The prevalent decreased self-esteem of the depressive contributes to lack of interest in appearance, cleanliness, and grooming.

☐ GOAL

The patient will resume self-care in grooming; will ingest adequate foods and fluids and establish adequate elimination; will achieve adequate sleep/rest/activity pattern.

☐ IMPLEMENTATION

- Assess activities of daily living (ADL) and vegetative signs.
- Identify problem areas and work out alternatives with patient and health team; taking care to consider individual preferences and needs; help patient do things for self and encourage independence in all ADL.
- Monitor food and fluid intake (may become necessary to record I&O).
- Weigh weekly (continued loss of weight may indicate deepening depression; weight gain may indicate decreased depression).
- Work with patient to find acceptable eating pattern; if anorexic and apathetic to food, find out when this lessens; determine favorite foods and provide when possible; foods not requiring energy to ingest should be used, e.g., fortified liquids and soft foods; offer smaller portions more frequently.
- Assess for overeating patterns and provide special diet if indicated; assist to adhere to dietary requirements and recognize efforts to do so.
- Monitor for urinary retention, take to bathroom if necessary; ensure sufficient fluid intake.
- Monitor for constipation that may be caused by medicines, lack of activity, improper diet; use of laxatives may be required for proper elimination.
- Observe sleeping habits; help patient establish a bedtime routine to promote rest and sleep (without enough sleep, exhaustion may occur and the mental state deteriorate); assist to mobilize patient during day to facilitate rest at night; set limits on the amount of time patient will be allowed to spend in bed during the day.
- Plan daily activities with patient; responsibility for ward maintenance tasks may help renew a sense of self-worth and purposefulness; simple tasks, such as emptying ashtrays, straightening chairs, putting away cards, games or crafts equipment with supervision may be appropriate for deeply depressed patients; more difficult tasks can be gradually assigned as tolerated.
- Assess for variations in mood and energy levels, scheduling activities and rest accordingly, the psychiatrically depressed patient usually feels low in the morning and better as the day progresses.
- Determine activities and interests enjoyed prior to depressed state (often depressed persons have few hobbies and have not participated in recreational or crafts groups since schooldays); use simple crafts that can be finished in one sitting to give a therapeutic sense of accomplishment; encourage group activity (e.g., singing, poetry reading, painting, working with clay) to assist to become more comfortable in groups and to establish community and group socialization; know that patient may need nurse's presence to tolerate group activities at first.
- Provide for regular exercise as tolerated by physical condition; increase as depression lifts, simple exercises, walks, may progress to group sports.
- Stress that using one's own resources to achieve activity will produce an elevation of mood and patient will feel better.
- Establish a routine for bathing, shampooing, and nail care; know that patient may require physical assistance/display resistance to using the energy required; monitor oral hygiene; assist with grooming and encourage whenever interest is shown in improving appearance; assist with clothing choice, maintenance and recognize progress in these areas.

☐ EVALUATION CRITERIA/DESIRED OUTCOMES

The Patient
- Has adequate nutritional intake, maintains appropriate weight
- Has satisfactory elimination pattern
- Sleeps 6 hours at night with no daytime naps
- Maintains adequate hygiene and grooming
- Participates occasionally in scheduled activities

NURSING DIAGNOSIS #3

Potential for violence related to feelings of anger, hostility, suicidal ideation

Rationale: The potential for expression of anger and hostility is present in all depressed patients. This may be manifested inwardly or outwardly to self/others. Freud believed that an individual who is unable to express angry feelings will direct the angry feelings inward rather than at the appropriate person or object. Suicide is considered to be an aggressive, hostile act against oneself.

GOAL

The patient will be safe from injury and will channel destructive impulses into constructive expression.

IMPLEMENTATION

- Refer to *The Patient who is Suicidal,* page 144.
- Assess impulse control by restricting patient to observable areas when first admitted; ask if patient has ever thought of hurting self or of suicide.
- Remove potentially harmful items such as razor blades, scissors, medications; allow sharp instruments to be used only with one-to-one supervision; continue to assess for suicidal risk; remember that when improvement of a severe depression occurs, the suicidal risk is increased.
- Assess for absence of reality testing; intervene prior to escalation of hostile behaviors.
- Establish a one-to-one relationship; assess potential for self-defeating acts; problem solve with patient for alternative behaviors; use role playing to practice new behaviors.
- Work out plan to be used when patient feels impending loss of control of own impulses (e.g., contract with patient to ask nurse to accompany him/her to exercise room when angry at self or others); to utilize alternate ways of expression (e.g., handball, racketball, throwing sponges or foam bags; shouting or confronting with words).
- Contract to spend time with patient when feelings of anger and hostility occur to permit expression of accumulated feelings, crying and rage.
- Give positive reinforcement by words and your presence when patient follows through on contract to control impulses ("You really were aware that you were losing control and took good care of yourself by asking me to stay with you".)

EVALUATION CRITERIA/DESIRED OUTCOMES

The Patient
- Identifies some causes of anger, hostility and new alternative behaviors
- Identifies when feelings of anger and hostility are imminent.
- Requests assistance for control by alternative, safe expressive methods
- States suicidal ideation is not present

NURSING DIAGNOSIS #4

Social isolation related to withdrawal, limited verbal communication

Rationale: The severely depressed individual feels that s/he has not had his/her expectations met in the past and wishes to avoid this in the future. Therefore, the person retreats into him/herself to avoid socialization that could produce additional losses or failure. The absence of social reinforcement contributes to further withdrawal and decrease in self-esteem. The limited energies of the depressed patient are also perceived as needed for self-preservation rather than for involvement with others.

GOAL

The patient will strengthen ability to relate to others by increasing social interactions and verbal communications with staff and other patients.

IMPLEMENTATION

- Assess interpersonal behaviors and help patient define problem areas in social relationships (e.g., patient who is hypercritical of self and others can discuss and practice a softer, more accepting approach).
- Help patient to look at situations where s/he may push people away out of fear of rejection (i.e., reject them before they reject him/her).
- Practice social skills, use role playing; give positive reinforcement.
- Work with patient to identify communication problems and assist in development of clear communication patterns.
- Assess for past and present interests and schedule activity with others whose interests are similar; peer group activities are especially helpful for adolescents and the elderly.
- Recognize the depressed patient is not usually able to decrease social isolation without assistance; be consistent in assisting the patient to obtain social contacts; remember that in the elderly, withdrawal from social situations may be the result of sensoriperceptual changes that can be alleviated by correcting visual or hearing problems.
- Explore the persons in patient's life with whom feelings can be shared; if there is no one, explore how this came about and what feelings result from this occurring; discuss what can be done to change the situation and how the patient can take action to do so; practice role playing to help initiate contacts and sharing of feelings.
- Set realistic goals with the patient, such as initiating one staff or patient contact per day, and then increase as tolerated.
- Strongly encourage regular group therapy attendance even if patient does not participate in the beginning.
- Recognize and praise sincerely any efforts made to increase social interaction/verbal communication.

EVALUATION CRITERIA/DESIRED OUTCOMES

The Patient

- Initiates one contact with staff member
- Identifies one acquaintance with whom contact could be made
- Identifies shyness as a problem and participates in role playing to improve social skills
- Attends group therapy regularly and occasionally contributes

---

NURSING DIAGNOSIS #5

Disturbance in self-concept: self-esteem related to real or threatened losses

Rationale: Low self-esteem is the result of a fragile ego that can be further damaged when the individual experiences a real or perceived loss. This may have a guilt component in which the person has unrealistic expectations of self and others, and these predispose to a pattern of failure. The prevalent denial of self-pleasure and inability to accept positive reinforcement also contribute to the perpetuation of poor self-regard. Since a disturbance in self-concept develops over a period of time, the development of the ability to view oneself more positively requires continuing attention.

GOAL

The patient will improve level of self-esteem.

IMPLEMENTATION

- Accept the patient as a person; develop a therapeutic nurse-client relationship that conveys respect and dignity (this positive approach is reassuring to the patient).
- Listen to what the patient is saying and observe nonverbal communication; convey interest, concern, empathy, and caring.
- Allow to describe doubts about self and respond honestly, presenting alternative facts without disputing patient perception; talking about doubts can help put them into perspective.
- Structure time and activities so that success is possible in all tasks; add more responsibility as patient improves and point out progress that is being made; if necessary, do activities along with patient to interrupt lethargy.
- Give sincere praise for accomplishments to reinforce patient capabilities.
- Assist to improve appearance as attention to hygiene, clothing, posture, etc., will improve self-concept.
- Do not use reassurance; instead assist patient to verbalize about low self-esteem and develop ways to express feelings appropriately outwardly rather than turning them inward.
- Focus on positive accomplishments and strengths; assist in identifying ways to change self-deprecating behavior.
- Allow rumination for only specific lengths of time and then encourage to proceed to present projects and future plans rather than focusing on the past.
- Encourage new interests and assist to reevaluate expectations; achievable goals will assist in promoting an improved self-concept and interrupt feelings of worthlessness.
- Encourage progress in social interactions and role play intimidating situations.
- Encourage regular attendance at group therapy, occupational therapy, and recreational activities with gradually increased participation.
- Convey feelings of optimism and confidence that the patient is a worthwhile person.

EVALUATION CRITERIA/DESIRED OUTCOMES

The Patient

- Displays fewer self-deprecating behaviors
- Increases participation in unit activities
- Demonstrates greater socialization
- Improves grooming and appearance
- Identifies one successful accomplishment

NURSING DIAGNOSIS #6

Alteration in thought processes related to misinterpretations of reality

Rationale: The patient who is moderately depressed may exhibit retardation of thoughts and inability to concentrate. As depression increases to the severe level, the patient may also exhibit rumination and loss of perspective although remaining in touch with reality. The severely depressed patient may display distortions of reality through delusional thoughts. These thoughts often enforce the feelings of worthlessness and guilt and are punishing in character. Hallucinations rarely occur and are usually transient, but may present as voices that reinforce the perceived negative characteristics of the patient.

GOAL

The patient will learn to trust others and define and test reality.

IMPLEMENTATION

- Establish reality with patient by identifying self; make contacts brief but frequent; demonstrate consistency and honesty; be aware of testing behaviors prior to allowing trust to develop; explain expectations and requirements clearly.

- Listen and observe carefully as distortions of reality are difficult to understand; take time to give patient feedback on what you understand; if you do not understand, ask patient to repeat until the meaning is clear to you.
- Ask patient to try and give you one idea at a time and to speak slowly so it is easier for you to understand; it may be possible to comprehend the emotions behind the verbal communication rather than what the patient is actually saying; use this information to try and determine the theme that is the basis for the delusion; remember that delusions are often symbolic in meaning.
- Refrain from arguing or agreeing with the patient regarding delusions; these are very real to the patient and will be defended if you attempt to discredit them; state that you know the delusions are real to the patient but they are not to you.
- Look for stressors that may precipitate a thought disturbance and attempt to identify and discuss these.
- Avoid laughing at disturbed thought processes; even though the patient may be psychotic, oftentimes there is an awareness of what is occurring in the environment.
- Use extreme caution in touching an individual who does not perceive reality accurately; it can be very frightening to the patient and hazardous for the care giver.
- Do not discuss delusions but reinforce reality; give positive reinforcement when reality is perceived accurately.
- Assist in the differentiation of reality and fantasy; provide and encourage validation of thoughts with others.
- Monitor for aggressive activities as a result of disturbed thinking and maintain a safe environment for the patient and others.

☐ EVALUATION CRITERIA/DESIRED OUTCOMES

The Patient
- Displays less retardation and fewer concrete associations in verbal communication pattern
- Expresses fewer delusional thoughts
- Identifies some environmental stressors
- Verbalizes more readily to staff
- Gradually perceives and describes reality appropriately

NURSING DIAGNOSIS #7

Knowledge deficit regarding successful management of the depressive state

Rationale: A severe depression may be alleviated through the use of appropriate support systems that contribute to the development of increased personal strengths and abilities. These may include the use of psychotherapy on an outpatient basis and/or group therapy in a therapeutic setting. The continued use of psychotropic drugs may require a change in drug or manner of usage, and patient information is vital. The involvement of family or significant others in education regarding the management of depression is also a major factor in the projected success of treatment.

☐ GOAL

The patient will achieve increased personal growth and develop and utilize beneficial support systems.

☐ IMPLEMENTATION

- Assist patient/family/significant other to understand that when depression is related to major loss, the grieving process must be experienced, with the stages requiring about 1 year for resolution; the patient may have had previous unresolved losses that now need attention and additional treatment may be necessary; conversely, some depressions may lift after a period of time, with or without treatment; refer to *The Patient Experiencing Grief and Loss*, page 80.
- Educate regarding the use of psychotropic medications (side effects, hazards, benefits); explain that sometimes these medications are required for a long period of time; ensure patient/significant other understand how the drug is to be used and the importance of continued compliance.
- Discuss the benefits of individual, family (especially for adolescents), and group therapy and ascertain the understanding of indicated referrals; involve as many significant others in follow-up care as possible.
- Utilize other members of the interdisciplinary team, e.g., social worker, for assistance in related areas requiring postdischarge referrals.
- Teach early symptoms of recurring depression so that assistance can be obtained promptly.
- Teach regarding effective management of stress (refer to Table 1, *Stress Management*, page 24), use of assertive techniques, productive use of time, and problem-solving skills so that situations contributing to the development of depression may be changed as well as achieving improvement in the effectiveness of coping skills.
- Prepare patient/family to cope more effectively after discharge by providing information regarding agencies that will be helpful for adjustment to the community and maintenance of patient outside the hospital (e.g., local mental health centers and Mental Health Association, Suicide Prevention Center, and Crisis Intervention Center); inform that assistance is provided based on an ability to

pay so that all patients have access to continuing treatment at government-supported agencies.

☐ **EVALUATION CRITERIA/DESIRED OUTCOMES**

The Patient/Family
- Expresses willingness to assist in follow-up care
- States understanding of need for continuing treatment and use of medication

- Has follow-up appointment at local mental health clinic
- Demonstrates visibly improved efficiency in accomplishment of ADL
- States hopefulness and plans for future

Table 3
Antidepressants

Action	Side Effects	Nursing Implications
Chemical agents that help lift depressions; used in conjunction with psychotherapy.	All of this group can produce a toxic psychosis; patient becomes confused, disoriented, and may hallucinate.	• Explain to patient that 3-4 weeks are required for onset of action; teach what side effects to be alert for, and to report to any physician/clinic. • Use cautiously with history of hypertension.
Heterocyclics This group of drugs is also effective in treating phobic symptoms in patients with severe anxiety. Tricyclics *amitriptyline (Elavil)* *imipramine (Tofranil)* *trimipramine (Surmontil)* *amoxapine (Asendin)* *nortriptyline (Pamelor, Aventyl)* *desipramine (Norpramin)* *protriptyline (Vivactil)* Tetracyclics *maprotiline (Ludiomil)* Triazolopyridines *trazodone (Desyrel)*	Blurred vision, dry mouth, ataxia, postural hypotension, tachycardia, palpitation, dizziness, fainting, nausea and vomiting, urinary retention, inability to sleep; profuse sweating, aggravation of narrow-angle glaucoma; stimulates CNS; potentiates alcohol. In large doses, has a sedative action, thus reducing need for sedatives at night. May cause confusion, especially in elderly.	• Patient will usually develop a tolerance to any side effects. Monitor pulse and blood pressure for irregularities. If postural hypotension present, instruct patient to sit up slowly, pause, and make a gradual change to being upright. • Check urinary output and bowel movements daily. Ensure adequate fluid intake. • Check with drug manufacturers for incompatible drugs. A dose of 50-100 tabs can be lethal; limit amount a patient has at any one time. • Contraindicated before surgery or with history of narrow-angle glaucoma, epilepsy, congestive heart failure.
Monoamine oxidase (MAO) inhibitors *isocarboxazid (Marplan)* *tranylcypromine (Parnate)* *phenelzine (Nardil)*	Orthostatic hypertension, blurred vision, constipation, dry mouth, urinary retention, sedation, sexual dysfunction. A Parnate (or Nardil) and cheese reaction is a hypertensive crisis (severe headache, dizziness, tachycardia, pallor, chills, stiff neck, nausea and vomiting, fear, restlessness, muscle twitching, chest pain, palpitation) that occurs when patients take Parnate or Nardil and then eat cheese; can occur when taking other MAO inhibitors as well; also have adverse reactions with other foods and certain drugs, including the tricyclic drugs.	• Advise patient not to eat cheese, yogurt, wine, beer, bananas, avocados, yeast products, broad (Fava) beans, chicken livers, or pickled herring (the drugs contain tyramine, which interacts with these foods). Also wise to avoid large amounts of coffee, tea, and chocolate. Do not give with psychomotor stimulants, epinephrine, ephedrine, or meperidine (Demerol), or tricyclic drugs.
CNS Stimulants Give feeling of energy and well-being; used to treat mild depression. Chemical and biological similarity to ephedrine and amphetamine. *methylphenidate (Ritalin)* *dextroamphetamine (Dexedrine)* *methamphetamine (Desoxyn)*	Tachycardia, hypertension, dry mouth, headache, jitteriness, insomnia, decreased appetite; increased susceptibility to accidents, addiction. Nervousness and insomnia; overcomes drug-induced lethargy caused by tranquilizers. High drug-abuse potential; masks warning signs of fatigue. Anorexia and weight loss, especially in children.	• Advise patient of potential side effects and observe for same; reduce dosage with side effects. • Teach safety precautions. Avoid using with dependent type persons. • Check for potentiation of other drugs and discuss with physician.

The Patient with a Developmental Disability

Definition/Discussion

Developmental disability, formerly mental retardation, refers to subaverage general intellectual functioning existing concurrently with deficits in adaptive behavior and manifested during the developmental period (American Association of Mental Deficiency). It is not a disease entity itself but a complex of symptoms from a variety of causes including

Before birth: genetic variations (Down Syndrome or Mongolism, Tay-Sachs), German measles or infection in mother during pregnancy, incompatible blood between mother and child (RH factor), glandular disorders, toxic chemicals, nutritional deficiencies, excessive drug use

During birth: birth injury due to long and difficult labor or very rapid delivery, abnormal position of fetus, difficult forceps delivery

After birth: inflammation of the brain from high fever due to childhood diseases, accident with trauma to head, glandular disturbances, inadequate stimulation in early childhood, postdrownings

There are 5 levels of retardation according to the American Association of Mental Deficiency.

- *Borderline/Level 0*: IQ range 68 to 83, with a potential adult mental age (MA) of 10 years, 11 months to 13 years, 3 months; usually capable of marriage and being self-supporting, probably at a low socio-economic living standard.
- *Mild or Educable/Level 1*: IQ range 52 to 67, with a potential adult MA of 8 years, 6 months to 10 years, 10 months; capable of working but needs some supervision in financial affairs. Fourth/fifth grade academic possibilities as well as vocational skills by adulthood; often has difficulty keeping a job in competitive market. School placement is usually in classes for the educable mentally retarded (EMR); can usually be maintained within a community setting.
- *Moderate/Level 2*: IQ range 36 to 51, with a potential adult MA of 6 years, 1 month to 8 years, 5 months; first to third grade academic potential. Vocational possibilities usually at sheltered workshop or neighborhood job; school placement is usually in classes for trainable mentally retarded (TMR).
- *Severe/Level 3*: IQ range 20 to 35, with a potential

adult MA of 3 years, 9 months to 6 years; training goals are largely the self-help skills (toilet training, dressing self) with minimal independent behavior; school placement is usually a developmental center for handicapped or TMR program; some are able to work in sheltered workshop.
- *Profound/Level 4*: IQ below 20, and adult MA potential is 3 to 8 years and below, often accompanied by damage to the CNS; may require total care.

Nursing Assessment

☐ **PERTINENT HISTORY**

Presenting physical illness, psychiatric illness; history of behavioral manifestations of retardation; level of retardation, developmental stage; prior history of physical/mental illness; treatment and medications; physical setting in which patient normally resides

☐ **PHYSICAL FINDINGS**

Symptoms of present illness; mental status, orientation to time, place, person; susceptibility to primary and secondary infection; associated health problems and handicaps; impairment of motor activity and control; perceptual deficits, hyperactivity, inadequate nutrition, poor hygiene, seizure disorders; physical problems requiring special care techniques

☐ **PSYCHOSOCIAL CONCERNS/ DEVELOPMENTAL FACTORS**

Regular patterns of interaction; developmental level; cognitive deficits (short attention span, poor impulse control, hypersensitivity to environmental stimuli, tendency to act out, impaired learning and poor retention of knowledge); inadequate social adjustment; labile emotions and lowered self-esteem; decreased abilities and limitations in activities of daily living (ADL); fear of hospitalization; strengths and abilities (e.g., able to ambulate, see, hear, communicate verbally/nonverbally)

☐ **PATIENT AND FAMILY KNOWLEDGE**

Developmental level and adaptive capacity of patient; schedule of medications, action, dosage, and side effects to report; symptoms of disease and prognosis; ability to recognize behaviors of anxiety or withdrawal

Nursing Care

☐ LONG-TERM GOAL

The patient will maintain or increase admission levels of functioning within the limitations imposed by current illness.

NURSING DIAGNOSIS #1

Impaired communication: verbal related to the impaired ability to speak words, aphasia

Rationale: The individual with impaired verbal communication manifests a decreased ability to speak appropriately or to understand the meaning of words. Aphasia results from cerebral deficits and is demonstrated by the individual's difficulty in verbal self-expression or by a difficulty in understanding, or by a combination of both. The developmentally disabled individual, due to impaired cerebral function, possible physical deformity, and speech pathology, may experience difficulties in verbal communication. Some may communicate more effectively using sign language.

☐ GOAL

The patient will demonstrate an increased ability to understand and improved ability to express self; will demonstrate decreased frustration with problems of communication.

☐ IMPLEMENTATION

- Assess patient's ability to understand, speak, read, and write.
- Identify a method for patient to communicate basic needs.
- Develop alternate ways of communicating with the patient (e.g., use gestures and pantomime when speaking slowly and distinctly, point at objects being discussed, make flash cards with pictures or words depicting frequently used phrases, nod or shake head).
- Consult with speech pathologist or other appropriate resource for assistance in acquiring flash cards or for help with sign language.
- Decrease external stimuli and distractions; face the patient and make eye contact.
- Use uncomplicated words and sentences, one-step commands and directives.
- Match words with actions, use pictures.
- Respond to all attempts at speech even when they are unintelligible.
- Acknowledge when you do understand but when you do not understand do not pretend; let the patient know.
- Allow patient time to express self and time to respond.
- Focus on the present and give opportunities to make minor decisions.
- Repeat/rephrase requests when necessary.
- Acknowledge when patient appears frustrated, allow the patient time to rest.
- Use patient's own words to teach simple words/concepts; break concept/procedure into small components and allow to practice/talk about each component giving positive reinforcement and constructive feedback with each practice.
- Use behavior modification techniques in teaching new task (i.e., give positive reinforcement for achievements, desired behavior).
- Maintain a calm, positive attitude and talk to the patient whenever with him/her.
- Be creative in adapting patient's life experience to learning experience.

☐ EVALUATION CRITERIA/DESIRED OUTCOMES

The Patient

- Communicates basic needs successfully
- Demonstrates increased ability to understand
- Relates/demonstrates reduced feelings of frustration and isolation
- Demonstrates/states specific procedure/information as taught

---

NURSING DIAGNOSIS #2

Self-care deficit related to impaired cognitive, motor, developmental function

Rationale: The developmentally disabled person may be unable to initiate and complete those tasks necessary to care for own personal hygiene, nutrition, and grooming. With hospitalization for physical illness, impairment in task performance may increase significantly.

☐ GOAL

The patient will perform self-care in hygiene, grooming, and other ADL as able and appropriate; will maintain admission levels of functioning (specify) in ADL.

☐ IMPLEMENTATION

- Ask family/caretaker to describe patient's usual abilities and routine.
- Adapt patient's ADL to hospital routine.
- Be aware regression may occur when the patient becomes acutely ill; minimize regression by encouraging self-care.

- Work with family to maintain good health habits and self-care patterns.
- Encourage patient to dress self in own clothing; if hospital clothing is necessary, some minor adjustments may help the patient to be independent; allow ample time for dressing and praise positive behaviors.
- Help set up convenient routine for bathing and brushing teeth, using equipment used at home; observe for cleanliness and assist only if necessary.
- Follow toilet procedures used at home, using usual words and time schedule; may need to remind every 2 hours or to get up at night; do not diaper.
- Assist in choosing foods patient likes and can manage on diet as ordered; encourage self-help and teach to attain understanding of well-balanced diet using simple terms, demonstration, and return demonstration of basic food groups; provide nutritious snacks; favored objects, music, etc.
- Explain hospital routine of sleep/rest and assist patient to relax during rest periods and to sleep at night by following usual sleep routine including snacks, favored objects, music, etc., as appropriate.

☐ EVALUATION CRITERIA/DESIRED OUTCOMES

The Patient
- Demonstrates skills taught
- Ingests adequate diet to meet body needs
- Participates in own care
- Performs ADL within identified limits

NURSING DIAGNOSIS #3

Anxiety related to unfamiliar environment, need for treatment, medication

Rationale: The developmentally disabled patient may desire to comply with the health-related regimen dictated by health care professionals but be unable to do so because of feelings of anxiety brought on by the hospitalization and by impairment in cognitive, emotional, and physical development. The patient may experience vague feelings of uneasiness manifested by somatic complaints, decreased orientation and understanding, decreased ability to perform activities and to follow directions, and withdrawn or acting-out behavior. Inaccurate perceptions of health status usually involve misunderstanding of the illness, resulting in psychologic manifestations of anxiety and denial. Teaching should be routinely incorporated into nursing care whenever a patient faces an unfamiliar situation. The individual with a developmental disability is less able to deal with change and will need fre-

---

quent repetition of teaching and understanding on the part of the staff.

☐ GOAL

The patient will verbalize/communicate fears and feelings of anxiety; will identify factors that contribute to the anxiety; will develop a relationship of trust with care givers; will participate in own care and treatments; will demonstrate increased understanding of own illness; will comply with the treatment plan; will accept and communicate understanding of reasons for medications and treatments as able.

☐ IMPLEMENTATION

- Assess level of comprehension about planned treatments/procedures.
- Do not take expressions of hostility personally.
- Speak slowly and clearly when communicating with patient; use alternative methods of communication as necessary.
- Validate patient's understanding of what is being said.
- Acknowledge patient's feelings and their appropriateness.
- Listen to expressions of fear and anxiety.
- Correct any misconceptions, give appropriate instructions.
- Encourage to talk about how the diagnosis and treatment affect patient.
- Teach how to perform specific tasks and procedures, keep explanations simple and graphic.
- Plan, structure, and sequence teaching according to patient's abilities.
- Use demonstration techniques and audiovisual aids.
- Reduce external stimuli when demonstrating or explaining a medication or treatment.
- Prepare patient for procedures and treatments by explaining ahead of time what to expect and when to expect it; use words the patient understands and ask to repeat instructions in own words.
- Listen to and learn what patient expects; correct misunderstandings.
- Teach importance of adhering to prescribed regimen.
- Allow as much self-determination as possible within patient limitations; complete tasks when patient is unable to do so.
- Give positive reinforcement, verbal and nonverbal, immediately upon successful completion of a task.
- Maintain uniformity in treatments/procedures and explain any changes.
- Give emotional support by remaining with patient during treatments/procedures
- Explain to patient/family necessary information

about each medication (including possible side effects); observe and chart observations; check patient's retention of information.

- Meet with patient/family to discuss ongoing care and utilize family to help with patient care.

☐ EVALUATION CRITERIA/DESIRED OUTCOMES

The Patient

- Identifies and shares feelings/anxieties with staff, family
- Participates in own care and treatments, takes medications
- Controls impulsive and inappropriate behavior
- Accepts nurse's closeness and interest
- Participates in prescribed treatments/procedures

NURSING DIAGNOSIS #4

Potential for injury related to sensory, motor deficits

Rationale: These patients may be at risk for injury because of increased demand upon impaired sensory or motor function. Such increased demands may be situational (unfamiliar setting, environmental hazards); pathophysiologic (sensory-perceptual problems, altered mobility, effects of medications); or maturational (self-care deficit, inability to make informed judgment).

☐ GOAL

The patient will learn and practice (selected specific) injury-prevention measures; will identify factors that increase the potential for injury; will comply with safety rules; will ask for help when needed.

☐ IMPLEMENTATION

- Identify level of awareness, alertness, signs of confusion, altered sense of balance.
- Identify use of or need for prosthetic devices (e.g., crutches, canes, walkers, wheelchairs, eyeglasses, hearing aids).
- Teach use of prosthetic device when needed; use simple concepts broken down into small specific components, allowing time for return demonstration.
- Supervise treatments and use of prosthetic devices.
- Assess need for safety devices (e.g., side rails, wheelchair, walker).
- Remove unnecessary loose and hazardous objects from environment (e.g., medications, razors, sharp implements, treatment liquids); these patients tend to put things in their mouth or do unpredictable things with loose objects.
- Explain hospital routine, do's and don'ts in simple

relaxed manner; use verbal and nonverbal communication; include use of call lights, side rails, oxygen, other equipment.

- Have patient repeat back information in own words to facilitate understanding.
- Encourage patient to ask for help when needed.
- Answer call light promptly at all times.
- Integrate family into treatment plan and care whenever possible.

☐ EVALUATION CRITERIA/DESIRED OUTCOMES

The Patient

- Demonstrates selected injury-prevention measures
- Utilizes safety measures to prevent injury
- Identifies factors (verbally or nonverbally) that increase potential for injury
- Follows identified safety rules and procedures
- Communicates needs to nursing staff
- Is free from injury

NURSING DIAGNOSIS #5

Disturbance in self-concept related to illness, hospitalization

Rationale: Self-concept is a dynamic process of the perception of self that begins at birth and continues throught the life-cycle. It is related to life experiences and has 4 components: body image, self-esteem, role performance, and personal identity. Self-concept is learned during development and involves the individual's feelings, attitudes, and values and affects reactions to all experiences. The developmentally disabled individual may have a relatively precarious sense of self, in which case the trauma of hospitalization will threaten all aspects of self-concept. The adaptive individual may still experience a threat to his/her sense of wholeness, judgment of own worthiness, and to the perception of body structure and function, depending on the reason for acute care.

☐ GOAL

The patient will adapt to the hospital setting; will develop and maintain/regain feelings of self-worth and a positive body image.

☐ IMPLEMENTATION

- Respect and consider the patient's life experience and chronologic age, regardless of IQ or retardation levels.
- Do not treat the adult person as a child even though the developmental stage is that of a child.
- Assess the meaning of the loss of any body part or body function for the patient/family.
- Assist to verbalize feelings; facilitate expression of

feelings and encourage the patient to share experience of the hospital with the nursing staff.
- Correct misconceptions patient may have (e.g., that s/he is being punished).
- Provide alternative ways for nonverbal patient to deal with fear, anxiety, grieving (e.g., role playing, play therapy, audiovisual aids).
- Consult with allied health professionals (e.g., speech therapist, for help with nonverbal aids).
- Give positive reinforcement for self-help behaviors and socially acceptable attitudes and behaviors.
- Praise healthy habits and attitudes.
- Encourage questions; whenever possible, assign permanent staff to patient to build trust and rapport.
- Be aware that patient/family may have an unusual degree of emotional interdependence because of the limitations of the retarded person in daily life.

☐ **EVALUATION CRITERIA/DESIRED OUTCOMES**

The Patient
- Expresses feelings and concerns as able and shares perceptions with staff
- Participates in learning experiences
- Maintains control of body and bodily functions
- Verbalizes good feelings about self, if able
- Interacts adaptively with staff

NURSING DIAGNOSIS #6

Knowledge deficit regarding treatment plan, rehabilitation therapies, follow-up care, community resources

Rationale: Upon discharge, the patient/family/residential facility will need follow-up care, treatment, and knowledge of resources to effect completely the return to adaptive day-to-day functioning. The developmentally disabled patient, with the increased risk of infection and trauma, needs a well-developed and comprehensive plan for follow-up, treatment, and education to maximize the potential for adaptive individual and family coping, the maintenance of health, and for physical and psychologic well-being.

☐ **GOAL**

The patient/family will discuss the treatment plan, plan for continued therapies, and follow-up care, including the medication schedule and side effects to watch for; will plan to maintain daily needs such as hygiene, grooming, diet, and exercise; will identify and demonstrate knowledge of community resources.

☐ **IMPLEMENTATION**
- Include family/residential care giver in discharge planning.
- Assess level of knowledge and ability to comply with treatment plan, therapy schedule, and medication regimen.
- Review medications, their use, schedule, side effects.
- Review ADL, provide written plan.
- Provide patient/family with written follow-up plan to include schedule of appointments, names, phone numbers, and addresses of physician/therapist/clinic; home care; and medication and therapy schedules.
- Encourage verbalization of feelings and questions about illness and discharge.
- Discuss community resources and support groups with patient/family, provide contacts and information as needed.

☐ **EVALUATION CRITERIA/DESIRED OUTCOMES**

The Patient/Family/Residential Care Giver
- Participates in discharge planning
- Receives and verbalizes understanding of written set of instructions regarding medications, diet, exercise, treatments, and therapies
- Has written schedules for therapies, follow-up care, and appointments with physician/therapist/clinic together with a written list with their names, addresses, phone numbers as well as community resources/support groups
- Verbalizes knowledge of all prescribed medications with name, dosage, administration times and directions, possible side effects
- Is referred for assistance (financial, vocational, home health care) as needed
- Verbalizes awareness that hospital/clinic is willing to collaborate with community agencies for reports, future care

The Patient who is Dying/Terminal

Definition/Discussion

The process of dying is the final stage of life and involves the patient, family, friends, and all members of the health care team. Although death is a universal experience, the feelings and attitudes each person has regarding death are unique and affect the way his/her life is lived and terminated. People will usually face death in a manner similar to how they dealt with other crisis situations throughout life.

Kübler-Ross has identified 5 psychological stages of grieving that are usually experienced when an individual is facing death.

1. *Denial* is an adaptive coping mechanism to delay the pain and shock until the patient is better able to deal with the reality. Patients go in and out of denial throughout the grieving process as a protection against the anguish and despair of the situation. "Oh, no. This can't be true. I don't believe it!" demonstrates denial.
2. *Anger and rage* are felt regarding the unfairness of the diagnosis. The question asked during this stage is "Why me?". These feelings are projected onto family and care givers who are able to continue with life and activities.
3. *Bargaining* is an attempt to postpone dying until certain tasks are complete (e.g., birth of a grandchild, a relative's graduation). These requests are usually made to God and provide a way for the patient to deal with the situation in small increments.
4. *Depression* occurs with the realization that many losses are imminent (e.g., family, job, control, lifestyle, life itself) and produces a profound sadness and depression.
5. *Acceptance* is a time of acknowledgement and recognition that death is inevitable, and the patient accepts it after having gone through all the other stages. S/he may become increasingly disengaged and project an attitude of "It is all right." Some patients never reach this stage and die in denial, with anger or sorrow.

The nurse's responsibilities include giving support, empathy, and compassion so as to facilitate dignity, growth, and peace in the process of dying. Support groups and/or professional supervision from specialists in thanatology are helpful to assist with appropriate management of grief and mourning.

Nursing Assessment

☐ **PERTINENT HISTORY**

Type of illness (e.g., length, character, progression), previous serious illnesses, previous experiences with losses and death

☐ **PHYSICAL FINDINGS**

Amount of pain or discomfort, confusion, level of consciousness, vital signs, ability to participate in self-care and activities of daily living (ADL), alterations in body image, fatigue, nausea and vomiting, alopecia, insomnia, restlessness

☐ **PSYCHOSOCIAL CONCERNS/ DEVELOPMENTAL FACTORS**

Past and present support system, patient's/family's previous responses to crises, cultural and ethnic beliefs and practices, religious requirements and preferences, personality characteristics (e.g., pessimism, optimism), usual coping mechanisms, psychiatric problems or diagnoses, suicidal ideation or attempts, symptoms of anxiety

☐ **PATIENT AND FAMILY KNOWLEDGE**

Disease entity and probable course of progression, options regarding treatment, acceptance of diagnosis and prognosis, intellectual capacity, alternatives to hospitalization, support or bereavement groups, community resources

Nursing Care

☐ **LONG-TERM GOAL**

The patient will experience physical comfort during the terminal process; the patient will die in a manner appropriate to and consistent with his/her values, beliefs, and philosophy of life. The family will assist in meeting the final needs of the patient; the family will progress toward acceptance of loss and toward adaptive grieving.

NURSING DIAGNOSIS #1

a. **Powerlessness** related to poor prognosis, inevitable death, loss of control/function
b. **Ineffective individual coping** related to inability to face death
c. **Anxiety** related to an unknown future

Rationale: Fear of the unknown, of pain, mutilation, rejection, being alone at time of death, dependency, loss of control, identity, self-esteem, and loss of the physical body contribute to decreased stamina and effectiveness of coping mechanisms. High anxiety and fear narrow perceptions and interfere with learning and coping. Usual coping mechanisms may not work during this time of crisis and the patient may resort to maladaptive coping strategies.

☐ GOAL

The patient will identify and develop effective and adaptive coping mechanisms to reduce anxiety and fear and facilitate normal grief.

☐ IMPLEMENTATION

- Identify the stages of the grieving and dying process on a continuing basis; remember that more than one stage may be evident at the same time, progression is not necessarily sequential and may arrest at any stage; coping will change with each stage and with the passage of time.
- Determine what the MD has told patient/family (it is MD's responsibility to inform patient/family of probable death); be present when diagnosis and prognosis are discussed with patient/family if possible to help in planning for future care.
- Allow patient to experience denial as needed without reinforcing denial; do not force the acceptance of truths patient is not yet ready to deal with; discuss the reality of the situation without stripping patient of all hope.
- Monitor presence of mutual avoidance between patient and family (pretending dying is not occurring in order to protect each other); this may persist until death occurs and could keep the patient isolated and unable to express wishes and feelings.
- Be alert for displacement of anger onto family/staff; assist to express feelings more directly by use of reflection (e.g., "It must be very hard for you to not be out of bed today.").
- Provide privacy for and encourage the expression of crying, screaming; provide alternative outlets to express anger (e.g., an extra pillow for punching) if energy permits.
- Assist patient to verbalize feelings regarding fears of the unknown, abandonment, etc.; explore their

meaning; be alert for spiritual needs and possibly psychiatric referral.
- Allow control of own care and ADL as possible to minimize fears of dependence and shame over decreased functioning.
- Be flexible with schedules to assist patient in accepting additional care required with less stress.
- Accept irritability and do not take personally or act defensively; be aware of own nonverbal behavior in communicating to patient.
- Demonstrate concern and caring by giving empathy and reflecting your observations (e.g., "You seem upset today.").
- Monitor the degree of hope present; do not encourage false or unrealistic hopes but allow patient's faith and hope to sustain him/her throughout the dying process.
- Show interest in patient's plans for the future and help adjust to the future as being "a day" or "a week" from now rather than longer periods of time.
- Assist patient to deal with guilt feelings by identifying what they feel guilty about; correct distorted perceptions; encourage making amends if possible (e.g., writing a letter, asking for forgiveness) and forgiving themselves so that peace and acceptance can occur.
- Encourage verbalization of feelings of depression and fears regarding the many losses associated with the loss of life; refer to *The Patient Experiencing Grief and Loss*, page 80
- Watch for clues to suicidal ideation (e.g., "It would be better to end this quickly."); provide a safe environment at all times and institute precautions as necessary; refer to *The Patient who is Suicidal*, page 144.
- Allow grief to be expressed in any way that is not detrimental to patient; know that silence may signify the beginning of acceptance and disengagement, and is normal.
- Use touch judiciously; know that some patients need to be held and touched and are unable to ask for it; other patients may prefer not to be touched.
- Show receptivity to what patient may be trying to explain (e.g., visions or conversations experienced in altered states of consciousness preceding death); question carefully to gain understanding of meanings but do not pry into the experience.
- Assist patient with life review; identify tangible and intangible legacies and fulfillments that have been achieved; encourage reminiscing with family/friends.
- Lend perspective that it is good to have others' lives go on even though his/hers is ending, that death is part of life and can be faced with courage to attain a sense of completion.
- Allow for individual differences in dying process as dictated by culture and lifelong patterns of liv-

ing; know that people face death in a manner similar to how they deal with other life crises.
- Be aware of patient/family wishes regarding death and assist with their being carried out; inform physician and other members of the health care team.

☐ EVALUATION CRITERIA/DESIRED OUTCOMES

The Patient
- Does not despair
- Has a reduced level of anxiety and fear
- Copes adaptively with the dying process
- Expresses feelings constructively

NURSING DIAGNOSIS #2

Alteration in comfort: pain related to trauma, advanced disease, dying process

Rationale: During the process of dying, many physical and psychologic changes occur that may produce pain and discomfort. These vary in severity, intensity, and duration but are a source of concern to the patient and to the family, and require attention by the nurse to provide comfort and peace at the end of life.

☐ GOAL

The patient will verbalize when discomfort, pain, and feelings of anxiety occur so they can be minimized and comfort provided.

☐ IMPLEMENTATION

- Ask patient to tell you when discomfort, pain, or anxiety is felt; ask family to watch for signs and report these as they develop; refer to *The Patient Experiencing Pain*, page 104, and *The Patient Experiencing Anxiety*, page 22.
- Keep patient dry, clean, and in comfortable surroundings; provide light, loose bed covers and circulating air; reposition patient frequently for comfort but do not move unnecessarily.
- Provide sufficient indirect light; do not draw shades as patient has decreased vision in darkness and can see only what is near; encourage visitors to sit near the head of the bed for better vision.
- Keep in mind that patients are often very anxious about going to sleep at night because they fear dying alone in the darkness; check on patient frequently and leave soft light on at all times.
- Monitor for elevated temperature; know that internal temperature may be elevated even though patient is cool to the touch.
- Speak in normal voice rather than a whisper; encourage family to continue talking to patient even

though comatose; do not discuss patient within his/her hearing.
- Use noninvasive measures (e.g., backrubs, soothing music) in conjunction with pain medications to increase comfort and therapeutic effects of the analgesics.
- Administer oral care as needed, suction gently; elevate head of the bed to 30°-45° to ease respirations if necessary.
- Inform family when analgesics are allowed and how they will be administered; know that maintaining a pain-free state is a goal for terminal patients though not all experience pain.

☐ EVALUATION CRITERIA/DESIRED OUTCOMES

The Patient
- Verbalizes occurrence of discomfort
- Accepts noninvasive comfort measures
- Responds to analgesics when administered
- Achieves adequate rest and sleep
- Remains pain-free as much as possible

NURSING DIAGNOSIS #3

Self-care deficit: feeding, bathing/hygiene, dressing/grooming, toileting related to decrease in physical and emotional strength

Rationale: The progression of the dying process creates increased fatigue and decreased interest and ability to perform self-care activities. There is also an increased need for physical care related to possible immobility, incontinence, fever, dehydration, and other manifestations of severe illness.

☐ GOAL

The patient will maintain as much control as physical condition permits over ADL for as long as possible; the family will contribute to the care of the patient whenever appropriate.

☐ IMPLEMENTATION

- Encourage participation in self-care as long as possible; ask for preferences (e.g., best time for bathing) to sustain patient interest in maintaining functioning; do not ask patient/family to perform tasks they are unable or unwilling to do.
- Protect from embarrassment over incontinence, altered body image, inability to eat neatly; provide privacy during times when shame over decreased abilities might upset patient.
- Provide accepting, nonjudgmental, concerned care; make sure patient knows s/he is still considered a part of the living and not "in limbo" or unimportant in the eyes of the care givers.

- Allow to wear own clothes if possible; encourage family to bring favorite clothing from home.
- Encourage family to assist with feeding, grooming, etc., to decrease isolation and occupy visiting time; teach as necessary to facilitate any care giving.
- Provide cosmetics, wigs, ribbons, etc. to encourage cheerfulness in patient's life and improve appearance and self-esteem.
- Monitor skin condition; encourage patient to participate with grooming as much as possible; provide for shaving and hair care regularly as patient/family desire.
- Refer to *The Patient Experiencing a Body-Image Disturbance*, page 27.
- Maintain a neat, comfortable environment for patient/family; allow presence of personal articles that are pleasing and meaningful to patient.

☐ EVALUATION CRITERIA/DESIRED OUTCOMES

The Patient
- Participates in ADL as strength allows
- Expresses personal preferences regarding grooming and environment

The Family
- Participates appropriately in patient care

NURSING DIAGNOSIS #4
a. **Social isolation** related to separation from family, friends, and confinement to hospital environment
b. **Diversional activity deficit** related to fatigue, immobility, withdrawal

Rationale: The patient who is terminal conserves failing strength and energy for the dying process and may be unwilling and/or unable to show interest in outside activities. Required occupations of family may prevent frequent visits, and the awkward feelings of friends regarding death may decrease social contacts. The increasing disengagement also contributes to feelings of abandonment.

☐ GOAL

The patient will participate in visits from others; will enjoy activities as strength permits.

☐ IMPLEMENTATION

- Arrange to spend time with patient even when care is not needed to promote feelings of acknowledgement and prevent feelings of abandonment and alienation.
- Discuss interests and activities that patient has enjoyed; determine what physical strength is available for diversion; make allowances for unscheduled pleasurable times when patient is able to participate.
- Encourage family/friends to visit; explore their feelings of discomfort regarding patient's terminal illness.
- Explain to family that the patient's silence does not necessarily mean rejection and that the presence of a loved one is helpful even if conversation is not continuous.
- Involve occupational/adjunctive therapist as appropriate to provide ideas and supervision for acceptable diversions.
- Discuss how much contact patient desires with others; consider possibility of appropriate roommate to help decrease the sense of isolation that is often felt.
- Remember loneliness is the greatest pain of all and that patients may not want to be removed from unit activities even though unable or unwilling to participate.

☐ EVALUATION CRITERIA/DESIRED OUTCOMES

The Patient
- Participates in activities as strength allows
- Anticipates and acknowledges visitors
- Has minimal level of withdrawal

NURSING DIAGNOSIS #5
Alteration in family process related to anticipatory grieving

Rationale: Family members experience the same stages of response to the dying process as the patient as defined by Kübler-Ross. These do not occur at the same time in all family members or simultaneously with the patient. If the spouse or another member of the family remains fixated at the denial stage, it may be difficult for meaningful communication regarding dying to occur. The family may experience ambivalence and guilt related to partial acceptance of the anticipated death.

☐ GOAL

The family will progress through stages of adaptation to impending death; will resolve feelings that may prevent expressions of timely grieving.

☐ IMPLEMENTATION

- Establish a trusting relationship with family members; encourage ventilation of feelings regarding patient's condition on an ongoing basis.
- Assess information given to family; determine whether it is the same as what patient knows; answer questions; ask what they do not understand

and clarify as needed; refer to other members of the health care team as appropriate.

- Listen carefully to what family members say; observe what information is imparted through non-verbal behavior; encourage them to share feelings with members of health care team.
- Monitor for destructive or inappropriate behavior caused by tension, anxiety, anger, or fear; do not argue with family but remain supportive and non-judgmental; remember family is sensitive to implied criticism due to feelings of guilt and anger; use empathic statements (e.g., ''This must be very painful for you.'').
- Assess dysfunction in family caused by imminent death (e.g., patterns of ineffective communication, lack of problem-solving abilities); encourage to function (e.g., ''What will you do about . . .?'').
- Monitor for development of pathologic grieving reactions; intervene with appropriate referrals as indicated.
- Utilize all health care team members in meeting needs of family (e.g., social worker, nurse therapist).
- Assist to obtain outside assistance as needed for financial problems, supplies (e.g., social service agencies, American Cancer Society).
- Explore role strain; assist family in changing roles as needed to minimize stress and maintain family cohesiveness.
- Encourage open communication and the sharing of feelings, concerns with each other; respect that some people do not wish to discuss grieving and feelings.
- Support progress of grieving through each stage; reassure that feelings are normal and resolve with appropriate expression and the passage of time.
- Encourage review of patient's life with family; help to integrate past into the present for increased acceptance of the dying process.
- Encourage normalcy in family life as much as possible to provide and maintain mutual support.
- Encourage family to maintain social relationships as much as possible to facilitate reinvolvement in usual activities following successful grieving.

☐ EVALUATION CRITERIA/DESIRED OUTCOMES

The Family

- Demonstrates progress in adapting to impending death
- Expresses feelings of grief
- Shows cohesiveness, tolerance, and support of each other
- Functions adequately in stressful situations
- Expresses knowledge regarding use of appropriate community resources

---

NURSING DIAGNOSIS #6

Spiritual distress related to a disturbance in belief system, hopelessness, or inability to participate in services

Rationale: The patient's religious beliefs and philosophy of life provide a source of strength, hope, and faith in life. A terminal illness can produce profound disturbances in the belief and value systems of patients and families that may result in feelings of anger, guilt, and fear. When a patient begins to question ''Why me?'' and ''What have I done to deserve this?'', spiritual distress may result.

☐ GOAL

The patient will express increased understanding and acceptance of death; will participate in religious practices as desired and as strength permits.

☐ IMPLEMENTATION

- Determine wishes of patient/family regarding pastoral care and services; remember that the actual offering of spiritual counseling may verify to patient/family that illness is terminal; obtain MD's order if required; contact spiritual advisor when requested.
- Respect right of patient/family to refuse participation of spiritual leader in dying process.
- Assess influence of cultural beliefs related to spiritual needs; become as knowledgeable as possible about the practices and requirements of various religions in care of the dying.
- Show acceptance of spiritual needs; remain nonjudgmental and understanding about patient's/family's search for meaning in suffering.
- Permit beneficial rituals as much as possible; provide privacy and seclusion as necessary.
- Consult health care team members to provide requested services; allow diet restrictions according to beliefs without endangering physical condition.
- Permit possession of religious or spiritual articles (e.g., Bible, rosary beads, clothing).
- Encourage spiritual rituals not damaging to physical condition; assist as necessary with positioning and provision of articles required for participation.
- Determine ritual care and arrangements required for the dying, dead, and for burial; involve physician and other staff as indicated.
- Respond with concern and empathy when patient/family discuss spiritual beliefs; do not attempt to change or influence religious affiliations.
- Continue to offer services of a spiritual leader if initially refused.
- Know that strong feelings of anger toward God, ambivalence toward the dying person, and guilt for having these feelings are natural (although usually temporary) in family members, and that

intervention by a religious professional may diminish these feelings.

☐ EVALUATION CRITERIA/DESIRED OUTCOMES

The Patient
- Expresses increased acceptance of death
- States increased spiritual peace
- Accepts and practices spiritual rituals indicated for specific beliefs

The Family
- Discusses concerns and feelings with appropriate spiritual leader
- Expresses understanding of guilt and ambivalence toward ill member

---

NURSING DIAGNOSIS #7

Knowledge deficit regarding terminal care in nonacute setting and resocialization of family following death of member

Rationale: As an alternative to death in an acute hospital, it may be possible to provide home or hospice care for the terminally ill. Utilization of community services and family members can provide more personal attention and allows family to experience less guilt and more positive adjustments to their grief.

☐ GOAL

The patient will accept nonacute care if indicated; the family will provide care in an outpatient setting that meets needs of patient; will utilize community services when needed to adjust to loss of member.

☐ IMPLEMENTATION

- Inform patient/family of options to acute hospital care (e.g., hospice, private home, own home); refer to *The Patient Receiving Hospice Care*, page 85.
- Ensure complete understanding of physical and psychologic requirements of the patient and the willingness and ability of the family to meet those needs.
- Refer to home health agency for predischarge visit; work with discharge planner to teach necessary skills to family and provide information regarding medications, and physical and emotional care.
- Refer to social worker for information regarding financial difficulties caused by extended illness; assist family to utilize social service agencies as needed.
- Inform care givers of available mental health services and how to set up an appointment.
- Provide family with phone numbers of agencies and people for questions and emergencies.
- Identify agencies which may be of value to family in coping with loss (e.g., support, bereavement, spouse groups) if indicated.
- Refer to appropriate community resources for assistance in terminal care in outpatient settings (e.g., American Cancer Society, Alzheimer's Disease Association).

☐ EVALUATION CRITERIA/DESIRED OUTCOMES

The Patient
- Indicates acceptance of nonacute care without anxiety

The Family
- Demonstrates understanding of requirements for care and abilities to provide it
- Expresses knowledge regarding community resources and appropriate support persons and groups available

The Patient Experiencing Fear

Definition/Discussion

Fear is an emotional response to a consciously recognized internal/external source that is perceived as dangerous.

Nursing Assessment

☐ **PERTINENT HISTORY**

Precipitating factors, length and severity of response, degree of restriction of life-style, usual methods of coping

☐ **PHYSICAL FINDINGS**

Changes in vital signs, sweating, pupillary dilations, trembling, tension, restlessness, insomnia, decreased ability to concentrate, crying, demanding behavior, somatic complaints

☐ **PSYCHOSOCIAL CONCERNS/ DEVELOPMENTAL FACTORS**

Childhood fears, nightmares, past experiences and memories, patterns of pessimism/persistent worry

☐ **PATIENT AND FAMILY KNOWLEDGE**

Previously learned responses and management, degree of disruption, perception and interpretation of fear-producing event(s), readiness and willingness to learn

Nursing Care

☐ **LONG-TERM GOAL**

The patient will interact with the environment in such a way that factors and situations that cause fearfulness are recognized and managed in an adaptive way.

NURSING DIAGNOSIS #1

Ineffective individual coping related to fearful response

Rationale: A decrease in control, objectivity, and judgment occurs when fear is experienced resulting

---

in personality disorganization and impaired ability to maintain activities of daily living (ADL).

☐ **GOAL**

The patient will identify the fear, its cause, and methods of effective coping.

☐ **IMPLEMENTATION**

• Attempt to identify the specific source of the fear.
• Use indirect, open-ended questions (e.g., "What is it about being in the hospital that concerns you most?").
• Go slowly in exploring fears; wait in silence; show willingness to get involved; remember the patient may not discuss the greatest fears as readily as those of less importance.
• Reassure that emotions felt are manageable.
• Give careful explanation of all that is to occur; following explanations, have patient tell you in own words what you said and what it means to him/ her; repeat this procedure as often as needed to ensure understanding.
• Encourage, when tolerated, the examination of the fears and different ways they can be managed; do not make decisions for the patient.
• If you are unable to reduce the fear (e.g., of dying during surgery) prior to the event, notify physician so appropriate corrective action can be taken (surgery may be cancelled).

☐ **EVALUATION CRITERIA/DESIRED OUTCOMES**

The Patient
• Identifies fear-promoting sources
• Verbalizes responses to fear
• Corrects distorted perceptions
• Defines alternative coping techniques

NURSING DIAGNOSIS #2

Alteration in comfort related to physical indicators of fear

Rationale: Physiologic changes that may cause discomfort occur during the emotional response of fear. The experience of pain is heightened when accompanied by fear.

Because fears change with circumstances, there is a continuing need for adaptation in management. It is useful to differentiate fear from anxiety as fear is often short lived in response to a specific threat, whereas anxiety is more vague and chronic.

☐ GOAL

The patient will discuss fears; will participate in measures to relieve fear and discomfort; will demonstrate increased relaxation and decreased physiologic behaviors of fear.

☐ IMPLEMENTATION

- Provide serene and safe environment; decrease disturbing stimuli.
- Encourage identification of specific discomforts and use indicated methods of alleviation (e.g., medication, back rub, bathing).
- Minimize muscle tension by proper alignment, positioning, and support.
- Encourage ambulation and exercise as indicated as a constructive use of energy.
- Teach relaxation techniques appropriate to age and condition (e.g., deep breathing, visualization).
- Use touch as indicated; be aware of individual variations in acceptance.
- Provide diversionary activities (e.g., music, books, TV, games, visitors).

☐ EVALUATION CRITERIA/DESIRED OUTCOMES

The Patient
- Has no complaints of physical discomfort
- Uses calm verbal communication
- Is free from visible muscle tension
- Utilizes diversionary activities

NURSING DIAGNOSIS #3

Knowledge deficit regarding management of fears

Rationale: Fears can be reduced through knowledge of causes and effective alternative controls.

☐ GOAL

The patient will differentiate between adaptive and maladaptive responses to fear.

☐ IMPLEMENTATION

- Spend at least 15 minutes with patient every day; direct the conversation towards responses to the hospital (e.g., "What thoughts are you having about the way your hospitalization is going?").
- Listen to and positively reinforce attempts to talk about decisions that involve dangerous procedures or major life changes; use clear and concise communication.
- Assist verbally and nonverbally in asking questions patient may have about the progress/outcome of diagnosis and treatment.
- Direct questions about diagnosis and treatment not appropriate to nursing to the physician and explain the reason the patient needs the answer (e.g., fear of the outcome of the illness).
- Involve and give explanation to other interested persons so they may reinforce the teaching you have done.
- Allow friends and family to express their fears so they will be comfortable and supportive; this intervention will be important in preventing the patient from realization of a fear of abandonment.
- Instruct parents that some fears occur throughout childhood and provide information for acknowledgement and management of fears in realistic ways.
- Refer, if indicated, to self-help, support, or information groups.

☐ EVALUATION CRITERIA/DESIRED OUTCOMES

The Patient
- Verbalizes those aspects of own body, health care, and environment that cause fear
- Utilizes situational supports to reduce fear
- States realistic goals in the adaptive management of fears

The Patient Experiencing
Grief and Loss

Loss is the removal of something/someone of great value to the person. Grief is the emotional responses that follow the perception, or anticipation, of a loss. Mourning is the psychologic process that results from a loss. The grief and mourning process is the process of coping with and adapting to the loss. There are three categories of loss

- *nurturing:* loss of a significant other through death, divorce
- *self-image:* loss of one or more aspects of usual self-image (e.g., self-respect; also includes loss of a body part or function such as a leg, bowel function)
- *sexual role identity:* loss of usual roles (e.g., family role, career role, sexual functioning, control over one's life)

An actual or anticipated loss in any of these categories will trigger the grief and mourning process. Although grief, loss, and mourning are most frequently associated with a death, they are present with all losses—such as the loss associated with a mastectomy (body part), with a colostomy (normal bowel function), or with paraplegia (normal body function plus usual role functions). According to Engel (1965), the grief and mourning process involves three stages: 1) shock and disbelief, 2) developing awareness of the loss, and 3) restitution. Full restitution may take a year or more and some people never completely recover. Each stage has its own adaptive responses and time frame.

Nursing Assessment

☐ PERTINENT HISTORY

Recency, causative or contributing factors of current loss(es); past experiences with loss and its successful/unsuccessful resolution

☐ PHYSICAL FINDINGS

Loss of body part/function; chronic pain; changes in physical status as response to loss (e.g., appetite, bowel habits, nausea, sleeplessness, fatigue, headaches, general malaise)

☐ PSYCHOSOCIAL CONCERNS/ DEVELOPMENTAL FACTORS

Developmental stage and tasks; recent change in lifestyle (e.g., childbirth, marriage, loss of significant other, change in economic state); social support system or lack of; multiple losses; category of loss (sexual role, self-image, nuturing); stage of grieving (Engel), individual's responses to loss: denial, shock and disbelief, anger, guilt, sadness, depression, acceptance, regression

☐ PATIENT AND FAMILY KNOWLEDGE

Adaptation to loss, plans for the future; self-help groups; professional counseling to enhance grief work or resolve past losses

Nursing Care

☐ LONG-TERM GOAL

The patient will cope with the loss experienced by completing each stage of the grief and mourning process.

NURSING DIAGNOSIS #1
a. **Grieving** (shock and disbelief) related to loss
b. **Self-care deficit** related to inability to perform activities of daily living (ADL) associated with overwhelming feelings

Rationale: Shock and disbelief comprise the first stage of the grieving process. The individual must work thorough denial of what is occurring. This is difficult to do in an unanticipated loss such as occurs in an auto or plane crash. Common behaviors are denying loss alternating with sadness, crying, screaming, and anger; these are considered adaptive behaviors. Almost any behavior is adaptive in this stage except homocidal or suicidal behavior. This stage usually lasts 1-7 days. The individual who has experienced psychogenic shock may for a time be physically or psychologically unable to care for own needs. There may be a decreased level of comprehension of the need to feed, bathe, dress, or otherwise care for self, coupled with alteration in the functioning of the neurologic, respiratory, circulatory, and musculoskeletal systems. Defense mechanisms such as regression also occur as a way of coping with the threat.

☐ GOAL

The patient will use nondestructive coping mechanisms to deal with the loss; will accept help with ADL; will resume management of own life in terms of ADL; will resume normal eating and hydration patterns with a caloric intake of (specify) cal/day and a fluid intake of (specify) ml/day.

☐ IMPLEMENTATION

- Accept any behavior that is not physically destructive; allow patient to cry, scream, pound fists, etc.; do not try to cut it off or limit it.
- Reinforce the occurrence of the loss while encouraging the patient to talk about it; do not support denial but elicit feelings (e.g., "It must be difficult to believe this is happening.")
- Spend at least 15 minutes/shift talking or just sitting and listening to the patient; allow the patient to direct the conversation.
- Assess level of ability to care for self, including comprehension, awareness, cognition, and affect.
- Be aware that patient may lack motivation to do anything for self, may be experiencing strong feelings of dependency.
- Tell patient it is acceptable to be dependent on others for a limited period of time to provide basic physiologic and psychologic needs.
- Provide a structured, consistent environment and routine.
- Assist with care; provide direction but offer choices; include patient in planning own care.
- Provide 1 consistent primary care giver to assist in developing/maintaining relationship of trust and safety.
- Provide with clear, firmly stated instructions when needed.
- Ensure that patient bathes or showers daily.
- Observe and chart actual diet consumed (e.g., solid and fluid intake).
- Ascertain favorite foods; plan diet with dietician and patient, considering patient's likes and dislikes.
- Offer small, frequent meals, fluids.
- Assess and chart patterns of elimination; provide balanced diet to promote regular elimination.
- Provide quiet environment, opportunity for rest.
- Observe physical condition and report problem to physician.

☐ EVALUATION CRITERIA/DESIRED OUTCOMES

The Patient
- Demonstrates adaptive first-stage grieving behaviors
- Accepts help with ADL
- Initiates own self-care with ADL
- Ingests adequate diet and hydration to compensate for loss due to stress and shock, and to meet present needs
- Has regular, adaptive sleep pattern; sleeps minimum of 4-6 hours/24 hours

---

NURSING DIAGNOSIS #2

Grieving (developing awareness) related to continued resolution of loss

Rationale: In the second stage of grief, loss is acknowledged ("Maybe I'll look OK with a prosthesis." "Do you think I'll be able to work with this?" "I'll never be able to cope."). Mood swings are common. Self-blame is a part of this stage (e.g., "If only I'd done . . ."). Adaptive behaviors of stage 1 may be interspersed with these new behaviors. This behavior can last from several weeks to months. When a loved one is lost, the length of this stage and the next seem to be dependent on the length and importance of the relationship. Reminiscing is an important part of this stage as is reliving the actual loss event.

☐ GOAL

The patient will express an awareness of the loss and its impact.

☐ IMPLEMENTATION

- Incorporate a discussion of the loss into your daily conversations with patient/family; appropriate questions might be "How do you see the effect of what has happened to you?" or "How is your family coping with what has occurred?"
- When patient begins to share feelings (i.e., anger, guilt, depression, sadness), encourage to do so; sit and listen.
- Reiterate that grieving is normal for this situation.
- When appropriate, tell the patient s/he is doing a good job of dealing with the loss.
- Involve in planning and doing some aspects of self-care.
- Restate questions the patient has asked so that s/he can explore the answers with your assistance.
- Ensure that patient has ongoing situational supports to help deal with the loss (e.g., friends, family, clergy).
- Adjust visiting hours for family/friends to stay as necessary; try to fulfill any patient requests.

☐ EVALUATION CRITERIA/DESIRED OUTCOMES

The Patient

- Talks about loss and its impact on life-style (e.g., wearing a prosthesis)
- Expresses feelings of anger, guilt, depression, sadness
- Develops/increases situational supports

NURSING DIAGNOSIS #3

Grieving (restitution) related to continued resolution of loss

Rationale: In the final stage of the grief process, the patient deals with the loss, structures new habits, and goes on with the business of living. Typical behaviors include making plans for the future, remembering both positive and negative aspects of life before the loss. Full restitution can take up to a year or more and some people never complete this stage. Behaviors from stage 2 may be observed periodically in this stage but lessen in frequency as time passes.

☐ GOAL

The patient will talk about the positive and negative aspects of the loss; will make plans for the future.

☐ IMPLEMENTATION

- Praise efforts to adapt to changed life-style; give positive reinforcement for making future plans.
- Allow the patient control over as much of own care and method of resolving the loss as possible.
- Refer for ongoing counseling, to community agencies as appropriate.

☐ EVALUATION CRITERIA/DESIRED OUTCOMES

The Patient

- Expresses both positive and negative impact of loss

- Makes plans for the future
- Increases situational supports over what was established in stage of developing awareness
- Resumes preloss roles and functions or modifications thereof.

NURSING DIAGNOSIS #4

Knowledge deficit regarding the process of loss resolution

Rationale: Many responses that the individual has to the loss may be frightening or confusing; simple information giving provides reassurance and structure.

☐ GOAL

The patient/family will understand typical grief responses.

☐ IMPLEMENTATION

- Discuss patient's/family's response to grief; point out how responses are common and necessary, that others experiencing a loss have many of the same responses.
- Tell what to expect next in the grieving process.
- Give positive reinforcement for all attempts to adapt to the loss.
- Explain that restitution will eventually occur and that frightening feelings/responses will diminish over time.
- Explain the benefits of expressing feelings and dealing with the loss now, and the dangers of unresolved grief leading to depression and stress-related diseases.

☐ EVALUATION CRITERIA/DESIRED OUTCOMES

The Patient/Family

- Verbalizes adequate knowledge of grief process
- States expectations for the future
- Explains that responses to grief are limited in time

The Patient Experiencing Guilt

Definition/Discussion

Guilt is a subjective feeling of remorse and self-reproach stemming from a belief that one has been responsible for wrong or losses, has transgressed the moral code/value system, or violated a principle of conscience.

Nursing Assessment

☐ **PERTINENT HISTORY**

Presence of situation(s) causing remorse or dishonor; details of situation (e.g., time, place, persons involved); perception of need for self-punishment; usual coping skills; compliance with health care plan

☐ **PHYSICAL FINDINGS**

Changes in vital signs, agitation, tension, restlessness, withdrawal, anxiety

☐ **PSYCHOSOCIAL CONCERNS/ DEVELOPMENTAL FACTORS**

Feelings of remorse or regret, disgrace and dishonor; expectation of reproach from family; self-punishment; preoccupation with situation; labels self in negative way; inability to forgive self; excessive stress level; substance abuse, erratic life-style, impaired judgment, low self-esteem, family dysfunction or violence; projecting blame onto others; compensation behaviors; desire to please others

☐ **PATIENT AND FAMILY KNOWLEDGE**

Past experiences, perception of situation, amount of disruption, readiness and willingness to learn

Nursing Care

☐ **LONG-TERM GOAL**

The patient will express and explore guilt feelings; the patient will develop alternative ways of coping with situations that produce guilt.

NURSING DIAGNOSIS #1
Potential for injury related to feelings of need for self-punishment

Rationale: Extreme feelings of responsibility for actual or potential physical or mental injury to self or others may produce suicidal ideation.

☐ **GOAL**

The patient will express feelings of guilt, remorse, and self-reproach without acting-out or self-destructive behavior.

☐ **IMPLEMENTATION**

• Make frequent intermittent contact with the patient, both verbal and nonverbal, to offer support and to build rapport and trust relationships.
• Observe for excessive stress level; assist to use adaptive coping mechanisms to obtain relief from stress; refer to Table 1, *Stress Management*, page 24.
• Offer self as nonjudgmental listener; encourage expression of feelings; reflect and summarize patient's words (e.g., "You seem to feel as though you could have prevented your stroke. Tell me more about that," or "You wish you hadn't spoken so sharply to your daughter?" or "Sounds like you can't forgive yourself for not going to the doctor when you first found the lump.").
• Assess for suicidal ideation; address issue with active suicide precautions if needed; provide controls for destructive behavior toward self or others; refer to *The Patient who is Suicidal*, page 144.
• Monitor acting-out behaviors; maintain a safe environment.
• Continue to assess for high stress levels and feelings of unresolved guilt.

☐ **EVALUATION CRITERIA/DESIRED OUTCOMES**
The Patient
• Verbalizes feelings of guilt
• States stress level is decreased

• Has no suicidal attempts or acting-out behaviors

NURSING DIAGNOSIS #2

Ineffective individual coping related to feelings of guilt

Rationale: Value systems and codes by which a person lives are learned. When a violation is imagined or recognized, guilt feelings occur, decreasing the effectiveness of usual coping abilities.

☐ **GOAL**

The patient will identify the perceived transgressions that cause feelings of guilt and ways to facilitate self-forgiveness.

☐ **IMPLEMENTATION**

• Allow patient to talk about transgression when ready.
• Allow time for rumination but assist in exploring the situation further to promote better understanding.
• Encourage to identify moral code or value system transgressed.
• Identify source of moral code or value in life experience (e.g., family, culture, religion).
• Explore present value system but do not become involved in "shoulds" and "should nots"; explain that there are many beliefs and value systems.
• Determine whether transgression was real or imagined.
• Support realistic assessment of the situation; offer other points of view regarding the incident.
• Explore ways to repent or apologize for real transgression (e.g., is patient willing to talk about incident to validate perceptions? is patient sorry? is patient willing to express sorrow and ask forgiveness? is patient willing to forgive self? patient may repent by being "good patient" and by cooperating with treatment plan, physical therapy, diet, medications).
• Explain that the process of repentance facilitates self-forgiveness.

☐ **EVALUATION CRITERIA/DESIRED OUTCOMES**

The Patient
• States causes of guilt resulting from perceived transgressions
• Evaluates realistically the need for repentance
• States ability to determine best course of action for self

NURSING DIAGNOSIS #3

Knowledge deficit regarding methods of managing guilt

Rationale: A realistic, problem-solving approach that examines alternatives and promotes rational behavior will diminish feelings of guilt and will produce a more efficient and positive approach to living. Differentiating between appropriate guilt in response to a transgression versus irrational guilt based on low self-esteem helps determine how to best intervene with patients experiencing guilt.

☐ **GOAL**

The patient will learn new and constructive ways to cope with feelings of guilt and alleviate guilt feelings.

☐ **IMPLEMENTATION**

• Assess patient for lack of knowledge about defense mechanisms and responses to loss and grief; teach as needed.
• Assist to identify other persons who may be available to share common problems of adult life; refer to community self-help, support, or informational groups.
• Encourage to discuss feelings and values with trusted person; help to reach out for emotional support; involve family as much as possible.
• Explain that self-forgiveness is important for mental health; emphasize the need for realistic expectations for self and others; one needs to accept his/her limitations and imperfections; refer to *The Patient Experiencing Shame/Embarrassment*, page 132, and *The Patient Experiencing a Threat to Self-Esteem*, page 127.
• Discuss and problem solve alternative ways of behaving in guilt-producing situations; explore pros and cons of these new ways, and encourage to anticipate response to them; refer to *Problem Solving*, page 248.
• Explore alternative ways to make amends (e.g., helping others, volunteer work).
• Suggest a limiting of "guilt time" to a specific amount of time a day (e.g., 10 minutes) when these feelings are addressed; instruct patient to focus attention on ADL, hobbies, and other feelings for the remaining waking hours.
• Teach assertive techniques to provide a positive self-image and ability to handle reproach, negative behavior of others.

☐ **EVALUATION CRITERIA/DESIRED OUTCOMES**

The Patient
• Identifies situations that stimulate guilt feelings
• Develops alternative ways of adaptively coping with guilt feelings

The Patient Receiving Hospice Care

Definition/Discussion

Hospice care is an interdisciplinary program of care with the philosophy of providing palliative and supportive services to meet physical, psychologic, social, and spiritual needs of dying persons and their families. Today hospice refers to a kind of care for the terminally ill that can be given in a variety of ways under different kinds of auspices. The services in one community differ from those of another as each determines it own needs, resources, and objectives. The family, as well as the patient, is considered to be part of the client unit of care and also receives nursing assessment and emotional support. Their contact with the patient is recognized as important to the family unit and is encouraged. On a home-care hospice plan, there must be a family member or individual who is able to be the primary care giver. Some experts feel that the home setting is ideal; most patients agree.

The objectives of hospice care are
- to provide a compassionate way of accepting terminal illness as a part of life
- to preserve the right of individuals to die with dignity
- to provide alternate ways to care for those in the hospital setting, in an independent facility, or in combination home-care and hospital units
- to supply a medically directed, multidisciplinary team of professionals and volunteers trained to meet the physical, emotional, and spiritual needs of the terminally ill and their families including
  - management of pain and other symptoms
  - emphasis on the quality of life
  - instruction and support for a family caring for a patient at home
  - coordinated care and support made available on a 24-hour basis
  - bereavement support

Unlike traditional care modalities, diagnosis and cure are not appropriate goals for the terminally ill; palliative care, defined as those measures that are designed to control symptoms and promote comfort, is prescribed.

☐ PERTINENT HISTORY

Specific disease; length of time since definitive diagnosis; prior experience with hospice care

☐ PHYSICAL FINDINGS

Related to specific disease process and therapeutic regimen; nausea, vomiting, diarrhea or constipation, fatigue, malaise, skin or mucous membrane lesions, pain

☐ PSYCHOSOCIAL CONCERNS/ DEVELOPMENTAL FACTORS

Disease-related changes in role/life style of patient/family; previous coping mechanisms; feelings about effects of illness and approaching patient death; spiritual strengths

☐ PATIENT AND FAMILY KNOWLEDGE

Diagnosis, prognosis, and plan of care including activities of daily living, treatments, medications, and supportive measures; strategies for dealing with the actual terminal event, readiness and willingness to learn

Nursing Care

☐ LONG-TERM GOAL

The terminally ill person will live meaningfully to the end of life and be free from pain and noxious symptoms. The family will receive emotional support to help them cope with this crisis.

NURSING DIAGNOSIS #1

Knowledge deficit regarding the difference between traditional medical care and the hospice concept

Rationale: The focus of the medical profession on cure and the advances in medical science, coupled with the caring relationship of patients and family, can make it difficult to choose palliative care. Full understanding of the hospice concept can help patients and families choose between hospital and hospice care when a cure is no longer a realistic choice. The nurse is in a position to give the information about hospice in the community. Hospice care is not for everyone.

85

GOAL

The patient/family will have sufficient information to understand the hospice concept and make an individual choice for the family.

IMPLEMENTATION

- Give the patient/family a working knowledge of prognosis, diagnosis, and plan of care.
- Discuss the concept of hospice care and assist in decision making regarding the most appropriate choice for patient/family.
- Recognize that lack of acceptance of impending death can be an obstacle for families in making a decision based on the true situation.
- Identify community resources and hospice contacts in the community; provide referral telephone numbers.
- Provide list of resource materials on death and dying that may be helpful.
- Suggest keeping a journal so that questions will not be forgotten but recorded during this stressful time.

EVALUATION CRITERIA/DESIRED OUTCOMES

The Patient/Family

- Expresses understanding of the hospice concept
- Makes an individual choice appropriate to the situation

NURSING DIAGNOSIS #2

Alteration in comfort: pain related to physical, emotional, spiritual aspects of dying

Rationale: Pain control is the cornerstone of hospice care. Physical pain is often associated with the terminal nature of the disease while emotional and spiritual pain are associated with the stages of coping with dying. Drug tolerance is reportedly rare. The patient's need for more medication is directly related to the progression of the disease, with the dying person undermedication is unnecessary.

GOAL

The patient will experience relief from or control of physical, emotional, and spiritual pain.

IMPLEMENTATION

- Assess the patient's experience of pain, listening for clues to alleviation; refer to *The Patient Experiencing Pain*
- Give oral forms of analgesics when possible (if the patient is unable to swallow or if uncontrollable vomiting is present, parenteral analgesics are acceptable).
- Know that morphine and methadone are most helpful for intractable pain; both can be administered in liquid form (oral dosages are 3-6 times the parenteral dose); an antiemetic, such as compazine is frequently included if nausea is a source of discomfort as well as pain.
- Administer pain medication around the clock, not PRN; awaken patients at night to take doses so that blood levels remain constant.
- Inform famiy that patients receiving morphine may initially be drowsy or sleep around the clock for 24-36 hours but then become alert; decrease dosage for those who do not become alert after 36 hours.
- Observe for respiratory depression, note rate and depth of respirations prior to administering morphine.
- If pain is due to muscular, skeletal, or joint pathology, aspirin may be indicated; advise the patient to take with meals, food, or an antacid; teach the patient to report side effects such as headache, dizziness, visual disturbances, stomach irritation, or tarry stools.
- If pain is not controlled, work with physician, patient, and family to devise a better regimen; include nonpharmacologic methods of pain relief (e.g., relaxation, imagery, massage).

EVALUATION CRITERIA/DESIRED OUTCOMES

The Patient

- Expresses relief or control of pain
- Takes pain medications regularly
- Remains alert to surroundings

NURSING DIAGNOSIS #3
a. **Self-care deficit: total** related to disease progression
b. **Impaired physical mobility** related to weakness
c. **Alteration in bowel elimination: constipation** related to pain medication, immobility, poor intake
d. **Alteration in nutrition: less than body requirements** related to anorexia
e. **Fluid volume deficit** related to poor intake

Rationale: The terminal patient may suffer from a variety of minor to severe discomforts related to the effects of the disease progression. Prevention or proper treatment of problems will promote patient comfort to the best possible degree.

GOAL

The patient will maintain acceptable level of comfort; will express relief from unpleasant symptoms.

☐ IMPLEMENTATION

- Provide environment conducive to patient comfort (e.g., well ventilated, temperature controlled, with suitable lighting).
- Observe patients on analgesics for decrease in large bowel function; stool softeners may be indicated; nausea and diarrhea may be controlled with appropriate medications.
- Encourage fluids as tolerated as terminally ill patients are prone to dehydration; enhance nutrition with a soft diet or anything that sounds palatable to the patient (food prepared by family members may be tolerated best).
- Assess for incontinence and work with the care givers for protection; report to the physician for alternative methods of control (e.g., Foley catheter).
- Promote comfort by regular turning of patients at least every hour; have family perform complete active or passive range-of-motion (ROM) exercises four times a day.
- Position for maximum comfort (e.g., Fowler's position if experiencing dyspnea).
- Encourage patients to be as active as possible: ambulating, sitting in a chair, turning, moving all extremities; or being turned and moved; know that each patient has an individual capacity for exercise and movement; patients who are free from pain and symptoms are more likely to want to move about.
- Observe closely for impaired skin integrity; attention to the skin is crucial for comfort since ill patients do not have optimal nutrition and exercise; frequent turning and movement change soft tissue pressure points and increase the speed of circulation; baths, lotion, back rubs, and gentle massage contribute to the patient's comfort.
- Provide mouth care after meals and as needed; use mouth swabs, soft toothbrush, and refreshing solutions.
- Keep clean and dry with fresh bed linens as needed.
- Offer assistance with hair grooming, nail care as desired by patient.

☐ EVALUATION CRITERIA/DESIRED OUTCOMES

The Patient
- Expresses acceptable degree of physical comfort
- Is free from dehydration, skin breakdown
- Evacuates soft formed stool at least every 3 days

NURSING DIAGNOSIS #4
a. **Anticipatory grieving** related to loss and fear of death
b. **Spiritual distress** related to loss of life and suffering

---

Rationale: *Medical treatment is not always successful in curing disease and as the patient/family come to the realization that the disease is terminal there is often fear of death and a sense of loss. Physical effects of disease may prevent the patient from participating in usual religious practices and may be a cause for concern. The patient/family may be discouraged at times and express questions about the meaning of life, death, and suffering.*

☐ GOAL

The patient/family will express feelings/concerns about approaching patient death; will relate resolution of spiritual disturbance; the family will identify strategies for adapting to anticipated loss.

☐ IMPLEMENTATION

- Refer to *The Patient who is Dying/Terminal*, page 72.
- Encourage the patient/family to talk freely; be a good listener, spend time, develop a trusting relationship.
- Do not avoid topics of conversation because they make you uncomfortable; seek support yourself from a knowledgeable peer.
- Encourage family members to meet other family members in hospice-support groups to share with each other.
- Encourage hobbies, crafts, interests as tolerated; children and pets provide a great sense of enjoyment and enrichment.
- Encourage patient/family members to talk about concerns, fears, anger, frustrations, and feelings of loss over their loved one; sharing one's own feelings is appropriate, too.
- Encourage family members to regularly engage in some pleasurable activity that does not involve the patient to provide respite for them; provision of child-care, housekeeping, patient-sitting, or transportation services may be necessary.
- Assist patient/family member to obtain the services of a minister, chaplain, rabbi, priest if clergy or pastoral care is desired.
- Listen attentively as the patient/family members talk about the positive aspects of their lives and the meaning of death.
- Provide bereavement counseling as needed; to die and lose a loved one is a difficult task; listen to the patient/family members and reassure them that these feelings are valid and expected; instruct them that the completion of the grieving process can vary in length for different people (1-2 years is usual); inform the patient/family that the hospice team will be available to the family while they adjust to the loss of the loved one and to life without that person; refer to *The Patient Experiencing Grief and Loss*, page 80.

☐ EVALUATION CRITERIA/DESIRED OUTCOMES

The Patient/Family

- Verbalizes acceptance of the inevitability of death
- States spiritual needs are being met
- Adjusts to the loss and to life without that person
- Takes up the tasks of living and resumes predeath activities

The Patient with a Manic-Depressive (Bipolar) Disorder

Definition/Discussion

Manic-depressive disorder is a major affective disorder usually characterized by recurring opposite emotional states of mania and depression. Mania may be characterized by an elevated, expansive, elated, euphoric, or irritable mood with associated symptoms of hyperactivity, inflated self-esteem, pressure of speech, decreased need for sleep, distractibility, flight of ideas, and excessive involvement in risk-creating activities. Depressive episodes are similarly severe and exaggerated. Prognosis of individual manic episode is good, even without treatment, provided patient does not suffer from complete physical exhaustion. The nursing care in this guide pertains to the manic phase of a bipolar disorder. For the nursing care of the patient in the depressive phase, please refer to *The Patient Experiencing Depression: Severe,* page 60.

Nursing Assessment

☐ PERTINENT HISTORY

Previous acute or chronic patterns of psychiatric problems, outpatient or hospitalization, treatment and medications; family history of psychiatric problems, depression, manic-depressive illness, loss, family history of affective disorders

☐ PHYSICAL FINDINGS

Poor hygiene, inadequate nutrition, physical exhaustion, sensorimotor impairment, hyperactivity, insomnia, signs of exhaustion, irregular menstrual periods, increased sex drive/energy/verbal activity

☐ PSYCHOSOCIAL CONCERNS/ DEVELOPMENTAL FACTORS

Mood swings, affect of euphoria and elation, loose associations with "flight of ideas" (thought sequence characterized by rapid, disconnected speech often incomprehensible to listener), delusions and grandiose ideas, inability to focus on needs, impulsive activities with disregard for consequences, dysfunctional interpersonal relationships, noncompliance with treatment plan

☐ PATIENT AND FAMILY KNOWLEDGE

Schedule of medications and side effects to report; symptoms of acute phase and prognosis; ability to recognize the individual's impairment in both social and occupational functioning; knowledge of community resources and support groups, readiness and willingness to learn

Nursing Care

☐ LONG-TERM GOAL

The patient will resume effective management of own life; the patient will identify those behaviors indicating an approaching manic or depressive episode.

NURSING DIAGNOSIS #1

Potential for injury related to sensory/cognitive deficits, verbal/motor hyperactivity

Rationale: *The individual with perceptual/cognitive deficits coupled with verbal and motor hyperactivity is at high risk for physical injury. These patients have a decreased ability to identify hazards within the environment and a decreased understanding of the need for health maintenance and preventive self-care. At the same time there is increased physical and mental activity depleting the body's store of energy and exhausting usual coping mechanisms. While medication may be used to control mania, nursing actions are also needed to manipulate the environment to meet the needs of a patient unable to assume control of self.*

☐ GOAL

The patient will accept external control of self and of environment; will demonstrate increased control of motor and verbal behavior.

☐ IMPLEMENTATION

- Monitor motor and verbal behaviors as unobtrusively as possible.
- Assess orientation and ability to communicate with others regularly.
- Provide one consistent primary care giver to supply external controls on physical activity.
- Set limits with staff participation and consensus; give rationale for limits (e.g., patient is upsetting self or others with behavior).
- Restrict from acting out physically; use physical restraints only when verbal intervention and seclusion have failed.
- Provide with clear, firmly stated instructions for all activities.
- Decrease external stimuli; remove from stimulating, exciting, noisy, disturbing influences as much as possible.
- Provide with time in separate, quiet (seclusion) room as needed.
- Continue to provide space for patient to move around and ambulate but limit excessive exercising; remain with patient but engage in as little conversation as possible; inform that plan is to provide a quiet, safe place.
- Provide large-motor-skill activities such as walks, movement therapy, specific program of exercise, while considering short attention span and easy distractibility.
- Administer lithium as ordered and observe for possible side effects; refer to Table 4.
- Assess patient for danger to self or others; do not respond to verbal abuse personally.
- Ask if patient has any homicidal/suicidal thoughts; if "yes" report immediately and ensure patient is cared for on a one-to-one basis.
- Be alert to patient's wish to leave hospital (most manic patients see no need for hospitalization); keep patient in sight of staff at all times.
- Remove hazardous objects and substances from the environment to protect patient from own uncontrolled impulses.

☐ EVALUATION CRITERIA/DESIRED OUTCOMES

The Patient
- Tolerates, accepts external controls and decreased environmental stimuli
- Decreases verbal, motor activity
- Is free from injury

NURSING DIAGNOSIS #2

a. **Self-care deficit: feeding, hygiene, grooming** related to hyperactivity, distractibility and the individual's inability to control own behavior
b. **Sleep pattern disturbance** related to hyperactivity

Rationale: *The individual experiencing a manic episode is unable cognitively to focus on purposeful activity such as caring for body hygiene and feeding oneself. The patient may have little or no appetite, no desire for rest, and an inability to perceive the need for either nutrition or sleep. Since the consequences of uninterrupted activity with neither adequate nutrition or rest can be life threatening, the patient must be involved in activities to promote self-care.*

☐ GOAL

The patient will manage own grooming, hygiene, and nutrition; will resume normal eating patterns with an adequate caloric intake; will drink adequate fluids; will sleep 4-6 hours/night without awakening.

☐ IMPLEMENTATION

- Ensure that patient bathes or showers at least every 1-2 days, dresses each day, and keeps own clothes clean (loose, comfortable clothing is preferable).
- Be aware patient may not be able to tolerate activities that are highly structured and confining.
- Provide with frequent flexible opportunities to shower and change clothes, groom nails and hair, perform oral hygiene.
- Work with patient to identify an acceptable time and place for grooming activities; give positive reinforcement for all appropriate grooming.
- Help patient to learn to use the washer-dryer.
- Observe and chart actual diet consumed (solid and fluid intake).
- Discuss dietary needs with dietician; ask patient for favorite foods; plan menu for patient with increased caloric intake, considering likes and dislikes.
- Provide high-caloric finger foods and drinks that can be consumed easily while standing or moving.
- Use creative ways to encourage patient to maintain adequate diet (e.g., juice, peanuts, milkshakes).
- Provide quiet environment, seclusion room, sedation if necessary, and the opportunity for frequent short naps to facilitate restoration of a regular sleep pattern.
- Promote rest and sleep (e.g., give warm bath,

back rub; give sedatives as ordered, monitor for desired effects).

☐ EVALUATION CRITERIA/DESIRED OUTCOMES

The Patient
- Demonstrates adaptive personal hygiene and grooming
- Initiates own self-care
- Maintains admission weight
- Has balanced fluid intake and output
- Sleeps minimum of 4-6 hours/24 hours

NURSING DIAGNOSIS #3

Alteration in thought processes related to high levels of anxiety, inability to cope with feelings

Rationale: Impairment in the process of reality testing is a cognitive alteration that may be manifested in the individual experiencing an episode of mania. The impairment is characterized by flight of ideas, pressured speech, and delusions (e.g., false, fixed beliefs that cannot be corrected by logic). Frequently these delusions are delusions of grandeur. Delusions may be the patient's method of coping with anxiety and feelings of powerlessness, and of being overwhelmed. The individual thus has an inability to differentiate own thoughts and feelings from the reality of the outside world, which, combined with physical and verbal hyperactivity, creates difficulties in communicating with others.

☐ GOAL

The patient will differentiate between reality and fantasy; will express realistic ideas and plans.

☐ IMPLEMENTATION

- Listen to and chart patterns, themes, and symbols used in verbal communication; validate meaning with patient before making an interpretation.
- Be aware that patient's conversation may be filled with both rational and psychotic statements; state to the patient those statements that are confusing to you as a way to help keep on the subject and facilitate communication and understanding.
- Assign a primary care giver to help develop a relationship of trust; spend specific minimum amount of time daily interacting with and listening to patient.
- Assist in validating what is/is not real; interpret reality by stating you do not believe or perceive as the patient does.
- Do not discuss the grandiose ideas/delusions (a nontherapeutic method that may allow the patient to become more out of control).

- Look for and identify the reality stimuli causing the stress and delusional thinking; explore this with patient.
- Address patient's feelings and interpret reality (e.g., "You must be feeling very anxious right now."); listen for patient's feeling tone and follow up on it.
- Explain the reality of the actual situation, do not argue; encourage patient to assume responsibility for clarifying own thoughts.
- Provide limits, with a quiet room, walking, talking with patient, staying aware of patient's anxiety level.
- Persevere and be consistent in one-to-one interactions.
- Direct the focus from delusional expression to discussion of reality-centered situations.
- Encourage validation of thoughts by sharing them with staff, other patients, significant others.
- Set limits for discussing repetitive delusional material.
- Assist to differentiate between needs and demands.
- Teach to focus attention on real things and people, and to set limits on own behavior.

☐ EVALUATION CRITERIA/DESIRED OUTCOMES

The Patient
- Expresses realistic ideas and plan; differentiates between reality and fantasy
- Speaks more slowly and uses complete sentences
- Communicates clearly and realistically with staff, patients, significant others

---

NURSING DIAGNOSIS #4

Disturbance in self-concept: self-esteem related to feelings of inadequacy, ineffective coping

Rationale: By projecting an image of competence and independence the manic individual protects the self from confronting underlying feelings of helplessness, vulnerability, and loss which, if acknowledged, would lead to loss of self-esteem. However, as the individual's mood escalates, the hyperactivity, extravagant spending, impulsive decision making, lack of self-care, and exhaustion ultimately require that others assume responsibility for the individual's care. It is generally believed that the elation of mania actually represents a massive denial of underlying depression so that the patient's projected air of independence masks an underlying need for dependence coupled with feelings of helplessness, hopelessness, and worthlessness. Disturbance in self-concept may be manifested by the refusal or inability to take responsibility for self, by self-destructive behavior, displays of hostility, re-

---

fusal to acknowledge the problem or to accept re-habilitation efforts, and by manipulative and acting-out behavior.

☐ GOAL

The patient will acknowledge and identify own dependency needs; will engage in problem solving to develop more adaptive ways of coping.

☐ IMPLEMENTATION

- Establish one-to-one relationship; demonstrate an accepting attitude.
- Plan convenient times to spend with patient; include both one-to-one interactions and ward activities.
- Use silence; share with patient your willingness to spend time without talking.
- Help identify situations that increase anxiety and discuss adaptive ways to cope with the anxiety.
- Be aware of when demands are being made and convey acceptance while refusing to comply with excessive irrational demands.
- State observations/themes about the dynamics of the patient's behavior; provide immediate feedback about behaviors that involve demandingness or dependency.
- Assist in developing alternate ways of seeking gratification.
- Assist in learning how to make decisions and to accept responsibility for self.
- Help to identify and acknowledge feelings and learn how to communicate these feelings appropriately to others.
- Refrain from defensive personal response to criticism, physical attack, or profanity.
- Avoid positive reinforcement of negative behavior by ignoring it or minimally responding to it, unless it threatens others.
- Identify where limit setting is needed (e.g., grandiose plans such as business deals and spending sprees); set limits on behavior, and follow through consistently.
- Enforce in an unambiguous, firm manner; provide a consistent approach by all staff; keep lines of communication open among team members and update care plan with team periodically.
- Reevaluate the need for limit(s) at regular intervals and review the impact of the inappropriate behavior on others; point out the effect of behavior on others.
- Give immediate verbal reinforcement for all positive behaviors and statements of realistic expectations of self and others.

☐ EVALUATION CRITERIA/DESIRED OUTCOMES

The Patient

- Identifies and verbalizes own dependency needs
- Recognizes and acknowledges feelings of self/significant others
- Sets own limits on manipulative and acting out behavior
- Identifies/utilizes new problem-solving behaviors

NURSING DIAGNOSIS #5

Knowledge deficit regarding treatment plan, schedules, medications, follow-up care, community resources

Rationale: *Inadequate preparation for discharge may lead to noncompliance with treatment plans; manipulative behavior towards staff, peers, and family, and reversion to previous maladaptive methods of interaction. To effect change in the patient who experiences episodes of mania, new, adaptive and personally rewarding behavior that increases the individual's positive sense of self must be used instead of the previously described maladaptive behavior.*

☐ GOAL

The patient/family will demonstrate knowledge of treatment plans and follow-up care, medication schedule, continued need for medication, and side effects.

☐ IMPLEMENTATION

- Teach side effects of each medication being given, including lithium, and interventions to minimize any side effects.
- Teach the importance of adhering to the treatment and medication schedule.
- Stress importance of continuing maintenance dose of lithium even when not experiencing a manic episode.
- Give the responsibility of requesting and taking own medications prior to discharge to patient.
- Emphasize need for periodic blood test to ascertain lithium levels.
- Detail signs of increasing euphoria/depression; devise a strategy for getting immediate attention.
- Review adaptive, nonmanipulative ways of dealing with day-to-day living, stress, anxiety, fear, and frustration.
- Ask patient to detail a plan to maintain grooming, hygiene, nutrition.
- Assess availability of family and include them in discharge planning whenever possible.
- Provide written directions, schedule of appoint-

ments, instructions, names, addresses, telephone numbers of physician/therapist/clinic.
- Discuss community resources and support groups available; give patient list of resources.

☐ EVALUATION CRITERIA/DESIRED OUTCOMES

The Patient/Family
- Has written list, schedule of medications and treatments; verbalizes importance of taking them, possible side effects and how to treat them
- Verbalizes need to monitor blood level periodically when taking maintenance doses of lithium
- States willingness to cooperate with treatment plan in a responsible, informed, active way
- Describes dangerous effects of poor health practices and of noncompliance with the medications, planned, prescribed health care regimen
- Demonstrates ability to employ adaptive coping techniques
- Knows and identifies community resources and support groups

Table 4
Lithium Carbonate

Action/Uses	Side Effects	Nursing Implications
Normalizes pathologic mood without sedation or impairment of intellectual functioning. Is used to treat acute mania and to prevent recurring manic-depressive episodes. Blood levels must be maintained within a narrow range (0.6–1.4 mEq/liter; toxicity is much more prevalent at levels greater than 1.5 mEq).	*Minor* side effects: fine tremor, nausea, diarrhea, ataxia, drowsiness, thirst, polyuria, sedation *Moderate* side effects: nausea and vomiting, ataxia, dizziness, slurred speech, blurred vision, increasing tremor, muscle irritability or twitching *Toxic* symptoms: severe tremor, marked drowsiness, confusion, nystagmus, oliguria, chorea, convulsions, coma, death	• Requires 1-2 weeks for onset of action. • Most patients experience some temporary side effects; reassure that tremor is common, nonhazardous, and may disappear completely. • If nauseated, instruct to take pills with meals. • Teach family potential side effects, to observe for signs of increasing untoward ones, and to report to physician. • Coordinate arrangements for monitoring patient's serum lithium levels (done weekly initially, then usually bimonthly for maintenance). • Draw blood levels at least 12 hours after last dose to prevent a "false" elevation. • Be especially alert to side effects/toxic symptoms in patients on diuretics, low-salt diet, thyroid extract, or those with impaired renal function or CHF.

The Patient Manifesting Manipulation

Definition/Discussion

Manipulation is the process of influencing another in order to meet one's own immediate needs and desires. Because of a lack of trust, others are exploited, controlled, and treated as objects without regard for their feelings. This produces feelings of dehumanization in others and ultimately in the self. Manipulative behaviors are immature and may include dependency, being demanding or controlling, attempts to secure a privileged status through flattery or the giving of gifts, bargaining, seductive actions or statements, splitting (playing staff and/or family against each other), low tolerance for frustration, anger and physical or verbal aggression, passive aggression such as forgetting or noncompliance, and denial of disease, problems or feelings. Although some of the behavior is unconscious, part of it is conscious and deliberate in order to avoid authentic ways of relating. Since some rewards are obtained through manipulative behavior, there may be decreased incentive to change.

Nursing Assessment

☐ PERTINENT HISTORY

Previous episodes of manipulative behavior (exploitation of interpersonal contact, acting-out behavior); substance abuse, abuse to self or others; emotional difficulties in person and/or family

☐ PHYSICAL FINDINGS

Physical illness, trauma, organic disorder, use of alcohol, prescribed or nonprescribed drugs/medications, inadequate nutrition, neglect in self-care

☐ PSYCHOSOCIAL CONCERNS/ DEVELOPMENTAL FACTORS

Life-style of manipulative behavior and/or continual crisis (pretended helplessness, insincerity, apparent feelings of distress and loneliness); hostility, mistrust towards others, expressed contempt for motivations of others; ineffective patterns of communication (unnecessarily demanding, acting-out behaviors); inadequate or underdeveloped socialization skills; dysfunctional family relationships; unmet dependency needs, chronic or acute anxiety, feelings of in-

adequacy, fear of loss of control, hostility towards self (or others), powerlessness

☐ PATIENT AND FAMILY KNOWLEDGE

Ability to recognize behaviors of anxiety, frustration, and powerlessness; identification of manipulative behaviors by family; ability to assess family interactions; patient's/family's socialization skills and interpersonal relationships; readiness and willingness to learn

Nursing Care

☐ LONG-TERM GOAL

The patient will express own needs and wishes directly; the patient will demonstrate responsibility for own actions; patient will accept "no" as an answer to unreasonable requests.

NURSING DIAGNOSIS #1

Ineffective individual coping related to inability to express emotions directly, get needs met

Rationale: Ineffective individual coping is manifested when an individual experiences an inability to adequately meet their needs on a regular basis. Reasons for failure to meet one's own needs can result from not clearly identifying the need, feeling unworthy of asking for help directly, and not trusting others will respond if asked. The individual develops manipulative patterns of behavior in an effort to gain control and get others to meet their needs without directly asking. This method of operating frequently annoys and alienates others. Thus, the manipulative behavior is unsuccessful in getting the underlying needs met.

☐ GOAL

The patient will verbally acknowledge that present behavior is unsuccessful in getting needs met; will identify own coping patterns, the consequences of the behavior that results, and accept responsibility for own actions; will collaborate with the health team to determine one or more alternative strategies for adaptive functioning.

☐ IMPLEMENTATION

- Confront the patient with his/her attempts at manipulation; describe the behavior and how it makes you feel, suggest alternative ways to ask for what patient needs, e.g., "This is the third time you said I am neglecting you. That makes me feel guilty. Can you tell me specifically what I can do for you while I'm here?"
- Ignore manipulative behavior when possible (avoid making a public issue out of manipulative behavior).
- Avoid attempts by the patient to focus on the behavior of the nurse or other patients; redirect attention to the meaning of own behavior.
- Define clear expectations and consequences if expectations are not met, communicate these positively.
- Be consistent in interactions, limit setting and role modeling; be aware that mistrust of others will be modified slowly.
- Set specific limits on destructive behavior; collaborate with all involved health staff in achieving consensus about behavior expectations and means of approach.
- Limit only those behaviors that clearly impinge on the health of the patient and/or the rights and interests of others, using only methods that can feasibly be carried through.
- Recognize signs of anxiety and teach methods of decreasing discomfort; refer to *The Patient Experiencing Anxiety*, page 22.
- Allow and encourage the verbal expression of angry feelings; do not engage in accusations, arguments, demands for justification from patient; refer to *The Patient Manifesting Anger*, page 13.
- Identify one specific incidence of manipulative behavior by the patient, have patient verbally describe the consequences that resulted; have patient state an alternative method of behaving and discuss any possible changes in consequences.
- Tell the patient to deal directly with you (or you will continue to confront him/her with the effects of manipulation).
- Plan nursing care plans and daily routine with patient, identifying individual responsibilities; communicate this arrangement to staff, both verbally and in a written plan.
- Accurately record the instructions and information given in the nursing notes and nursing care plans; accompany physician on rounds to discourage the patient from changing, ignoring, or distorting the communication.
- Emphasize to staff the importance of clear, consis-

tent communication among staff at all levels regarding the patient's manipulative behavior and the approach to be utilized.
- Evaluate results of nursing care with the patient.
- Verbally reward and praise efforts in carrying out own responsibilities.
- Educate patient, through role playing, in ways to improve communication skills; assist in the identification of problem areas and clarification of unmet needs.
- Promote clear and assertive communication so that patient develops willingness to deal with own feelings as well as becoming aware of the feelings of others.
- Keep family informed of what you are doing and why; include them in the plan of action.
- Praise staff/family members for their efforts at reducing the manipulative behavior of the patient.

☐ EVALUATION CRITERIA/DESIRED OUTCOMES

The Patient
- Acknowledges and identifies own manipulative behavior and that the behavior is unsuccessful in getting one's needs met
- Acknowledges responsibility for own actions
- Identifies personal strengths and accepts the positive responses of others
- Asks directly for needs to be met
- Operates within the behavioral criteria for patients on the unit, ceases manipulative behaviors
- Makes decisions and follows through with appropriate actions to change provocative situations in personal environment

---

NURSING DIAGNOSIS #2

Disturbance in self-concept: self-esteem related to feelings of unworthiness and lack of trust

Rationale: Self-concept is a dynamic process of the perception of self that begins at birth and continues throughout the lifecycle. It has four components, body image, role performance, self-esteem, and personal identity. A positive self-concept is based on the knowledge of being loved, the acceptance of love, and the ability to love others. To develop and maintain self-esteem and a positive personal identity, an individual needs to feel worthwhile, lovable, and in control of his/her life. A child learns to see him/herself the way s/he is seen by parents/family members. The child who feels rejected, deceived will in turn develop a pattern of rejection and/or deception of others. Manipulative patients do not trust others to give them what they need if they ask for it directly.

GOAL

The patient will accept nurse concern and attention; will demonstrate one adaptive behavior; will identify and learn stress reduction activities for control; will acknowledge and accept positive feedback and praise from others; and will discuss feelings about self with staff/family.

IMPLEMENTATION

- Listen to patient, observe for nonverbal behaviors.
- Spend specific amount of time with patient each shift; use silence; share with patient that you are willing to spend time without talking; encourage to express feelings during this time, recognize that manipulative behavior is utilized to get one's needs met.
- Assist patient to acknowledge mistakes made, state what has been learned, and move on; educate how thoughts and beliefs shape behavior.
- Role play adaptive alternative methods of behaving; how to ask directly for what one wants, how to communicate one's feelings and negotiate.
- Teach assertive techniques.
- Assist to identify those problems that s/he cannot control directly and help to practice stress-reducing activities for control; refer to Table 1, *Stress Management*, page 24.
- Give consistent positive verbal feedback for all adaptive behavior.

- Assist patient to identify strengths and positive relationships and activities; refer to *The Patient Experiencing a Threat to Self-Esteem*, page 127.
- Encourage verbalization of feelings regarding hospitalization and/or illness; acknowledge that powerlessness can precipitate feelings of fear and anxiety, which intensify manipulative behaviors; refer to *The Patient Experiencing Powerlessness*, page 115.
- Contract for behavior change by having patient write out and implement one adaptive, short-term goal; assist to implement one adaptive method of behavior in a specific situation; refer to *Behavior Modification*, page 250.
- Maintain a stable physical environment when possible and assist with external controls when needed.
- Assist in adaptive social interaction with other patients.

EVALUATION CRITERIA/DESIRED OUTCOMES

The Patient
- Demonstrates methods for reducing stress
- Accepts and acknowledges positive feedback
- Discusses feelings about self with nurse
- Communicates more directly thoughts, feelings and requests
- Begins to verbalize more realistic self-perceptions

The Patient Manifesting Noncompliance

Definition/Discussion

Noncompliance in a health care setting means not adhering (or only partially adhering) to a prescribed therapeutic or disease-prevention regimen. The individual may desire to comply but is prevented from doing so by certain factors.

Nursing Assessment

☐ PERTINENT HISTORY

Previous unsuccessful experience with advised regimen, increasing amount of disease-related symptoms despite adherence to advised regimen, concurrent illness of family member; health beliefs that run contrary to professional advice; lack of understanding of diagnosis and treatment plan; history of forgetting appointments, medications, treatments

☐ PHYSICAL FINDINGS

Physical illness, duration, trauma, organic disorder; severe symptoms from prescribed treatment; impaired ability to perform tasks (sensory, motor deficits); degree of pain

☐ PSYCHOSOCIAL CONCERNS/ DEVELOPMENTAL FACTORS

Difficulty in changing personal habits, desire to remain ill and dependent for secondary gains; negative attitude toward health care providers; feelings of being manipulated by health care providers, denial of illness, low self-esteem, high stress level, life-style of continual crisis, financial and cultural factors; belief that compliance will not affect outcome, support of patient by family during illness

☐ PATIENT AND FAMILY KNOWLEDGE

Ability to recognize behaviors of anxiety and frustration; ability to recognize negative symptoms due to prescribed treatment; degree of understanding of diagnosis and treatment plan; costs of treatment; beliefs about illness, treatment, outcome; readiness and willingness to learn

Nursing Care

☐ LONG-TERM GOAL

The patient will comply with the prescribed treatment or disease-prevention regimen in a responsible, informed, and adaptive manner; the patient will participate in self-care to optimum level and achieve maximum health potential.

NURSING DIAGNOSIS #1

Noncompliance related to anxiety

Rationale: The patient experiencing uneasiness and apprehension about present illness or hospitalization may attempt to control this anxiety by overtly or covertly refusing to participate in the health care regimen. Causes of such anxiety may be negative experiences with the disease or with the health care system itself, or a lack of understanding regarding the value of treatment. Other stressors such as financial concerns, family, work, personal relationships can contribute to noncompliance. Since noncompliance as a diagnosis has a highly subjective component the nurse must identify causative and contributing factors and not make value judgments.

☐ GOAL

The patient will verbalize anxiety and fears related to the illness; will identify the factors contributing to anxiety; will identify adaptive alternatives to present coping patterns.

☐ IMPLEMENTATION

- Assess level of anxiety; ask patient to describe feelings and concerns, and discuss what precipitated this state.
- Establish one-to-one relationship; encourage expression of feelings and experience of being ill and hospitalized, and disruptions occurring in life.
- Summarize and reflect back expressions of feel-

ings (e.g., "It makes you feel out of control not knowing what and when tests are scheduled.").

- Use open-ended questions; talk with patient about health care experiences (e.g., "Tell me about your last hospitalization.").
- Ask for concerns directly regarding treatments, drugs, costs of illness, diet.
- Assess knowledge of the diagnosis, disease process, and treatment plan (e.g., "What have you been told about your diagnosis?" "Do you know what an EKG is?").
- Explain and discuss the treatments and medications being given.
- Explore the effects of behavior of noncompliance on self/family.
- Assess for recent changes in life-style (personal, work, financial, health, family); discuss how these changes are affecting behavior.
- Explore and discuss with patient the effects of anxious behavior on the illness and on the treatment plan.
- Discuss fears and anxieties about the illness and the treatments being received.
- Encourage to discuss fears and concerns with family.
- Make referrals to appropriate agencies as indicated (e.g., dietician, support group, social services, home health care, counselor, other community agencies).

☐ EVALUATION CRITERIA/DESIRED OUTCOMES

The Patient
- Identifies feelings of anxiety
- Discusses fears and anxieties
- Identifies factors that are contributing to anxiety
- Makes adaptive plan to deal with anxieties with the assistance of the nurse

---

NURSING DIAGNOSIS #2

Noncompliance related to negative side effects of prescribed treatment

Rationale: The patient for whom the prescribed treatment plan causes discomfort, inconvenience, or severe physiologic or psychologic symptoms may respond by altering the treatment plan or by discarding it completely. The patient may choose to do this rather than to communicate problems to the health care team.

☐ GOAL

The patient will verbalize and describe those experiences that have caused him/her to alter or discontinue the prescribed plan of treatment; will receive appropriate treatment for side effects of medication

or treatments; will develop adaptive alternative coping patterns.

☐ IMPLEMENTATION

- Identify medications and treatments patient is receiving.
- Have patient describe side effects, feelings, and any change in sensory perception experienced in response to the treatments and medications; assess onset and duration of patient's complaints.
- Evaluate motivation and attitude toward continuing treatment; empathize with discomfort and difficulties; lend perspective on necessity of compliance; ask what would convince patient to adhere to treatment plan as prescribed; discuss other possibilities, modifications and expected outcomes.
- Identify possible adverse interactions among drugs and establish whether toxicity is present (review blood level of drug).
- Assess other contributing factors of prescribed therapies (e.g., requires prolonged period of administration; unsupervised, complex, and special equipment needed; involves change in life-style, inconvenience in terms of time, place, route, side effects, cost; culturally unacceptable, against religious beliefs).
- Discuss revised plan of care with patient including home health care and referral to social services if needed.
- Assist in reducing causative factors of continued side effects of medications.
- Teach importance of adhering to revised care plan and review effects of drugs and treatments with patient.

☐ EVALUATION CRITERIA/DESIRED OUTCOMES

The Patient
- Describes experiences that caused alteration in prescribed regimen
- Identifies treatments and medications and possible side effects
- States/uses methods discussed to reduce causative factors
- States rationale for treatments and medications
- Demonstrates/implements revised plan of care

NURSING DIAGNOSIS #3

Noncompliance related to unsatisfactory relationship with care givers

Rationale: The patient who is unable to communicate effectively with the care giver or who feels devalued by the care-giving environment may respond with noncompliant behavior toward the health care plan. Such factors as personnel shortages, lack of privacy, cultural differences, seeing a

---

variety of care givers, long waits in crowded and impersonal waiting areas, overbooked schedules, difficulty of access, and complex/costly treatments all contribute to the patient's feelings of frustration and confusion.

☐ GOAL

The patient will express feelings (e.g., anger, frustration, confusion) related to clinical care; will discuss situations in which s/he has been noncompliant; will be accepted and valued as an individual; will identify sources of dissatisfaction; will accept information about prescribed therapeutic plan; will be an active participant in self-care.

☐ IMPLEMENTATION

- Assess causative or contributing factors and discuss these with the patient (e.g., referral process, physical setting, method of scheduling dietary planning); reduce contributing factors where possible.
- Assess and discuss cultural differences between patient and clinical setting.
- Listen attentively to patient's ideas and concerns; allow patient to describe situation from own point of view; assess reality perception.
- Treat in respectful way; approach in unhurried, relaxed manner; avoid negative criticism.
- Encourage expression of feelings (e.g., "Tell me more about your concerns with the side effects of your blood pressure medication.").
- Summarize and reflect back expressions of feelings (e.g., "So you're saying you were really upset/scared/angry when you heard the results of your blood test.").
- Encourage to define and discuss own needs; refrain from forcing treatments.
- Assess for stress level, stage of loss, anxiety, negative attitudes toward health professionals, self-esteem.
- Refer to *The Patient Manifesting Anger*, page 10, *The Patient Experiencing Anxiety*, page 22, *The Patient Manifesting Denial*, page 52, and *The Patient Experiencing Fear*, page 78.
- Encourage mutual problem solving and interdependence; explain team approach as an important part of care.
- Assess problem-solving skills and teach as needed; refer to *Problem Solving*, page 248.
- Invite patient to ask questions; provide reliable information; refer to *Guidelines for Teaching Patients and Families*, page 229.
- Discuss and explain procedures in advance; prepare for new situations by anticipating situation and utilizing role playing, problem solving, and behavior modification.

- Give verbal and nonverbal positive reinforcement for adaptive coping and appropriate compliance.
- Involve in active participation in activities of daily living (ADL) in own way; praise for participation in self-care.
- Be aware that cost of medication or treatment is often a problem for the elderly, adolescents, and heads of household; make appropriate referral to social service as needed.
- Discuss revised plan of care with physician; encourage use of generic drugs for person with financial constraints.
- Consult with physician and other health team members to explore problems and plan care.
- Refrain from performing nonessential procedures.
- Introduce patient to other persons who have had similar experiences but who have had positive reactions.

☐ EVALUATION CRITERIA/DESIRED OUTCOMES

The Patient
- Expresses feelings (anger, frustration, confusion) freely regarding clinical care
- Identifies sources of dissatisfaction and discusses modifications
- Participates actively in planning own care and in self-care

---

NURSING DIAGNOSIS #4

Knowledge deficit regarding treatment plan, schedules, medications, follow-up care, community resources

Rationale: *Inadequate preparation for discharge may lead to noncompliance with treatment plans and a reversion to maladapative coping mechanisms.*

☐ GOAL

The patient/family will be involved in discharge planning and plans for follow-up care and treatments, including medications, their side effects, and how to have prescriptions refilled; will know and have written copy of scheduled appointments, transportation schedules, physician/clinic/therapist/hospital names, telephone numbers and addresses, and list of community resources; will assist in completing a written plan for self-care, and care with the assistance of others; will continue interpersonal interactions and effective communications with family members/members of the health care team.

☐ IMPLEMENTATION

- Assess patient's/family's level of knowledge and ability to comply with the medication and treatment plan.

- Teach side effects of medications and interventions to minimize side effects where present.
- Teach the importance of adhering to the treatment and medication schedule.
- Give responsibility of requesting and taking own medication prior to discharge.
- Teach how to take own medications and do self-treatments; obtain return demonstration.
- Discuss follow-up schedule of care; develop a specific written plan and provide written directions and instructions as needed.
- Discuss adaptive ways of dealing with feelings of anxiety, fear, confusion, frustration.
- Assess availability of family members and include them in discharge planning whenever possible.
- Discuss community resources and support groups available; give patient list of resources.

☐ EVALUATION CRITERIA/DESIRED OUTCOMES

The Patient/Family

- Approaches health care team for consultation in health maintenance
- Has list, schedule of medications and treatments; verbalizes importance of taking them
- Can ask for information about treatment plan and express feelings and concerns
- States intention to cooperate with treatment plan in a responsible, informed, active way
- Describes dangerous effects of poor health practices, and of noncompliance with planned, prescribed health care regimen
- Knows and identifies community resources and support groups

The Patient with an Obsessive-Compulsive Disorder

Definition/Discussion

An obsessive-compulsive disorder is characterized by a pattern of symptoms that includes repetitive thoughts that the individual is unable to control (obsession), an impulse or urge to act that cannot be resisted without extreme difficulty (compulsion); much psychic effort is needed to control the impulse to keep it from becoming an irrational act. Treatment includes individual or group psychotherapy, behavior modification, desensitization, tranquilizers. The *DSM-III-R* classification is Anxiety Disorders.

Nursing Assessment

☐ PERTINENT HISTORY

Ritualistic behaviors (e.g., compulsive cleanliness, handwashing, dressing and undressing, placing belongings a certain way) with extreme anxiety and discomfort if routine is disrupted, perfectionism (need for rigid and purposeful activity), many self-imposed "shoulds" and discomfort during relaxation and pleasurable activities

☐ PHYSICAL FINDINGS

Poor hygiene, inadequate nutrition, side effects of medications, inability to rest and sleep, increased motor behaviors

☐ PSYCHOSOCIAL CONCERNS/ DEVELOPMENTAL FACTORS

Thinking processes characterized by indecision and an intellectual, rigid, and task-oriented focus, which limits creative thought, spontaneity, and expression of feelings; traits of hoarding, critical self-righteous aggression, and stubbornness or persistence; ritualistic speech (i.e., repeating the same story or belief constantly in an automatic response to anxiety that is caused by interpersonal relationships); ability to carry out own activities of daily living (ADL)

☐ PATIENT AND FAMILY KNOWLEDGE

Treatment plan, symptoms of acute phase/prognosis, schedule of medications, strategies to cope with anxiety, community resources and support groups, readiness and willingness to learn

Nursing Care

☐ Long Term Goal

The patient will limit ritualistic acts and participate in adaptive activities; the patient will cope with anxiety in adaptive ways; the patient will express feelings as they occur.

NURSING DIAGNOSIS #1
a. **Alteration in thought processes** related to high levels of anxiety, anger
b. **Self-care deficit: feeding, bathing/hygiene, dressing/grooming, toileting** related to ritualistic behavior

Rationale: The onset occurs from 10-40 years of age; acute attacks are often precipitated by a stressful incident. Dynamics include an unconscious attempt to relieve anxiety with ego defense mechanisms such as isolation of affect, displacement, and undoing (i.e., displacement of anger onto an unrelated act such as compulsive cleanliness in an attempt to undo unacceptable angry feelings and impulses).

☐ GOAL

The patient will spend progressively more time each day in adaptive ADL and less time doing ritualistic behaviors.

☐ IMPLEMENTATION

- Approach in quiet, calm manner; respect autonomy and patient's need to control.
- Accept patient as an individual; use empathetic responses and avoid judgmental or disapproving responses.
- Use verbal interaction to assist patient to gain control of overwhelming feelings and impulses (e.g., nurse to patient who is pacing the hall and wringing hands before lunch: "You seem upset about going into the dining room. Let me walk with you and we can talk about what's going on with you.").
- Plan ADL with patient, allowing patient to make choices and to include time for ritualistic behavior; assist with hygiene, grooming, and meals until patient is able to participate in own care.
- Do not confront patient with ritualistic behavior or interrupt behavior abruptly (anxiety will increase and patient may decompensate or panic).
- Set reasonable limits on ritualistic behavior and give patient adequate time to prepare for next activity.
- Join patient in constructive activities such as quiet, detailed hobbies (e.g., sewing, ceramics, artwork) or games such as cards, dominoes, checkers, chess.
- Give positive reinforcement (e.g., your time, conversation, attention) when patient is engaged in constructive activities; avoid reinforcing ritualistic behaviors (by limiting conversation about and not giving attention to them).
- Assist patient to set limits on own behavior; refer to *Behavior Modification*, page 250).

☐ EVALUATION CRITERIA/DESIRED OUTCOMES

The Patient
- Increases adaptive behaviors of ADL
- Decreases time spent in ritualistic behaviors and compulsive acts
- Increases time spent on constructive leisure-time activities

---

NURSING DIAGNOSIS #2

Ineffective individual coping related to anxiety, inability to express feelings directly

Rationale: Coping with anxiety and intense feelings is a learned behavior; anticipatory guidance can assist the patient to learn to identify and cope with anxiety and feelings.

☐ GOAL

The patient will learn effective methods to cope with anxiety; the patient will identify and express feelings.

☐ IMPLEMENTATION

- Assist patient to express feelings and concerns; listen empathetically and assist patient to name feelings as they occur; observe patient's verbal and nonverbal expressions of feelings; share your observations in nonjudgmental ways (e.g., "I notice you have just started pacing the floor and talking to yourself. I'm wondering what you are feeling right now." or "You've been scrubbing that table top for a long time. I'm wondering what your thoughts and feelings are as you scrub.").
- Explore new ways to help the patient express feelings (e.g., role playing, assertive techniques, poetry, music, dance, sports).
- Discuss patterns of behavior with patient, especially events that occur before the ritualistic behaviors; work with patient to identify stressors and develop alternative adaptive ways to cope with stress and anxiety; refer to Table 1, *Stress Management*, page 24.

☐ EVALUATION CRITERIA/DESIRED OUTCOMES

The Patient
- Identifies and expresses feelings
- Demonstrates effective methods of coping with anxiety

NURSING DIAGNOSIS #3

Knowledge deficit regarding disorders, coping with ritualistic behaviors, effective coping strategies for stress and anxiety, follow-up care, treatment, and medications

Rationale: The tendency toward obsessive-compulsive behavior recurs with stress of everyday life; anticipatory guidance assists the patient to prevent recurrence of acute episodes.

☐ GOAL

The patient/family will discuss treatment plan and follow-up care, including medication schedule and side effects to watch for; will maintain ADL, limit ritualistic behaviors, and discuss community resources.

☐ IMPLEMENTATION

- Assess patient's level of knowledge and ability to comply with medication and treatment plan.
- Teach the importance of taking medication daily; discuss their effects; as patient improves, shift the responsibility of getting and taking medication to patient, as preparation for discharge.
- Discuss a follow-up care schedule, and develop a plan to use in case patient feels anxious, compulsive, or out of control.

- Assess availability of significant others; include them in discharge planning if possible.
- Plan with patient ways to maintain self after discharge (e.g., caring for clothing, transportation, food shopping and meal preparation, recreation and work/school); help set personal goals and offer support in these.
- Encourage verbalization and questions; ask patient to describe in own words: medication, treatment plan, follow-up care, and symptoms to report to MD.
- Discuss community resources such as support groups, rehabilitation and vocational training, day-care centers.

☐ **EVALUATION CRITERIA/DESIRED OUTCOMES**

The Patient
- Has appointment for follow-up care with MD, clinic, or day care center, and can state how to contact them before appointment if necessary
- States actions, dosage, and possible side effects of medications; knows when to report the latter to MD or clinic; has prescribed schedule for taking medications.
- Has plan to maintain ADL and to limit ritualistic behaviors.

The Patient Experiencing Pain

Definition/Discussion

An unpleasant sensory and emotional experience resulting from the perception of noxious stimuli. Chronic pain is pain that continues for longer than 6 months. Techniques to manage pain include

- *pharmacologic:* use of narcotic or non-narcotic analgesics administered orally, parenterally, rectally, or intrathecally
- *noninvasive:* applications of heat or cold, massage, topical anesthetics, hypnosis, relaxation, guided imagery, distraction
- *neurologic:* acupuncture, nerve block, cordotomies, transcutaneous electrical nerve stimulation (TENS).

Nursing Assessment

☐ PERTINENT HISTORY

Cause of pain; location (e.g., deep, superficial, referred); severity; duration, rhythmicity of episodes; quality; what time of day it is worse; precipitating, aggravating, alleviating factors; duration in weeks/months/years; fatigue, irritability; change in appetite or sleep patterns; decreased interest in living, recreational activities; rubbing of affected area; previous treatment; effect on activities of daily living (ADL); general health history

☐ PHYSICAL FINDINGS

Level of consciousness; changes in vital signs; diaphoresis; nausea and vomiting; muscle tension, weakness, spasms; changes in skin color; restlessness, agitation; change in facial expression (e.g., frown); apathy or withdrawal; crying, whimpering, moaning, screaming; clenching of fists or jaw

☐ PSYCHOSOCIAL CONCERNS/ DEVELOPMENTAL FACTORS

Attitude of family; concerns (e.g., diagnosis, prognosis, finances); perception of what will be helpful in management; amount of disruption; secondary gains; past experience with pain and coping efforts used, personality style, cultural influences or practices; meaning of pain, fears, perceptions regarding pain

and pain relief; chronic pain: depression, guilt, hopelessness, level of anxiety

☐ PATIENT AND FAMILY KNOWLEDGE

Cause of and ability to manage pain; strategies to tolerate chronic pain, readiness and willingness to learn

Nursing Care

☐ LONG-TERM GOAL

The patient will be free from pain OR the patient will cope adaptively with chronic pain.

NURSING DIAGNOSIS #1

Alteration in comfort: pain related to injury, recent surgery, specific stimulus (specify)

Rationale: *Acute pain is of short duration; complete resolution is anticipated with treatment of the underlying etiology.*

☐ GOAL

The patient will experience reduction in or relief of pain.

☐ IMPLEMENTATION

- Assess the level of discomfort using a 0-10 point self-rating scale to obtain an objective measure of the pain.
- Encourage to talk about previous experience with pain.
- Attempt to understand the religious, cultural, and psychologic influences on this particular patient's reaction.
- Administer prescribed analgesics promptly PRN; know the time of onset and duration of effect of drug ordered.
- Utilize knowledge of patient's present reaction and tolerance to pain in addition to physician's orders to make your decisions about giving medication; do not withhold medication just because

you feel the patient's pain is not real or should be adequately tolerated; remember that it is the patient who is feeling the pain; there is little fear of addiction to medication when given for acute pain over a short period of time.

- When giving pain medication, tell the patient about the medication and its expected effect; talk positively about it.
- Evaluate the effect of pain medication: did it eliminate or reduce the pain? If the latter only, consider changing medication as not all patients will respond in the same way to the same drug; consult with physician.
- Monitor for and take steps to prevent side effects of analgesics (e.g., respiratory depression, sedation, nausea, constipation).
- Medicate patient prior to participation in activities that will cause discomfort (e.g., coughing, turning, deep breathing).

☐ EVALUATION CRITERIA/DESIRED OUTCOMES

The Patient

- Rates pain less than 4 after pain medication
- Is free from side effects of drugs
- Demonstrates decreasing need for medication as days pass.

NURSING DIAGNOSIS #2

Alteration in comfort: chronic pain related to neurologic injury, metastatic cancer, altered body function

Rationale: Chronic pain differs from acute pain in duration (over 6 months), physiologic indicators (the patient may exhibit none of the vital signs/behavioral responses to acute pain because of adaptation), and emotional reactions (e.g., anxiety, depression, withdrawal, anger or apathy, helplessness, hopelessness). The chronicity of the pain can make it much more difficult to manage.

☐ GOAL

The patient will engage in ADL without preoccupation with pain; will achieve a satisfactory measure of pain control.

☐ IMPLEMENTATION

- Plan with patient the kinds and timing of activities that can reduce, eliminate, or minimize the suffering; educate regarding modification of activities (e.g., walk rather than jog).
- Allow as much time as needed to accomplish the task (patients in pain cannot tolerate being rushed) when patient is caring for self; assist only when necessary.

- Provide opportunity for adequate rest as fatigue will increase perception of pain.
- Allow to talk intermittently, but not constantly, about the pain and suffering; finding the cause of the suffering often relieves or reduces it.
- Give positive feedback to efforts to share feelings and to cope with the suffering.
- Have friends/family/staff available when patient needs to see them.
- Ensure all staff is aware of the patient's usual response to pain; allow patient to participate in planning for management; ask what ideas the patient thinks might be effective.
- Do not reinforce the focus on pain; instead begin to reward non-pain-focused behavior.
- Utilize activities and conversation (e.g., distraction) to help the patient focus on something other than the pain; find out what patient likes to talk about, activities s/he enjoys.
- Hold patient care conferences to discuss responses to pain; plan approaches and write them in nursing care plan; be consistent in use of plan but be alert for new approaches.
- Take a few seconds and inwardly ask yourself, "What would I be like if I were suffering like this?"; identification of how we feel and respond increases our understanding of the variety of ways other people respond to situations, particularly painful experiences.
- Facilitate family understanding of the suffering by giving careful explanations to them of how and why the patient responds as s/he does.
- Instruct in proper use of heat or cold applications when ordered by physician.
- Encourage regular exercise if tolerated.
- Teach body relaxation techniques (see Table 1, *Stress Management*, page 24) not only for pain reduction but also to use during periods of tension and anxiety (tension and anxiety can increase the perception of and reaction to pain).
- Teach effective use of analgesics, side effects, efficacy; that pain should be managed, not endured.
- Help patient to be realistic in expectations of effects of medications; know that often pain medications can be reduced in frequency and amount as pain control is achieved or enhanced with other pain management modalities.
- Consider with the physician the preventive approach if pain is expected to occur consistently; regular, rather than PRN pain medication may be more effective.
- Be alert to symptoms of depression (e.g., withdrawal, sad affect, suicidal ideation).
- Teach to use support systems and diversional therapy to cope with pain.
- Tell patient about outside resources (e.g., pain clinics, reputable hypnotists, acupuncturists, family/individual psychotherapists).

☐ EVALUATION CRITERIA/DESIRED OUTCOMES

The Patient

- Describes events and conditions influencing the occurrence and level of pain
- Identifies a pattern of medication use, diversional and relaxation activities that assist in the reduction or elimination of pain
- Demonstrates use of relaxation techniques and distraction methods to manage pain
- Acknowledges utilization of outside resources for selected circumstances
- Requests information regarding noninvasive methods of pain relief

---

NURSING DIAGNOSIS #3

a. **Fear** related to pain, anticipation of pain, possible addiction
b. **Anxiety** related to pain, anticipation of pain, possible addiction

Rationale: *Fear about the return of pain can potentiate the patient's experience of it, making it more difficult to control. The patient may have specific fears concerning pain or may experience nonspecific anxiety and dread when pain occurs. When the patient's pain is not adequately relieved, a vicious cycle begins: unrelieved pain causes increased anxiety, which in turn increases the sensitivity to pain and diminishes the patient's confidence in the drug. Many patients will misuse analgesics because of unfounded fears of addiction.*

☐ GOAL

The patient will experience a lessening of fear and anxiety caused by pain; will employ adaptive coping mechanisms to keep the level of anxiety manageable.

☐ IMPLEMENTATION

- Refer to *The Patient Experiencing Anxiety,* page 22.
- Inform prior to tests or surgery when and where the pain can be expected to occur, possible severity, and how long it may last; instruct in measures to manage the pain; reassure that medication will be available.
- Be alert for denial of pain (e.g., saying everything is OK while grimacing, never complaining of pain or asking for pain medication).
- Encourage verbalization of past experiences, expectations, and perceptions of pain.
- Utilize pain-relief measures before pain becomes severe (they will be more effective).
- Encourage verbalization of feelings when pain is relieved to dissipate reactions to the stress; recognize that physiologic manifestations (e.g., shaking, chills, vomiting) may occur; attend to physical needs.
- Be supportive; the presence of the nurse is very effective in reducing fear and anxiety and encouraging development of trust.
- Reassure regarding addiction possibilities as necessary; encourage patient not to suffer because of an unfounded fear of becoming drug-dependant.

☐ EVALUATION CRITERIA/DESIRED OUTCOMES

The Patient

- States when feelings of fear and anxiety occur
- Verbalizes fears and concerns regarding the experience of pain
- Requests medication appropriately
- Acknowledges that addiction is unlikely

The Patient with a Phobic Disorder

Definition/Discussion

A phobia is an intense irrational fear of a situation or object that interferes with the individual's ability to function in everyday life. Major types of phobias are

- *agoraphobia:* Fear and avoidance of going out into public places, especially going out alone; person may not be able to go out at all or may be able to go out only with a trusted companion
- *social phobia:* Fear of being embarrassed or humiliated while eating, drinking, speaking, or being in the presence of others; may also involve depression and an inability to cope with anxiety
- *specific phobia:* Fear of one specific object or situation (e.g., zoophobia: fear of animals; claustrophobia: fear of closed spaces; hydrophobia: fear of water); patient may have fear of airplanes, cats, dogs, lightning, doing math, public speaking, etc.

The *DSM-III-R* classification is Anxiety Disorders.

Treatment includes psychotherapy, behavior modification, desensitization, relaxation exercises, biofeedback, tranquilizers.

Nursing Assessment

☐ PERTINENT HISTORY

Previous experience of fear and anxiety related to anticipation or contact with a specific object or situation; assess patient's feelings, perceptions, and concerns

☐ PHYSICAL FINDINGS

Physiologic changes associated with anticipation of or actual contact with feared object (e.g., changes in pulse, respiration, skin color; sweating; fainting); history of a panic attack with symptoms of fight-flight reaction (e.g., rapid heartbeat, increased respirations, weakness of knees, inability to problem solve or function); general anxiety level (mild, moderate, severe, panic)

☐ PSYCHOSOCIAL CONCERNS/ DEVELOPMENTAL FACTORS

Adaptive/maladaptive coping methods, strengths and weaknesses; family dynamics and secondary gains (e.g., attention, nurturing, dependency, control); ability to carry out own activities of daily living (ADL)

☐ PATIENT AND FAMILY KNOWLEDGE

Schedule of medications and side effects to report, ability to recognize and cope with behaviors of acute phobic response, community resources and support groups, readiness and willingness to learn

☐ LONG-TERM GOAL

The patient will accept and participate in treatment to reduce phobic responses; the patient will demonstrate an ability to cope adaptively with phobic response; the patient will realistically evaluate situations, objects, and own strengths and weaknesses.

NURSING DIAGNOSIS #1

Self-care deficit: feeding, bathing/hygiene, dressing/grooming, toileting related to acute anxiety, inability to perform self-care

Rationale: *As anxiety increases in response to the phobic stimuli, functioning decreases and the individual cannot concentrate, problem solve, or effectively participate in ADL. Defense mechanisms such as regression also occur in response to the perceived threat.*

☐ GOAL

The patient will independently perform ADL (e.g., eating, dressing).

☐ IMPLEMENTATION

- Approach in quiet, calm manner.
- Accept patient as an individual; avoid judgmental or disapproving responses.
- Utilize interventions to decrease anxiety from moderate, severe, or panic levels to a mild level;

refer to *The Patient Experiencing Anxiety*, page 22; administer medications as ordered to decrease anxiety.
- Adjust patient's initial ADL routine to minimize contact with feared object or situation (e.g., if phobic about eating with others, allow to eat in own room; if phobic about elevators, allow to use stairs).
- Offer choices in planning ADL and allow patient to make independent decisions about ADL (e.g., time and method of hygiene, exercise, meals, projects).
- Offer hope that treatment will reduce phobic response and increase ability to cope.

☐ EVALUATION CRITERIA/DESIRED OUTCOMES

The Patient
- Performs ADL
- Experiences decreased anxiety

NURSING DIAGNOSIS #2
a. **Fear** related to phobic stimulus
b. **Ineffective individual coping** related to phobic response

Rationale: Anticipation of or actual contact with the feared object results in painfully uneasy feelings, apprehension, and an activation of the autonomic nervous system. The ego-defense mechanism used is displacement (unconscious discharge of feelings upon an object other than the one that elicits feelings). When the fear and anxiety bind (are displaced on) to a specific object, they become manageable, and the patient is able to cope with most aspects of daily life. There is often a history of a specific fear of the object or situation since childhood. Severe feelings of powerlessness and inability to control response or control situation result in ineffective coping.

☐ GOAL

The patient will cope with specific fear and anxiety reactions; will accept and participate in treatment to reduce phobic response; will reduce phobic response.

☐ IMPLEMENTATION

- Review *The Patient Experiencing Fear*, page 78.
- Assist the patient to describe fearful experience(s); identify factors that increase or decrease fear such as size, color, distance, or motion of the feared object (e.g., large dog may be more feared than small dog).
- Identify physiologic changes associated with anticipation or contact with feared object or situation.
- Ask open-ended questions (e.g., "What else bothers you about this situation?"); accept feelings and concerns without agreeing or disagreeing with patient.
- Explore pattern of usual coping with fear and anxiety; identify and point out adaptive and maladaptive coping patterns; reinforce adaptive ones and strengths.
- Teach to recognize the fear response in its early stage and to acknowledge fear rather than to deny or avoid it.
- Discuss alternative coping mechanisms to keep the fear manageable, instead of avoiding the feared situation or object.
- Practice alternative coping mechanisms (e.g., relaxation techniques, behavior modification, assertion, stress management, biofeedback, guided imagery, anticipatory role playing); refer to Table 1, *Stress Management*, page 24 and *Behavior Modification*, page 250.
- Utilize "reframing" to alter perceptions of feared situations or objects (e.g., with patient who has phobic response to taking tests: assess the patient's perception and beliefs [how patient perceives the problem], identify pattern to be changed and any positive aspects of the fear response, and offer another frame of reference, such as
  - Patient: "I blank out and hyperventilate if I have to take a test" [patient perceives mind and body working against self when taking a test, i.e., patient blanks out and hyperventilates]
  - Nurse: "Sounds as if your mind and body are working very hard to prepare you to take a test and may be overdoing it. Would you be willing to learn and practice relaxation exercises to help you take the test?").
- Create alternative behaviors to substitute for phobic response (e.g., teach to do progressive relaxation, positive affirmations, timed practice and rehearsal of actual test taking); offer suggestion of trial run approach ("Think of the first time you take a test as a trial run. As you take the test, be aware of test-taking strategies that work for you and those that need to be modified next time you take a test.").

☐ EVALUATION CRITERIA/DESIRED OUTCOMES

The Patient
- Participates in the treatment plan to decrease phobic response
- Acknowledges specific fears
- Begins to cope with specific fear and phobic response

NURSING DIAGNOSIS #3
Knowledge deficit regarding coping with phobic response in adaptive way.

> **Rationale:** *The tendency towards a phobic response recurs with acute stress; anticipatory guidance assists the patient to prevent reoccurrence of a phobic response*

☐ GOAL

The patient will identify behaviors and stimuli of phobic response; will participate in problem solving to develop strategies to cope effectively with stress and anxiety; will plan for follow-up care.

☐ IMPLEMENTATION

- Determine patient's ability to comply with medication and treatment plan.
- Teach the importance of taking medications daily; discuss their effects; shift the responsibility of getting and taking medication to patient as improvement is noted, in preparation for discharge.
- Reinforce strategies to cope effectively with anxiety and fear.
- Include family in discharge planning if possible.
- Plan with patient ways to maintain self after discharge (e.g., caring for clothing, transportation, food shopping and meal preparation, recreation and work/school); help set personal goals and offer support in these.
- Plan productive activity (e.g., occupational or art therapy) daily; ask what patient would like to achieve and help with this goal.
- Encourage verbalization and questions; ask patient to describe medication, treatment plan, follow-up care, and symptoms to report to physician.
- Discuss community resources (e.g., support groups, rehabilitation and vocational training, day-care centers).

☐ EVALUATION CRITERIA/DESIRED OUTCOMES

The Patient

- Develops plan to cope with phobic response in adaptive way; describes stressors and ways to cope effectively with stress and anxiety
- States doses, actions, schedule, and possible side effects of medications to report to MD
- Has appointment for follow-up care with physician, clinic, or day care center and knows how to contact them before appointment if necessary

The Patient Experiencing Post-Traumatic Stress Disorder

Definition/Discussion

Post-traumatic stress disorder is the human response to a psychologically traumatic event or stressor that is usually outside the range of human experience, such as natural or man-made disasters, rape, or military combat. Symptoms may be experienced soon after the event/stressor, or delayed for 6 or more months, and may persist for varying lengths of time.

Nursing Assessment

☐ PERTINENT HISTORY

Military history; past or present traumas, losses, accidents, illnesses, stressors, catastrophies; environmental changes; suicidal or homicidal attempts or ideation; drug or alcohol abuse; social or cultural isolation; legal or authority problems; ideation of rage or violence; alteration in interest and ability to manage activities of daily living (ADL); persistent intrusive recollections, reexperiencing trauma; depression; avoidance of situations or activities that may produce feelings resembling traumatic event

☐ PHYSICAL FINDINGS

Sleep disturbances with recurrent dreams, nightmares; hypervigilance; increased startle response; anxiety or panic; decreased concentration; muscle tension; restlessness or agitation; apathy; somatic complaints; tremors; altered vital signs; inappropriate affect

☐ PSYCHOSOCIAL CONCERNS/DEVELOPMENTAL FACTORS

Usual coping mechanisms; guilt, alienation or detachment, numbness, powerlessness, life-style; significant relationships; socialization; personality characteristics; level of self-esteem and ego strengths; school and employment adjustment; patterns of pessimism, fears, worries, dependency; family dysfunction or violence; communication patterns

☐ PATIENT AND FAMILY KNOWLEDGE

Experience of trauma by patient/family, severity of trauma and resulting disruption, degree of involvement of patient/family, perception of importance of traumatic event(s), acceptance of assistance, involvement of community agencies, readiness and willingness to learn

Nursing Care

☐ LONG-TERM GOAL

The patient will effectively manage thoughts and behaviors concerning the traumatic event or stressor; the patient will reconstruct life to achieve optimal adjustment for the future.

NURSING DIAGNOSIS #1
a. **Ineffective individual coping** related to decrease in control over self/environment as a response to a traumatic event
b. **Powerlessness** related to intensity of stressor

Rationale: Usual coping mechanisms may be ineffective when a severe stressor is experienced, and a feeling of powerlessness may result.

☐ GOAL

The patient will develop alternative adaptive coping mechanisms; will verbalize a measure of control.

☐ IMPLEMENTATION

- Encourage to identify and describe situations that cause feelings of powerlessness and inability to influence events.
- Employ active listening techniques to build trust and decrease feelings of alienation and isolation.
- Show interest in patient's concerns and feelings;

encourage verbalization regarding fears of inability to regain control of life.

- Encourage identification of areas of control and ways to broaden these areas; refer to *The Patient Experiencing Powerlessness*, page 115.
- Promote realistic differentiation between situations where control is possible and those where it is not; allow patient to discuss and explore these issues.
- Assist to work on developing internal locus of control to increase motivation.
- Monitor level of anxiety and intervene as indicated; refer to *The Patient Experiencing Anxiety*, page 22, and *The Patient Requiring Crisis Intervention*, page 49.
- Encourage patient's perception of self as able to cope with stress and find meaning in the traumatic event.
- Promote objectivity in perception of trauma and provide new information as needed so past and present events may be better understood.
- Teach skills in priority setting, effective communication, decision making, socialization, and ability to obtain appropriate assistance; use role playing to promote understanding and knowledge.
- Teach how to manage persistent intrusive thoughts or images of the trauma or stressor
  - use desensitization where indicated
  - limit time allowed for rumination
  - substitute positive memories and positive mechanisms (e.g., sublimation, humor) for those causing stress
- Encourage hope for the future by developing new, realistic life goals where indicated; assist in broadening gains made in adapting to stress after trauma.
- Encourage awareness of experiences relating to stressors or trauma that have previously been avoided so that patient can integrate trauma into rest of life experience.

☐ EVALUATION CRITERIA/DESIRED OUTCOMES

The Patient
- Verbalizes feelings of being in control
- Demonstrates appropriate appearance and affect
- Demonstrates adequate coping skills
- Uses appropriate support systems
- Understands and continues to resolve traumatic event

NURSING DIAGNOSIS #2

Disturbance in self-concept: self-esteem related to guilt associated with traumatic experience

Rationale: *The belief that one has been responsible for harm to self or to others, or has violated a principle of conscience produces guilt and an alteration in the perception of self-worth.*

☐ GOAL

The patient will identify and express causes of guilt feelings; will develop effective ways of managing guilt feelings to achieve improvement in self-esteem.

☐ IMPLEMENTATION

- Encourage to verbalize feelings of perceived guilt and consequences of actions; support in expressing these feelings.
- Demonstrate positive regard for patient at all times despite ruminations, recriminations, and self-defeating attributes.
- Avoid telling patient "shoulds" and "should nots."
- Avoid reinforcing patient's devaluation of self and abilities; refer to *The Patient Experiencing a Threat to Self-Esteem*, page 127.
- Assist in identifying type(s) of guilt (e.g., guilt of the survivor, guilt of omission/commission); support realistic assessment of situation.
- Encourage to reappraise situation and work on assimilation of experiences.
- Plan needed changes in goals to prevent repetition of behaviors that produce failures.
- Assist to identify positive aspects of life, relationships, and successes that have been obtained.
- Promote constructive ways of changing relationships where it is needed; role play to increase expertise in effective communication.
- Discuss concept of alienation of others through repetitive expressions of self-blame.
- Discuss self-forgiveness concept as necessary for improved mental health.
- Plan specific time for guilt and negative feelings and limit attention to these the remainder of the time.
- Encourage attendance and participation in group therapy so patient can obtain additional support and understanding through the concept of universality.
- Assist in problem solving and in determining how past experiences can relate to present life.
- Teach assertive techniques to improve positive self-image and ability to handle negative aspects of the behavior of others.

☐ EVALUATION CRITERIA/DESIRED OUTCOMES

The Patient
- Verbalizes and identifies causes of guilt feelings
- Expresses guilt appropriately
- Verbalizes forgiveness of self
- Describes self in positive terms

- Demonstrates realistic perceptions and goals for the future

---

NURSING DIAGNOSIS #3

Social isolation related to feelings of alienation, withdrawal, depression

Rationale: Severe trauma, an unusual experience, can produce feelings of isolation and alienation; the individual tends to withdraw from contact with others and become increasingly isolated and depressed.

☐ GOAL

The patient will seek out relationships; will increase participation in activities with others.

☐ IMPLEMENTATION

- Establish a caring, empathic, and supportive relationship with patient.
- Employ active listening techniques to decrease isolation; show interest and caring (e.g., "I know I haven't had the same experience you have, but I can help now with problems that are the result of that trauma.").
- Encourage verbalization about the trauma that produced the wish to withdraw.
- Teach about the process of recovery from stress trauma so patient will realize that many others have had similar post-traumatic experiences.
- Recognize that numbness is a way of coping with painful feelings; allow to work through experiences of trauma gradually so they can be put in proper perspective.
- Assist with physical care as needed so patient will appear acceptable to others.
- Increase exposure to others gradually so patient can overcome withdrawal.
- Communicate in easy-to-understand terms; introduce only 1 new person or activity at a time.
- Encourage participation in group therapy to utilize the concept of universality.
- Teach strategies to improve social skills; role play to improve communication techniques and self-confidence.
- Introduce appropriate outside support systems that may be of value in assisting recovery (e.g., Veterans Outreach, Victims of Violent Crimes).

☐ EVALUATION CRITERIA/DESIRED OUTCOMES

The Patient
- Identifies causes of withdrawal and strategies for decreasing isolation
- Exhibits improved affect and appearance

- Discusses effective ways to cope with alienation and depression
- Demonstrates improved ability to communicate
- Attends a group for survivors of violent experiences

NURSING DIAGNOSIS #4

Potential for violence related to intense feelings of anger, betrayal, or fear

Rationale: Extreme feelings of betrayal, rage, fear, or perception of actual or potential injury to self or others may produce violent behavior.

☐ GOAL

The patient will experience a reduction of violent feelings; will verbalize rather than act upon violent thoughts or feelings.

☐ IMPLEMENTATION

- Provide regular, frequent contact to build rapport and promote a trusting relationship.
- Encourage expression of feelings and offer support and encouragement when verbalization is appropriate.
- Determine what causes an increase in acting out or impulsive, aggressive behavior; maintain vigilance to prevent precipitating events.
- Assess for suicidal ideation; maintain a safe environment at all times with suicide precautions as needed; refer to *The Patient who is Suicidal*, page 144.
- Identify and utilize ways of coping with feelings of rage without resorting to violence (e.g., exercise, punching bag, foam balls, recreational activities, sports); refer to *The Patient Manifesting Aggression*, page 10.
- Contract with patient to notify others when feelings of loss of control are imminent in order to prevent escalation and acts of violence to self or others.
- Know history of previous violent behaviors and how they were most effectively managed.
- Set limits and provide controls for all violent or aggressive behaviors toward self or others; explain reasons for doing this.
- Maintain distance so patient does not feel cornered; remember that patient may have very different perceptions of the surroundings than you do.
- Restrain or isolate patient if necessary.

☐ EVALUATION CRITERIA/DESIRED OUTCOMES

The Patient
- Verbalizes feelings of violence toward self and others without acting upon them

- Identifies precipitating factors that cause thoughts of violence
- Utilizes alternative behaviors rather than acts of violence
- Notifies staff when violent impulses are experienced

NURSING DIAGNOSIS #5

Sleep pattern disturbance related to anxiety caused by stressful event(s)

Rationale: Psychologic and physiologic alterations as a result of a severely stressful occurrence may be reflected in nightmares, recurrent dreams, and other impairments in sleep patterns.

☐ GOAL

The patient will achieve a restful sleep pattern appropriate to individual needs and free from disturbances.

☐ IMPLEMENTATION

- Determine reasons for impaired sleep patterns (e.g., nightmares, insomnia).
- Encourage verbalization about anxieties and fears and patient's perception of their effect on sleep.
- Attempt to decrease or remove factors that contribute to inability to achieve restful sleep.
- Reassure patient that surroundings are safe; provide comfort and serenity, especially during night hours.
- Arrange for attendant if needed until nightmares or frightening dreams are under control; breaking the cycle of fearful night episodes will help patient progress in other areas of trauma management.
- Allow night lights if needed and prevent shadows from causing episodes of stress.
- Be alert to exaggerated startle reflex that may precipitate flashbacks or recurrence of traumatic recollections.
- Provide structure of activities and regular routine at bedtime to promote rest.
- Prevent noises that might be interpreted as threatening.
- Do not wake patient unnecessarily.
- Decrease daytime naps and dozing to improve nocturnal rest.
- Encourage physical exercise to improve rest patterns.
- Administer medication as ordered.
- Teach relaxation techniques (e.g., deep breathing) to assist in keeping anxiety manageable; refer to Table 1, *Stress Management*, page 24.

☐ EVALUATION CRITERIA/DESIRED OUTCOMES

The Patient
- Demonstrates appropriate amount and improved quality of sleep
- Identifies causes of anxiety that result in sleep disturbances
- Utilizes techniques to decrease anxiety and stress and to promote relaxation prior to sleep
- Participates in the promotion of bedtime routine to promote rest

---

NURSING DIAGNOSIS #6

Knowledge deficit regarding the effective management of severe stress caused by trauma

Rationale: The patient/family will adapt more effectively to past trauma with adequate understanding of the event(s) and the stress syndrome resulting from it.

☐ GOAL

The patient will understand the stress syndrome following trauma; will make necessary adaptations to achieve equilibrium.

☐ IMPLEMENTATION

- Determine level of understanding of the syndrome, any misinformation present, attitudes and beliefs about the traumatic event, involvement of family members, and their perception of the problem.
- Assess level of cognitive functioning; determine what ways of teaching have been successful in the past and adjust teaching plan to appropriate level; take into account the physical as well as emotional states of those involved; remember that teaching may not progress steadily but may have to be readjusted frequently to be most effective; refer to *Guidelines for Teaching Patients and Families*, page 229.
- Teach necessity for compliance with drug regimen if indicated; give information regarding dosage, side effects, and indications.
- Encourage continued group therapy and use of community support groups so patient will achieve further adaptation through support from others and the concept of universality.
- Continue to work with patient on stress management, problem solving, and assertive techniques to improve adaptation to traumatic experiences and the quality of life.
- Make community referrals as indicated for sources of information and support; assist to understand

the purpose and role of organizations and groups that may be appropriate for assistance.

☐ EVALUATION CRITERIA/DESIRED OUTCOMES

The Patient/Family
- Verbalizes information regarding stress syndrome following trauma
- Utilizes problem-solving and stress-management techniques
- Attends group therapy in community
- Exhibits increased adaptation to life after trauma

The Patient Experiencing Powerlessness

Definition/Discussion

Powerlessness is a perceived lack of personal power or control over life events, experiences, or environment in a specific situation.

Nursing Assessment

☐ **PERTINENT HISTORY**

Identifiable causes, recognition, length and extent of loss of control; stresses or environmental changes; problems with family, significant others, or authority figures; legal or financial difficulties, illness, or losses; depression in family

☐ **PHYSICAL FINDINGS**

Abnormal vital signs, apathy, depression, withdrawal, confusion, crying, decreased concentration, inability to manage activities of daily living (ADL), restlessness, hostility

☐ **PSYCHOSOCIAL CONCERNS/ DEVELOPMENTAL FACTORS**

Usual coping patterns, life-style, school and work history, locus of control, family dysfunction, dependency patterns, anxiety/fear, discouragement, indecision

☐ **PATIENT AND FAMILY KNOWLEDGE**

Perception of problem, past experiences and management of similar situations, degree of disruption, readiness and willingness to learn

Nursing Care

☐ **LONG-TERM GOAL**

The patient will experience an increased sense of power and control over life events, experiences, and environment.

NURSING DIAGNOSIS #1

Ineffective individual coping related to perceived decrease in ability to control self, environment

---

Rationale: Usual coping mechanisms may be ineffective when changes in environment/status occur, resulting in a feeling of powerlessness.

☐ **GOAL**

The patient will identify situations that produce feelings of powerlessness; will strengthen existing functional coping methods; will utilize opportunities to develop new and effective strategies.

☐ **IMPLEMENTATION**

- Build a trusting relationship by making frequent verbal and nonverbal contact; be consistent and dependable (refer to *The Patient Manifesting Anger*, page 13, *The Patient Experiencing Confusion*, page 43, *The Patient Experiencing Denial*, page 52, and *The Patient Experiencing Fear*, page 78).
- Encourage patient to identify and describe situations producing feelings of powerlessness; remember the patient's perception may be quite different from yours.
- Listen to patient's feelings and concerns, show interest and concern for patient's welfare.
- Ask for patient's opinions, likes, dislikes, and wishes; utilize these in making care plan.
- Ensure environmental powerfulness by putting call light, telephone, bedside stand, urinal, and other desired items within reach; be aware that hospital room and objects in it are personal territory and respect patient's right to exert control over it.
- Promote active participation in simple and appropriate decision making in ADL (e.g., diet preferences, time and type of hygiene measures, arrangement of physical surroundings).
- Provide situations in which the patient can take control by making choices (e.g., "Would you prefer to have your dressing changed before or after lunch?" or "Would you like us to block the telephone until you're ready to receive calls?" or "How would you like your bedside stand arranged?").
- Give verbal and nonverbal positive reinforcement

and acknowledgment for active participation in planning care in ADL, goal setting, and alternative behaviors that increase sense of power and control (e.g., verbally acknowledge that patient made a list of questions to ask physician, asked the questions, and clarified information; or, "I see you can do your own colostomy care; how do you feel about that?" or "You have some good ideas on how to manage at home; would you like to discuss them with the discharge planning nurse?").

- Assist to direct and plan own care within the medical treatment plan; as much as safely possible, allow patient to decide how the nurse and other health team members will participate.
- Encourage questions; be able to say, "I don't know, but I'm willing to find out" or "I don't know; this is where you can find out."

☐ **EVALUATION CRITERIA/DESIRED OUTCOMES**

The Patient

- Identifies situations that produce feelings of powerlessness
- Describes own behaviors that enhance sense of power and control
- Utilizes situational supports to increase involvement in own health care
- Verbalizes feelings realistically

NURSING DIAGNOSIS #2

Anxiety related to perceived loss of control

Rationale: Anxiety is produced when an individual feels threatened by inability to control self or the environment.

☐ **GOAL**

The patient will identify and verbalize feelings of anxiety caused by powerlessness.

☐ **IMPLEMENTATION**

- Spend time with patient; show empathy and caring.
- Encourage to verbalize feelings of anxiety caused by loss of control and discuss management of these feelings.
- Maintain therapeutic, safe, and nonthreatening environment.
- Teach manageable relaxation techniques (e.g., deep breathing).
- Point out that as more control over life is achieved, anxiety will decrease.
- Give as much information as possible prior to treatments, procedures, daily care; increased

knowledge regarding the predictable outcome decreases anxiety.

☐ **EVALUATION CRITERIA/DESIRED OUTCOMES**

The Patient

- Recognizes and verbalizes feelings of anxiety
- Increases interest in regaining control of life
- Demonstrates use of relaxation techniques
- Realistically appraises causes of anxiety

NURSING DIAGNOSIS #3

Disturbance in self-concept: role performance related to feeling of powerlessness

Rationale: If significant alterations occur that require an alteration in how one performs in the various roles, feelings of powerlessness can result (e.g., if a carpenter can no longer use his hands, he cannot perform his role as breadwinner as a carpenter, and may feel he is powerless to support his family).

☐ **GOAL**

The patient will identify and make necessary adaptations to altered role.

☐ **IMPLEMENTATION**

- Assist patient to identify alterations in role performance that s/he has perceived.
- Encourage realistic appraisal of situations causing feelings of powerlessness that resulted in a changed self-concept.
- Allow verbalizations of concerns; give information when needed; if loss or alteration in role is permanent, permit to grieve.
- Support in efforts to adapt to altered role; discuss alternative methods of performance and role play to improve self-confidence.
- Refer to outside agencies for support, self-help, or information.

☐ **EVALUATION CRITERIA/DESIRED OUTCOMES**

The Patient

- States realistic perceptions of changes in role
- States adaptive possibilities to control changes
- Progresses through grieving process
- Contacts community agency

NURSING DIAGNOSIS #4

Knowledge deficit regarding how to problem solve, make decisions, become involved in self-care activities

Rationale: *A sense of power and control is increased with knowledge. Knowing what to expect lessens anxiety and encourages the development of alternative coping strategies. Knowing what choices are available and the probable outcomes increases the ability to problem solve.*

☐ GOAL

The patient will learn to problem solve; will develop alternate adaptive behaviors to increase sense of control and power.

☐ IMPLEMENTATION

- Assess patient for learning needs and provide appropriate information; refer to *Guidelines for Teaching Patients and Families,* pages 229, and *Problem Solving,* page 248.
- Assess for readiness to assume more complicated decision making; influencing factors include severity and stability of coping mechanisms, ability to problem solve, and personality traits (passive or nonassertive persons may not know how to problem solve or make decisions).
- Utilize chart information, family, and significant others to facilitate situations in which patient can achieve increased power and control.
- Determine patient's ability to problem solve and teach as needed; include family as indicated.
- Assess patient's perception and knowledge of treatment program, diagnosis, and symptoms; encourage expression of views before giving information, explanations, or reassurance (e.g., "What has your doctor told you about your new medication?" "How do you feel about taking it?" "What do you expect to happen in x-ray tomorrow?").
- Determine communication patterns; assist to identify preferences, feelings, needs, values, and attitudes; reinforce clear assertive communication of preferences and feelings to appropriate listeners.
- Teach assertive techniques, ensure that patient/significant others understand appropriate usage; role play to develop expertise.

☐ EVALUATION CRITERIA/DESIRED OUTCOMES

The Patient

- Demonstrates understanding of assertive techniques
- Makes decisions affecting self/family when appropriate

The Patient with
Rape Trauma Syndrome

Definition/Discussion

Rape **is any forced sexual activity.** The legal definition refers to forced vaginal or anal penetration without consent of the individual. Other forced sexual acts may be referred to as sexual assaults. *Rape trauma syndrome* includes both an acute phase (disorganization of life-style) and a long-term phase (reorganization of life-style). *Unresolved sexual trauma* occurs when the feelings of the rape are not dealt with adequately, resulting in compound silent reaction.

Victims of rape may be male or female; male victims rarely seek treatment.

Nursing Assessment

☐ PERTINENT HISTORY

Sexual assault (e.g., time, place, identity and description of assailant, type of sexual contact, witnesses); post-rape activities that may have altered evidence (e.g., bathing, douching, urinating, changing clothing), sexual history (e.g., date of last menses, contraceptives used, date of last sexual contact)

☐ PHYSICAL FINDINGS

Types of injury (e.g., ecchymoses, lacerations, abrasions), areas of injury (e.g., gastrointestinal [GI] system, skeletal muscle system, genitourinary [GU] system); symptoms of shock; pain, nausea and vomiting

☐ PSYCHOSOCIAL CONCERNS/ DEVELOPMENTAL FACTORS

Usual coping methods (e.g., level of anxiety, perception of event, emotional response); acute phase: emotional shock, denial, detachment, guilt, fear, anger, panic; long-term phase: continuation of acute responses together with phobias, nightmares, sleep disturbances, anxiety, depression, mistrust of opposite sex, and a change in sexual behavior

☐ PATIENT AND FAMILY KNOWLEDGE

Understanding of the event, ability to cope; acceptance of victim's need for love and support; perception of the patient as victim, not as participant; readiness and willingness to learn

Nursing Care

☐ LONG-TERM GOAL

The victim will regain emotional, physical, social, and sexual equilibrium; the patient will return to the precrisis level of functioning.

NURSING DIAGNOSIS #1

Rape-trauma syndrome (acute phase)

Rationale: Rape is an act of physical violence and power, not one of sexual passion. It is a crime of violence usually carried out under threat of death and harm; thus, feelings of fear of bodily harm, mutilation, and death continue after the assault is over. Initial reactions of rape victims may be "controlled" (e.g., outward calm, denial, shock, and disbelief with a delayed reaction of fear and anxiety) or "expressed" (e.g., crying, laughing, nervousness, anger, guilt). Heightened emotional reactions can cause the victim to feel out of control. The acute phase may last from a few days to a few weeks and may carry over into the long-term phase.

☐ GOAL

The patient (victim) will acknowledge situational support from staff/family; will begin adaptive coping with situation in own way; will seek appropriate medical treatment; will regain a measure of control over own life.

☐ IMPLEMENTATION

- Always provide a private examining room and stay with patient or arrange for other support person to stay.
- Do not alter the appearance or condition of the victim's body until physical evidence is collected

for the police; assist with collection of physical evidence with medical team responsible for this task.

- Explain hospital procedures in advance; help patient see the physical exam as important to well-being and not further intrusion.
- Give concrete and brief explanation about police procedures to provide a sense of control.
- Listen to and believe what the victim is saying; acknowledge the assault, encourage her to talk, and be supportive (e.g., "It must have been a terrifying ordeal for you . . ."); express warmth, interest, respect, and a nonjudgmental attitude; allow open ventilation of feelings, especially anger at the rapist; be aware that this anger may be directed at staff.
- Ask what is the most difficult thing for her right now and discuss it, refraining from giving advice of "You should have . . ." or "Why did you . . .?" (such statements will not be helpful); if victim says "It was my fault," or "I should have . . .," reinforce that the attack was not patient's fault, but the fault of the rapist, and that s/he did what s/he was forced to do in order to save his/her life (many victims "pay" the rapist for their life with the sexual act, then feel guilty, unclean, ashamed, self-critical).
- Accept and attend to the victim's ambivalence about family reactions (e.g., "What will I tell my husband?").
- Encourage victim to express feelings about the experience (usually of overwhelming terror), but do not dwell on the sexual aspects; victim may not wish to talk/may look undisturbed, or seem to be coping extremely well in order to deny or minimize the attack; allow to cope in this way but tell her that at a later date she may experience feelings of anger, fear, or sadness, and that this would be a normal reaction.
- Do all interviewing sensitively and with consideration for victim's feelings; while it will be necessary (for court records) to know the explicit sexual acts involved, only one person needs to gather this information *once*.
- Have a female staff member be with victim at all times to be an advocate, especially during any examination or interrogation; if a rape team is available, a member may fulfill this function; if a female victim asks for a female police officer, make all attempts to comply with request.
- Express your belief in patient's ability to deal with problems/decisions she will face in next few days; be sure she takes an active role in making and carrying out plans (e.g., reporting to police, returning to work).
- Describe and demonstrate nursing measures to relieve somatic symptomatology
  - *anorexia:* record intake, advise small, frequent meals
  - *bruising and edema:* avoid constricting garments,

elevate edematous body part, apply cool compress first 24 hours and then warm compress to edematous area
  - *headache:* pain-relieving measures
- Provide referral as needed for somatic difficulties.
- Allow to discuss treatment and experience of being interviewed and examined; express empathy.
- Explore support system; involve partner in counseling if appropriate.
- If victim is alone and she consents, call her family/friends and ask them to bring a change of clothes for her; if she has no one to call, develop a safety plan for her (e.g., transportation home, assistance from social services).
- Provide with information about available counseling services, option, rights, and follow-up treatments; allow patient to use telephone to call crisis/rape center.
- Give information about police investigations, court appearance, pregnancy, disease, and need for follow-up care.
- Arrange for rape crisis counseling sessions prior to departure from hospital.

☐ EVALUATION CRITERIA/DESIRED OUTCOMES

The Patient
- Experiences decreased symptoms of anxiety, fear, guilt
- Utilizes support persons and is able to trust them
- Does not leave ER alone
- Has written instructions for follow-up medical care, rape counseling telephone number

---

NURSING DIAGNOSIS #2

Rape-trauma syndrome (long-term phase)

Rationale: Reorganization of life-style following rape may take months or even years. This phase involves regaining a feeling of physical well-being and safety, completing the grieving process regarding loss of trust and self-esteem, and working through feelings so as to readjust to the normal routines of life.

☐ GOAL

The patient will return to the precrisis level of functioning; will experience optimal physical, psychologic, social, and sexual adjustment to the rape-trauma event.

☐ IMPLEMENTATION

- Encourage verbalization of thoughts/feelings/perceptions of the event.

- Explore strengths, resources, usual coping mechanisms.
- Assist to develop specific actions to overcome feelings (e.g., change in telephone number, taking trip, engaging in diversional activities).
- Discuss relationship with partner and help to identify positive responses and support from partner/family.
- Explain that the period of reorganization takes time and gradually the experience will be integrated and become less painful.
- Assist to verbalize anxiety and fears about sexual relationship and intercourse, discuss partner's response and concerns.
- Educate patient/partner about the grief process; grieving takes time and involves a variety of emotions, which need to be expressed.
- Give specific, written instructions regarding follow-up medical appointments, crisis and rape counseling phone numbers, and symptoms to report.

☐ EVALUATION CRITERIA/DESIRED OUTCOMES

The Patient
- Discusses feelings about the event
- Demonstrates minimum of one adaptive coping mechanism in dealing with the event
- Discusses perception of the event with therapist/family/partner
- Engages in precrisis activities in home/job/community

NURSING DIAGNOSIS #3

Alteration in family process related to rape crisis

Rationale: *A normally supportive family, when confronted with the rape of a family member, experiences stressors that challenge its previously effective functioning ability. A family may react by blaming themselves or by blaming the victim, and there may be moral and cultural conflict with reality. Frequently, they will develop a "conspiracy of silence" to protect the victim. This approach is nonproductive because family members need to express their reactions and feelings, and the victim only feels intensified guilt and shame.*

☐ GOAL

The family will verbalize an understanding of the victim's experience; will give the patient situational support; will maintain an adaptive system of mutual support for each family member.

☐ IMPLEMENTATION

- Assess family's reaction to the victim's situation; be aware that they often tend to blame the victim, to be nonsupportive, and to isolate her; reinforce that the attack was not the victim's fault or responsibility and that it was a terrifying experience where she feared she would be killed; that whatever her response to the rapist, it was to try to save her life or prevent bodily harm to herself/others.
- Know that family often feels responsible because they weren't there to protect victim and thus feel guilty and vulnerable; again, emphasize that the responsibility lies with the attacker.
- Discuss ways they can be supportive to victim (e.g., by listening to and believing what victim says; encouraging and allowing victim to talk; helping victim to resume her usual life activities; not overprotecting her; letting victim make the decision to prosecute or not; not dwelling on the sexual part of the rape, but on the victim's feelings); stress that victim needs to be held and stroked just as she would in any stressful situation, and not to withhold touch (otherwise may reinforce victim's feelings of being unclean, ruined).
- Share that it is typical for rape victims to have increasing fear and anxiety during the initial 48 hours and to want to talk at length about the experience; that victim may then "seem" to adjust, but may reexperience the feelings of the attack at a later date; if victim does not want to talk about the assault, family should not press but continue to provide caring and support.
- Instruct to work out with victim ways to be and feel safe (e.g., locks on windows, new lights, not walking alone at night); some action may need to be taken immediately (e.g., changing locks).
- Assess victim's equilibrium after seeing family.

☐ EVALUATION CRITERIA/DESIRED OUTCOMES

The Family
- Offers acceptance and emotional support to victim
- Expresses feelings and reactions to the rape

NURSING DIAGNOSIS #4

Knowledge deficit regarding potential physiologic and psychologic difficulties

Rationale: *Rape trauma can cause severe dysfunction in both the individual's and the family's equilibrium. Dysfunctions may not always be apparent initially but may occur later. Providing information regarding possible emotional and physiologic responses that indicate unresolved sexual trauma can assist the victim and family to recognize a compound or silent reaction, which is dysfunctional.*

GOAL

The patient/family will demonstrate an understanding of potential physiologic and emotional symptoms; will use adaptive coping mechanisms in dealing with feelings regarding the rape.

IMPLEMENTATION

- Educate patient/family to behavior that would indicate a compound or silent reaction
  - increased use of alcohol/drugs
  - continued somatic complaints (e.g., GI irritability, GU discomfort, skeletal muscle tension, migraine headaches)
  - persistent phobic symptoms (e.g., fear of being alone, going out at night)
  - extreme changes in sexual behavior or avoidance of members of the opposite sex
  - increased feelings of anxiety, guilt, lowered self-esteem
  - increased nightmares
  - recurrence of rape trauma symptoms in response to minor events (e.g., anniversary date)
  - withdrawal, lack of verbalization of rape, silence
  - negative behavior toward family and friends (may be displaced anger)
- Educate patient/family that recovery may be delayed and prolonged if any of the following factors are present
  - victim's first sexual experience
  - victim is young
  - prior victimization within 2 years
  - prior low self-esteem
  - lack of social support
  - chronic life stressors
- Instruct to seek long-term counseling to prevent dysfunctional reactions if they are in a high-risk group for delayed recovery (see above).
- Identify community resource centers available to victim and family.

EVALUATION CRITERIA/DESIRED OUTCOMES

The Patient

- Has an appointment for follow-up care with physician/clinic and knows to contact them if needed before the appointment date.
- Has an appointment with rape crisis center/counselor, knows to contact them before appointment date if needed; can state behaviors of increased psychologic difficulty that should be reported to the therapist.
- Has a daily plan that provides for adequate diet and rest, maintaining personal grooming, and interacting with others.

The Patient/Family

- Discusses emotional and physiologic responses to rape and treatment plan
- Has a written list of community resources and support groups, including sexual counseling groups

The Patient with Schizophrenia

Definition/Discussion

Schizophrenia is a psychotic reaction manifested by disturbed thinking processes, such as delusions and hallucinations, and extensive withdrawal of the individual's interest from other people and the outside world.

Nursing Assessment

☐ PERTINENT HISTORY

Previous acute or chronic patterns of psychiatric problems, hospitalization, treatment and medications

☐ PHYSICAL FINDINGS

Poor hygiene, inadequate nutrition, side effects of medications, decreased motor ability

☐ PSYCHOSOCIAL CONCERNS/ DEVELOPMENTAL FACTORS

Self-destructive, impulsive, or bizarre behaviors; withdrawal, mistrust, inability to communicate thoughts and feelings clearly, inability to do self-care (e.g., hygiene, grooming, nutrition, sleep), delusions, hallucinations; disorganized or bizarre thoughts, affect; regression to previous level of functioning, dependency, dysfunctional family relationships, noncompliance with treatment plan.

☐ PATIENT AND FAMILY KNOWLEDGE

Schedule of medications and side effects to report, symptoms of acute phase and prognosis, ability to recognize behaviors of acute anxiety or withdrawal, community resources and support groups, readiness and willingness to learn

Nursing Care

☐ LONG-TERM GOAL

The patient will regain some measure of independence in self-care, take own medicines, and demonstrate increased ability to communicate with others.

NURSING DIAGNOSIS #1

Disturbance in self-concept: self-esteem, personal identity, role performance, body image related to inability to trust, withdrawal from contact with others

Rationale: Self-concept is a dynamic process of self-perception that begins at birth and is related to life experiences. The schizophrenic may experience alterations in areas of self-esteem, personal identity, body image, and role performance. As impairment with reality testing increases, there is a retreat into fantasy and a withdrawal from social contact and the outside world. Mistrust and ambivalent feelings about self and other people contribute to disturbance in self-concept.

☐ GOAL

The patient will learn to tolerate nurse's closeness and interest; will withdraw fewer times from contact with other persons; will discuss difficulty trusting others.

☐ IMPLEMENTATION

- Establish dialogue in order to be able to spend time, talk, and plan with patient; demonstrate an accepting attitude.
- Plan with patient convenient times to spend together; include one-to-one as well as ward activities; listen and observe for nonverbal behaviors.
- Use silence; share that you are willing to spend time without talking.
- Observe pattern of social interaction and attendance at ward activities.
- Support with words and with your presence during activities that patient finds frightening or difficult.
- Discuss alternate ways to spend the day; describe behaviors in a nonthreatening way and indicate that you realize patient's difficulties in interacting with others.
- Explore patient's experiences of trust or mistrust

for others; offer hope for increasing ability to trust and relate to others.

- Provide anticipatory guidance for discharge (e.g., if patient is experiencing withdrawal from social situation, role play the situation); encourage patient to explore and pursue social situations where s/he feels most comfortable.

☐ EVALUATION CRITERIA/DESIRED OUTCOMES

The Patient

- Tolerates nurse's closeness and interest for short periods
- Withdraws fewer times from contact with others
- Discusses difficulties trusting others

NURSING DIAGNOSIS #2

Alteration in thought processes related to inability to evaluate reality

Rationale: Impairment in the process of reality testing is a cognitive alteration that is manifested by
- *hallucination: sensory perception that does not result from an external stimulus*
- *illusion: misinterpretation of an actual sensory experience*
- *delusion: false, fixed belief that cannot be corrected by logic*
Hallucinatory voices occur in situations where the person is anxious and expects to hear voices. Hearing voices may take away the painful/frustrating realities of interchange and relationships with others, or put the patient in a "listening mode" to be receptive to suggestions of the voices.

☐ GOAL

The patient will learn to define and test reality; will learn to control impulsive behavior dictated by hallucinations; will dismiss the internal voices s/he hears.

☐ IMPLEMENTATION

- Deal with and support reality: tell patient your name, remind patient where s/he is; be clear and concrete in your statements.
- Listen carefully; tell patient what you do and do not understand.
- Keep in mind that the patient is experiencing feelings of being overwhelmed and anxious; look for the reality stimuli causing the anxiety (e.g., a visit from a family member might trigger a thought disturbance).
- Help identify situations that increase anxiety and precede the development of hallucinations; discuss adaptive ways to cope with anxiety; refer to *The Patient Experiencing Anxiety*, page 22, and Table 1, *Stress Management*, page 24.

- Look for and chart behaviors and environmental stimuli that precipitate/relate to patient's withdrawing into fantasy (when reality is too threatening, fantasy provides a comfortable retreat that will lower anxiety); accept patient's need for fantasy without supporting the context of it.
- Determine when patient is hallucinating by observing nonverbal behaviors (e.g., talking to the TV or to no one in particular).
- Interpret reality by saying that you do not see or hear or believe these things if patient is experiencing hallucinations, illusions, delusions, or ideas of reference, and that s/he must be feeling very anxious right now.
- Do not talk to patient about the delusions (that is nontherapeutic and patient may become more out of control); rather, provide limits with a quiet room, walking or talking with patient, explore the basis for feeling s/he is the subject of others' conversations, and explain the reality of the actual situation.
- Do not try to convince the patient that the delusions are false; this only serves to strengthen the fixed belief.
- Observe for inappropriate behaviors associated with hallucinations; choose a time when patient is calm, and discuss how inappropriate behaviors affect and alienate others.
- Observe for behavior indicating patient is hearing voices (e.g., nodding head or tilting it to side, talking to people who are not present); when this occurs, ask patient what is going on at this time (if you ask if s/he is hearing voices, s/he is apt to say "no"); if s/he is hearing voices, discuss what hearing voices does (e.g., "Right now, you'd rather listen to the voices than talk with your wife."); help patient focus on things in the immediate environment; do not give status or recognition to the voices.
- Ask if patient has control over the voices; if not, supply controls with one-to-one support, or medications (controls will make patient feel more secure); assess need for one-to-one staff supervision (if danger to self or others); monitor safety needs; remove potentially harmful objects (e.g., razors, belts, glass, cigarettes, matches); refer to *The Patient Who is Suicidal*, page 144, and *The Patient Who is Violent*, page 149.
- Know that patient must dismiss the voices, and that s/he may be very anxious after this; when this occurs, alert staff so they can provide extra support as temporary replacements for the voices.
- Have patient sing, dance, play games, and tell the voices to "shut up" or "go away."

☐ EVALUATION CRITERIA/DESIRED OUTCOMES

The Patient

- Demonstrates reality testing
- Controls impulsive and inappropriate behavior

- Dismisses internal voices
- Discusses adaptive ways to cope with anxiety

NURSING DIAGNOSIS #3

Impaired social interaction related to alteration in thought processes resulting in incoherent/illogical thoughts and inability to express thoughts clearly

Rationale: *Schizophrenics have difficulty making correct associations, so it is difficult for them to communicate with others. Symbols, themes, and patterns of thought recur and have special meaning related to patient's inner fantasy life. The patient may have learned dysfunctional communication in family relationships.*

☐ **GOAL**

The patient will make his/her thinking understandable to others; will initiate conversation with staff or other patients.

☐ **IMPLEMENTATION**

- Listen to and chart patterns and symbols used in verbal communication; validate meaning with patient before making an interpretation.
- Look for patterns or themes in the patient's verbalization (e.g., "lovely princess in a tower;" "the dragons are trying to get me;" "I'm hooked up to all the TV stations and they control me . . .").
- Be aware that patient's conversation can be filled with both rational and psychotic statements out of sequence; define for the patient those statements that are confusing to you, as a way to help keep on the subject and facilitate communication and understanding.
- Validate clear communication (e.g., "You sound very sure of your feelings on this," or, "You made up your mind to participate in volleyball.").
- Talk about concrete realities (e.g., ward environment, eating, sleeping, and feelings about being in the hospital) if patient is having disassociated thoughts.
- Assign a permanent staff member to spend time each day interacting with and listening to the patient.
- Discuss and practice communication skills and goals of interactions and dialogue with other patients, staff, visitors.

☐ **EVALUATION CRITERIA/DESIRED OUTCOMES**

The Patient
- Communicates thoughts and feelings in logical, clear manner

---

NURSING DIAGNOSIS #4

Impaired communication: verbal and nonverbal related to inability to identify and express feelings

Rationale: *Cognitive disturbances contribute to sensory overload and confused feelings. The patient becomes overwhelmed with feelings and responds with inappropriate behaviors. Dysfunctional parent-child relationships may contribute to inability to identify, express, and cope with feelings, and to ambivalent feelings (contradictory feelings of love, hate, fear). Flat affect related to blunting of emotions makes it difficult for the patient to connect emotionally with others.*

☐ **GOAL**

The patient will identify and share feelings with a staff/family member, or another patient; will discuss ambivalent feelings; will plan alternative ways to express and use feelings.

☐ **IMPLEMENTATION**

- Explore feelings, accepting patient's right to feel as s/he does, no matter how illogical the feelings seem to you.
- Give positive reinforcement for any expression of feeling and stay with patient during this time.
- Work with patient to explore new ways to express feeling (e.g., to express anger, try handball, racketball, hitting a punching bag or bed, shouting, singing, confronting with words, swearing, batacas, tearing up phone books, throwing sponges or bean bags).
- Expect exaggeration of expression combined with uncomfortable feelings when practicing this new behavior or expressing feelings.
- Plan alternate ways to use feelings both within hospital and after discharge.
- Observe verbal and nonverbal behaviors that may indicate any interest in activities; give support to any expression of interest; discuss patient's feelings about activities.
- Work with family to continue facilitation of patient's expression of feelings after discharge.
- Observe verbal and nonverbal expressions of feelings; share your observations in a nonjudgmental way (e.g., "This is what I notice and I'm wondering what you're feeling right now?" or "You don't seem upset right now, but if someone spit at me, I'd be mad.").
- Observe for ambivalent feelings and attitudes; validate your observations (e.g., "Sometimes you hate your roommate and sometimes you love her; that's how you feel.").
- Discuss ambivalence as a normal state of being in all persons that doesn't have to immobilize; accept

patient's feelings of confusion or immobilization while continuing to work towards acceptance.

☐ EVALUATION CRITERIA/DESIRED OUTCOMES

The Patient
- Identifies and shares feelings with staff, family and others
- Discusses ambivalent feelings
- Plans other ways to express and use feelings

NURSING DIAGNOSIS #5

Self-care deficit: dressing/grooming, feeding, bathing/hygiene related to lack of interest in body and appearance

Rationale: Impaired cognitive functioning with poor reality orientation may cause decreased ability to be aware of and meet basic needs such as hygiene, dressing, grooming, nutrition, and sleep. Schizophrenics may be disorganized, dependent on others for care, regressed to an earlier stage of development, negative, or apathetic, decreasing the level of functioning in motor areas.

☐ GOAL

The patient will maintain good personal hygiene; will learn to manage own life in terms of personal grooming, hygiene, and nutrition.

☐ IMPLEMENTATION

- Ensure that patient bathes or showers at least every 1-2 days, dresses each day, and keeps own clothes clean; have patient use washer-dryer as necessary.
- Provide an opportunity for patient to groom nails and hair, clean teeth; work with patient to find an acceptable time and place for grooming activities; give positive reinforcement for good grooming and dress.
- Observe and chart diet actually consumed; assess learning needs for balanced diet and teach as indicated; use creative ways to encourage patient to maintain adequate diet (e.g., juice, peanuts, milkshakes, cookie-baking sessions).
- Observe physical condition and report problems to physician.

☐ EVALUATION CRITERIA/DESIRED OUTCOMES

The Patient
- Demonstrates good personal hygiene
- Initiates grooming
- Ingests adequate diet to meet body needs

NURSING DIAGNOSIS #6

Knowledge deficit regarding medications, treatment plan, follow-up care, symptoms to report to doctor, community resources

Rationale: The course of schizophrenia varies. Adherence to the prescribed medications is very important, since psychotic symptoms tend to reappear with cutback in medication. Inadequate preparation for discharge leads to noncompliance with treatment plan, resulting in an increase in acute episodes.

☐ GOAL

The patient/family will discuss treatment plan and follow-up care, including medication schedule and side effects to watch for; will maintain daily needs such as hygiene, grooming, diet and interaction with others; will utilize community resources.

☐ IMPLEMENTATION

- Determine patient's/family's ability to comply with medication and treatment plan.
- Teach the importance of taking medications daily; discuss their effects; shift the responsibility of getting and taking medications to patient as improvement is noted, to prepare for discharge.
- Discuss a follow-up care schedule, and develop a plan to use in case patient feels depressed, out of touch with reality, or spaced out.
- Assess availability of significant others; include them in discharge planning if possible.
- Plan ways patient will maintain self after discharge (e.g., caring for clothing, transportation, food shopping and meal preparation, recreation and work/school); help set personal goals and offer support in these.
- Plan for daily outlets for productive activity (e.g., occupational, industrial therapy); ask patient what s/he would like to achieve, and help with this goal.
- Encourage verbalization and questions; ask patient to describe in own words medication, treatment plan, follow-up care, and symptoms to report to doctor.
- Discuss community resources and support groups such as half-way houses, rehabilitation and vocational training, day-care centers.

☐ EVALUATION CRITERIA/DESIRED OUTCOMES

The Patient
- Has a list and schedule of medications, verbalizes the importance of taking them as prescribed, knows potential side effects and how to obtain refills
- Has an appointment for follow-up care with doc-

tor/clinic/day-care center; knows to contact them if s/he feels a need before the appointment date
- States behaviors of increased anxiety or withdrawal that should be reported to doctor

- Has a plan to maintain self on a daily basis that includes eating an adequate diet, maintaining personal grooming, and interacting with others
- nows community resources and support groups

Table 5
Antipsychotics (Neuroleptics, Major Tranquilizers)

Drug	Side Effects	Nursing Implications
Action: The action of this group of drugs is to ameliorate psychotic symptoms and normalize behavior. *Phenothiazines* *chlorpromazine (Thorazine)* *thioridazine (Mellaril)* *fluphenazine (Prolixin)* *mesoridazine (Serentil)* *perphenazine (Trilafon)* *promazine (Sparine)* *trifluoperazine (Stelazine)* Uses: Most effectively used in treatment of schizophrenia; may be beneficial in treatment of other functional psychoses, mania, agitated depression, and behavioral disorders resulting from organic brain disease. Drug effects are similar in this group; specific drug is chosen to increase or decrease side effects.	All of the antipsychotic drugs produce essentially the same side effects although the severity is variable; dangerous ones occur rarely. Side effects may be grouped as *autonomic*: dry mouth, stuffy nose, blurred vision, postural hypotension, urinary retention, constipation; or *extrapyramidal*: 1. *dystonia*: bizarre, involuntary movements of arms, legs, face and neck, often painful; may have difficulty talking and swallowing; onset may be sudden 2. *Parkinson-like syndrome*: mask-like facies, tremor rigidity, shuffling gait 3. *akathisia*: restlessness, pacing, rocking, shifting weight from 1 foot to another; subjective complaints that "I feel like I'm jumping out of my skin"; often difficult to differentiate from psychotic agitation 4. *tardive dyskinesia*: involuntary movements of the lips or jaw *Other*: jaundice, agranulocytosis, allergic skin reactions, photosensitivity, drowsiness, sedation, decreased mental alertness, breast engorgement, decreased libido, increased appetite, reduced convulsive threshold. Potentiates alcohol.	• Teach patient potential side effects, to be alert to them, and to report any occurrence. • Rinse dry mouth with water; avoid candy, gum, etc. as prolonged use may contribute to dental caries and fungal infections; sugarless gum is acceptable. • Teach to sit up slowly, pause, and make gradual change to being upright if patient has dizziness or postural hypotension. • Reassure that extrapyramidal symptoms are common and usually temporary. • Advise patient to report fevers or sore throats promptly. Avoid sunlight if photosensitivity or skin discoloration present. May drive car, but use extra caution if experiencing side effects. • Explain rationale for avoiding alcohol. • With all antipsychotic drugs, symptoms of psychosis often return when patient stops taking meds; stress value of daily meds as ordered. • Contraindicated with narrow-angle glaucoma. • Use cautiously with history of convulsive disorder or heart disease.
Butyrophenones *haloperidol (Haldol)*	Same effects as phenothiazines but less prone to stimulate appetite, less apt to produce orthostatic hypotension.	• As above; particularly good for aged patients. May cause depression after manic phase.
Thioxanthenes *chlorprothixene (Taractan)* *thiothixine (Navane)*	Chemically related to phenothiazines, and have similar effect.	• As above.

The Patient Experiencing a Threat to Self-Esteem

Definition/Discussion

Self-esteem is the perception or evaluation of self based on the quality of relationships with significant others, life experiences, and body image. Body image is an inner sense of identity that includes body functions, abilities, and limitations. A threat to self-esteem can be any event that negatively alters the individual's perception or evaluation of self. Common events that can threaten self-esteem are loss of significant others, change in body function or loss of part, role change, chronic illness, and aging.

Nursing Assessment

☐ **PERTINENT HISTORY**

Past coping style in dealing with threats to self-esteem

☐ **PHYSICAL FINDINGS**

Physical changes related to aging or pathophysiology

☐ **PSYCHOSOCIAL CONCERNS/ DEVELOPMENTAL FACTORS**

Loss of significant other, body-image disturbance, role change in family/work or from well to sick role, anxiety level, negative labeling of self, devaluing of self, withdrawal, powerlessness, passivity, aggression, self-derogatory verbal comments, hesitancy to ask for help, avoidance of direct eye contact when communicating, social isolation, self-consciousness

☐ **PATIENT AND FAMILY KNOWLEDGE**

Specific situation(s) that threaten self-esteem, how patient responds to threat to self-esteem, referrals for mental health interventions, readiness and willingness to learn

Nursing Care

☐ **LONG-TERM GOAL**

The patient will cope adaptively with a threat to self-esteem; the patient will maintain/regain a realistic perception of self.

NURSING DIAGNOSIS #1

Ineffective individual coping related to threat to self-esteem, inadequate psychologic resources

Rationale: As the individual experiences a negative evaluation of the self, there is a tendency to withdraw and become passive and depressed. The patient feels powerless and is unable to see choices or make decisions and thereby cope effectively.

☐ **GOAL**

The patient will explore feelings, perception of self, and source of threat.

☐ **IMPLEMENTATION**

- Provide openings for patient to express feelings by validating your observations (e.g., "You look upset . . . what is happening with you?").
- Accept feelings and explore further; focus on patient's perception of self and events; do not challenge defensive behaviors, but correct unrealistic perceptions.
- Listen for and assist to identify the sources of threats; utilize reality testing to evaluate the perception of the threat (e.g., does patient have correct information?); identify and explore distortion of reality.
- Validate own knowledge of the components of the threatening situation (e.g., prognosis, treatment, side effects) with health team, patient, physician, chart, and textbooks.
- Offer safe, supportive atmosphere of respect and calm attentiveness; provide for basic needs and activities of daily living (ADL).
- Assess anxiety level and facilitate coping with anxiety.
- Assess for knowledge of appropriate behaviors of current health role and health teach as needed; refer to *The Patient Experiencing the Sick Role*, page 134, and *The Patient Experiencing Chronic Illness*, page 38.

☐ EVALUATION CRITERIA/DESIRED OUTCOMES

The Patient

- Expresses feelings
- Identifies source(s) of threat to self-esteem

NURSING DIAGNOSIS #2

Knowledge deficit regarding coping with threat to self-esteem

Rationale: New ways of dealing with threat(s) to self-esteem must be learned for effective coping both now and in the future. The patient can learn to identify threats to self-esteem and typical responses to such threats and can devise a plan to deal with them.

☐ GOAL

The patient will explore own strengths and past coping mechanisms; will plan ADL.

☐ IMPLEMENTATION

- Explore past coping mechanisms and abilities; assist to generalize from past, successful coping to present threat situation; focus on strengths and assets.
- Allow to make as many decisions in ADL as possible (e.g., planning time of treatments, ambulation, hold visitors/phone, selecting menu).
- Give positive reinforcement, using words and active listening, as patient explores strengths and makes decisions on ADL.
- Involve family in support of adaptive coping with threat by nonjudgmental listening, acceptance, hopeful attitude, and touch.
- Assess patient's knowledge of relaxation techniques and teach as needed; encourage diversionary activities, hobbies, exercise as appropriate to physical condition.

☐ EVALUATION CRITERIA/DESIRED OUTCOMES

The Patient

- Identifies past coping mechanisms
- Participates in ADL
- Modifies past successful coping mechanisms to deal with current threat

---

NURSING DIAGNOSIS #3

Disturbance in self-concept related to threat to self-esteem

☐ GOAL

The patient will problem solve for alternative options to cope with threat to self-esteem.

☐ IMPLEMENTATION

- Problem solve to explore pros and cons of alternative coping responses; refer to *Problem Solving,* page 248; role play to practice alternative behaviors in small units so the patient can select most adaptive coping responses and experience success.
- Explore negative expectations; focus patient on questioning: Why do I have this expectation? Where does it come from? What person in my past (e.g., mother, father, friend) would agree with this negative expectation? What purpose does it serve? Does it realistically describe my here-and-now experiences?
- Facilitate anticipation of possible future threats; use role playing and behavioral rehearsal to assist patient to cope effectively in behavioral trial runs.
- Reinforce with words and behavior, realistic, positive anticipation of coping effectively with threat.
- Assess learning needs for communications of feelings and ideas, for asking to have needs met; teach communication skills and assertion techniques as needed.
- Teach to use positive self-affirmations (e.g., "I am flexible and calm," "I am a person who can learn and grow," "I am growing stronger and healthier," "I can learn from difficult relationships and situations.").
- Refer to community resources, clinics, therapists as necessary for continued mental health counseling.

☐ EVALUATION CRITERIA/DESIRED OUTCOMES

The Patient

- Identifies options for dealing with threats to self-esteem
- Identifies possible future threats to self-esteem and develops plan to deal with threats
- Practices positive affirmations about self
- Describes realistic perception of self

The Patient Experiencing Sensory Alteration

Definition/Discussion

Sensory alteration occurs when environmental stimulation (input) is inadequate, overwhelming (overload), meaningless, or monotonous to the individual. Typical responses to inadequate, meaningless, or monotonous stimuli are daytime sleeping, confusion, and hallucinatory behaviors. Responses to overload are increased anxiety, confusion, and "ICU syndrome," simulating psychosis. Sensory alteration occurs in all acute care settings. With the advent of critical care units, life-saving equipment, protective environments, and medical and nursing specialization, the intrusion on a person's environment/lack of stimuli has increased and even contributed to morbidity rates.

Sensory disturbances can occur through any or all senses (touch, smell, visualization, hearing). Causes can include confinement in a small room; lack of or excessive touching; no verbal input or too much verbalization around the patient; confinement in a windowless room; lack of new or meaningful stimuli; placement in isolation; change in external environment (e.g., new room, change in placement of equipment, personal supplies); semiconsciousness/movement through different levels of consciousness causing a distortion (misperception) of what is heard, felt, seen, or touched; separation from family; sleep deprivation; the approach of the evening/night hours.

Nursing Assessment

☐ PERTINENT HISTORY

Past experiences with sensory disturbances

☐ PHYSICAL FINDINGS

Acuity of all senses, level of activity, age, response to approach of evening and night, amount/type of sensory input used to at home, present pathophysiology, metabolic state, oxygen deprivation, mobility restrictions

☐ PSYCHOSOCIAL CONCERNS/ DEVELOPMENTAL FACTORS

Support system; availability of family; hobbies and interests; personal toiletries, pajamas, robe, pictures, and other belongings; coping strategies for dealing with confinement; layout of immediate environment and stimulation offered; social isolation; pain; stress

☐ PATIENT AND FAMILY KNOWLEDGE

Hospital routine; sounds, sights experienced and meaning of them; need for visitors and personal belongings, definition of sensory disturbance and ways of coping with it; medical regimen/treatment plan, diagnosis and prognosis, nursing treatment plan; level of knowledge, readiness and willingness to learn

Nursing Care

☐ LONG-TERM GOAL

The patient will regain and maintain sensory equilibrium.

NURSING DIAGNOSIS #1

Sensory-perceptual alteration: visual, auditory, kinesthetic, gustatory, tactile, olfactory related to amount (e.g., overload, monotony) and meaningfulness of environmental stimuli

Rationale: Patients are at risk for sensory-perceptual alteration when they are out of their usual, known environment or are not able to use their coping mechanisms for controlling and changing stimuli. The aged are especially vulnerable. A frequent response is confusion. Sufficient and meaningful sensory input must be introduced.

☐ GOAL

The patient will perceive and describe the components of the environment in an oriented, nondisturbed manner; will demonstrate optimal contact with reality.

☐ IMPLEMENTATION

- Assess at least once every shift for sensory status.
- Talk directly to patient; make eye contact.

- Use touch (e.g., give back rubs, massages, change position, stroke hair).
- Give frequent, intermittent attention; do not isolate patient physically or emotionally; speak to patient each time you enter or leave the room.
- Be aware of environmental monotony; use clocks, calendars, books, newspapers, television, radio, pictures, patient's personal possessions to stimulate and encourage patient to explore surroundings and maintain orientation.
- Give several periods of rest intermixed with stimulation throughout the day.
- Identify what you are going to do each time you see the patient; consider and utilize safety precautions as needed.
- Provide opportunities for the patient to sit, stand, or be partially upright; give passive or active exercises (some disturbances are caused by recumbent position alone).
- Approach patient often and reassure; do not increase fear and confusion by avoiding the patient; know that confusion that is physiologic in nature cannot be controlled by behavioral approaches.
- Control light, noise, odors, sights to tolerable levels; provide change of scenery, walks, rides, conversations with other patients, recreational or occupational therapy, and social activities as appropriate and possible.
- Have staff observe how patient is responding to them and the care they are giving (remember, the patient's response is a mirror of needs, not a response to take personally).
- Ensure that staff/family are aware of the patient's need for intermittent rest and stimulation; sensory overload mixed with sleep deprivation does not allow the patient to cope adequately with the hospitalization.
- Provide stimuli in quiet forms (e.g., conversation, playing games, reading to patient).
- Ensure that blind/deaf patients have the opportunity to express their special needs and have them met; communicate to staff the sensory facilities the patient may be lacking (e.g., blind or without glasses; deaf and without a hearing aid); increase input to other senses if one is nonfunctional.
- Refer patients with long-term sensory impairments to the appropriate community resources (e.g., Society for the Blind).

☐ EVALUATION CRITERIA/DESIRED OUTCOMES

The Patient
- Is oriented to environment, self
- Participates in plan of care to the extent possible

NURSING DIAGNOSIS #2

Knowledge deficit regarding sensory status (overload/monotony)

Rationale: Most individuals are unaware of the importance of receiving optimal level of stimulation for orientation and a sense of well-being. The patient must know that s/he has a responsibility to identify and communicate when meaningful stimuli are absent, or if there is overload or sensory restriction. Giving the patient responsibility aids greatly in supplying meaningful stimuli.

☐ GOAL

The patient will identify stimuli conducive to treatment and recovery; will identify risk factors or stimuli that increase fear, anxiety, and restlessness; will devise a plan to make incoming stimuli optimal and meaningful.

☐ IMPLEMENTATION

- Inform patient that being away from familiar surroundings will tend to produce feelings of isolation and monotony resulting in sensory alterations; it is helpful to bring in familiar pictures, radios, tapes and other items from home to facilitate orientation.
- Explain that the patient also has a responsibility for maintaining sensory equilibrium, and how to facilitate this specifically.
- Ask the patient to tell you when the stimulus is too little or too much (e.g., "It's so noisy." "I would like to rest."); attempt to reduce or increase the stimuli to meet the patient's needs.
- Instruct to vary activities frequently during the day (e.g., read, watch television, listen to radio); help devise a written plan to be kept at bedside as a guide/reminder.
- Involve family in the plan for introducing meaningful stimuli; educate family to the hazards of sensory deprivation and overstimulation, and how to minimize factors that cause disturbances.

☐ EVALUATION CRITERIA/DESIRED OUTCOMES

The Patient
- States importance of optimal sensory input
- Assumes responsibility as possible for level and type of stimuli
- Identifies and utilizes sources of support to deal with sensory overload/deprivation

---

NURSING DIAGNOSIS #3

Sleep pattern disturbance related to inability to fall asleep within 20 minutes of bedtime, sleeping during day and staying awake at night

Rationale: The individual experiencing a sensory alteration may experience a sleep disturbance man-

ifested by inability to fall asleep at bedtime or a reversal of sleep time, such as sleeping during the day and staying awake at night. This first pattern may occur as a result of too much input; the second pattern occurs when sensory input during the day is insufficient to maintain the patient at an alert, awake level of consciousness.

☐ GOAL

The patient will discuss feelings and concerns about sleep pattern; will experience a balance of rest and activity during day; will sleep 6-7 hours (or specific time) at night.

☐ IMPLEMENTATION

For the individual with an inability to fall asleep within 20 minutes at bedtime

- Provide comfort measures such as back rub, positioning; medicate for pain.
- Determine usual bedtime routine and establish it as much as possible during hospitalization.
- Provide periods of rest during the day to control buildup of effects of sensory overload as the day progresses.
- Intervene to reduce stress and anxiety; refer to *The Patient Experiencing Anxiety* , page 22.
- Allow to engage in interesting but nonstimulating activity during periods of restlessness.
- Increase physical exercise during the day as much as possible.

For the individual who sleeps during the day

- Provide an increase of stimulation during the day so that the patient remains alert and awake
  - visits from family members or hospital volunteers
  - physical exercise within reasonable limits
  - making or receiving phone calls
  - engaging in hobbies/activities of interest
- Monitor the fatigue level during the day and provide short rest periods when necessary.
- Awaken the individual who is sleeping except during arranged rest periods.

☐ EVALUATION CRITERIA/DESIRED OUTCOMES

The Patient
- Falls asleep and continues to sleep during the night for a specified amount of time
- Remains alert and awake during the day

NURSING DIAGNOSIS #4

Potential for injury: trauma related to sensory defects, reduced ability to protect self from hazards

Rationale: *Perceptual or physiologic defects that reduce the ability to protect oneself may include kinesthetic deficits resulting from paralysis or weakness, visual or auditory deficits, decreased hearing, tactile deficits (e.g., numbness or lack of ability to discriminate pain/extremes of heat or cold), or problems with balance. These deficits tend to increase with age. Patients with perceptual/physiologic defects are at risk for accident and injury and need preventive nursing measures to assure safety.*

☐ GOAL

The patient will remain free from injury; will acknowledge specific sensory defects and assistance needed; will utilize specific assistive devices.

☐ IMPLEMENTATION

- Determine effect of deficit on patient's ability to function safely, type of assistance needed from the nursing staff or family, teaching needed regarding the deficit, safety measures.
- Ensure that prescribed aids (e.g., hearing aids, eye glasses, braces, orthopedic shoes, walkers, canes) are utilized and in good working condition.
- Control hazards in the environment
  - keep the furniture and other items in the same place all of the time
  - keep the bed at the lowest position with wheels locked
  - answer the call light promptly when the patient requests help
  - provide description of the environment and remind patient of safety measures and hazards as needed

☐ EVALUATION CRITERIA/DESIRED OUTCOMES

The Patient
- Remains free from injury
- Utilizes specific aids/appliances
- Requests assistance with activities of daily living or ambulation as needed

The Patient Experiencing Shame/Embarrassment

Definition/Discussion

Shame is a subjective feeling of painful self-consciousness and embarrassment, ranging from mild to intense humiliation; it is excited by a consciousness of guilt, shortcoming, or impropriety.

Nursing Assessment

☐ **PERTINENT HISTORY**

Recent stress, loss of control or function; environmental changes; life-style

☐ **PHYSICAL FINDINGS**

Age, abnormal vital signs, loss of body part or disfiguring surgery, tremors, agitation, restlessness, fidgeting; voice/speech changes; poor eye contact

☐ **PSYCHOSOCIAL CONCERNS/ DEVELOPMENTAL FACTORS**

History of coping methods, rigidity of personality, self-esteem patterns, cultural perspectives

☐ **PATIENT AND FAMILY KNOWLEDGE**

Perception of problem, outside agency involvement, amount of dysfunction, reaction to previous similar situations

Nursing Care

☐ **LONG-TERM GOAL**

The patient will share feelings of shame; the patient will participate in problem solving to decrease and effectively manage these feelings.

NURSING DIAGNOSIS #1

Disturbance in self-concept: self-esteem related to perceived loss of control, function, or propriety, resulting in feeling of humiliation

---

Rationale: Self-concept is threatened by situations that decrease capabilities and expectations, which may result in embarrassment and loss of self-esteem.

☐ **GOAL**

The patient will maintain self-respect and dignity.

☐ **IMPLEMENTATION**

- Maintain respectful and courteous relationship with patient/family; call patient by name, knock on door, respect privacy.
- Monitor for behaviors indicating embarrassment (e.g., withdrawn, lack of eye contact, fidgeting).
- Encourage individuality and respect differences; assess individual preferences and note on care plan; assist to make decisions regarding care and environment to increase sense of control.
- Encourage to anticipate new situations and explore concerns and questions; support positive actions and attempts to adapt to changes.
- Role play potential threatening situations and develop new responses.
- Spend time with patient listening to concerns, assisting with activities of daily living (ADL), and building a trusting relationship; assist with reality testing to evaluate threats to self-esteem objectively.
- Know that most feelings of shame can be prevented.

☐ **EVALUATION CRITERIA/DESIRED OUTCOMES**

The Patient
- Participates in planning for care
- Requests changes in circumstances to decrease situations perceived as embarrassing
- Makes fewer negative statements regarding self
- Displays fewer "embarrassed" mannerisms

NURSING DIAGNOSIS #2

a. **Ineffective individual coping** related to feelings of shame and embarrassment, personal vulnerability

b. **Knowledge deficit** regarding effective management of feelings of shame/embarrssment

Rationale: Difficulty in adapting to situations perceived as humiliating may cause a decrease in the usefulness of existing coping mechanisms. Frequently people experience shame and embarrassment due to naiveté about how to handle a situation. Once the proper etiquette or appropriate behavior is known, potentially embarrassing situations can be handled differently.

☐ GOAL

The patient will acknowledge shame/embarrassment and maintain self-respect; will develop new effective ways of coping with situations that evoke shame or embarrassment.

☐ IMPLEMENTATION

- Determine patient's perception of self and situation; do not challenge if unrealistic, but do clarify misconceptions.
- Assess for lack of experience or skills in communication, assertiveness, or interpersonal relationships; patient may not know how to ask for privacy or how to negotiate for special needs or wants; use problem solving, behavior modification, and practice of desired behaviors (refer to *Problem Solving*, page 248, *Behavior Modification*, page 250, and *Guidelines for Teaching Patients and Families*, page 229.

- Encourage acknowledgment of feelings to 1 other person.
- Accept patient's feelings and validate him/her as a unique person.
- Explore shame situation: in what way does the patient feel embarrassed? humiliated?
- Encourage verbalization of feelings of shame; what has been previously experienced?
- Determine if hospital procedures or staff behaviors caused experience of shame; if so, make amends and manage environment to prevent causes.
- Explore "shoulds" (e.g., what the patient thinks s/he should do); refer to *The Patient Experiencing Guilt*, page 83; support realistic expectations and correct unrealistic ones (e.g., patient may not know expected behaviors for sick role and may feel shame at being dependent on others, sharing a bedroom with other people, exposing body for examinations, or experiencing intense feelings of fear or loss, grief and mourning).
- Teach that shame/embarrassment is common and normal and often can be anticipated and prevented.
- Problem solve with patient to restore self-respect and to avoid or change situation that evoked the shame.

☐ EVALUATION CRITERIA/DESIRED OUTCOMES

The Patient
- Verbalizes distressing feelings readily
- Identifies situations causing feelings of embarrassment
- Recognizes and accepts uniqueness of own feelings
- Makes valid realistic requests to have needs met
- Uses assertive techniques to prevent previously embarrassing situations

The Patient Adapting to the Sick Role

Definition/Discussion

Sick role behaviors are defined by society as those appropriate to the patient's stage of illness and position on the health-illness continuum. There are 3 stages of role change in the health and illness cycle: transition from health to illness, the period of actual illness, and convalescence. In the process of becoming a patient, stress and negative feelings may occur. The family, business, and social roles are abandoned for a new set of expectations defined by hospital and care givers. Regression to a point where nurturing is accepted contributes to the conservation of energy that can be utilized to promote health. The sick role is to be abandoned as soon as the patient improves and is able to care for self. Adaptive and maladaptive behaviors characteristic of the sick role are shown in table 6. Refer to *The Patient Experiencing Chronic Illness*, page 38, for patients whose former level of health will not be regained.

Nursing Assessment

☐ **PERTINENT HISTORY**

Previous experience or knowledge of sick role, expected behaviors; past illnesses, course, outcome; previous physical/mental health status: depression, stressors, crises, losses, mental illness

☐ **PHYSICAL FINDINGS**

Pathophysiology resulting in sick role, insomnia, excessive sleeping or crying, anxiety, fear, apathy, withdrawal, agitation, restlessness, hostility, anger, irritability

☐ **PSYCHOSOCIAL CONCERNS/ DEVELOPMENTAL FACTORS**

Feelings of powerlessness, effects of sick role on self-esteem, developmental level, support system, role changes (e.g., wife/husband employer, parent, child), cultural influences, usual coping patterns, life-style, personality style, patterns of communication, secondary gains for continuing the sick role

☐ **PATIENT AND FAMILY KNOWLEDGE**

Symptoms, prognosis, treatment plan; expectation of care givers of sick role behaviors; projected course of convalescence; availability of private or community supportive organizations, readiness and willingness to learn

Nursing Care

☐ **LONG-TERM GOAL**

The patient will take on behaviors appropriate to the current stage of illness and thereby facilitate the recovery process.

NURSING DIAGNOSIS #1

Anxiety related to transition from health to illness

Rationale: Illness and hospitalization are usually perceived as a threat to life and functioning. In addition, the patient is separated from family and friends, is in unfamiliar and sometimes frightening surroundings with strangers in attendance. There is also concern over financial cost, loss of independence, and depersonalization. The patient feels extremely vulnerable and anxiety increases.

☐ **GOAL**

The patient will move adaptively from health to illness by recognizing and reporting symptoms to health care worker; overcoming shock and disbelief to seek help; telling symptoms, problems, concerns to health care worker; accepting need for treatment as indicated.

☐ **IMPLEMENTATION**

- Establish self as a concerned and helpful professional who wants to understand patient/family and their concerns; encourage patient to describe symptoms and share feelings, fears.

- Orient patient/family to immediate environment; answer questions; explain medical regimen.
- Assess knowledge of procedures and teach as needed, giving descriptions with simple, nontension-producing words; include what the patient will feel, hear, see, taste, and experience.
- Assess patient/family for behaviors of anxiety and fear (e.g., excessive demands, refusal to cooperate, withdrawal, asking excessive questions); refer to *The Patient Experiencing Anxiety*, page 22, and *The Patient Experiencing Fear*, page 78.
- Assess for behaviors of shock and disbelief, denial, and other behaviors of loss; listen and give emotional support, accepting patient's need to cope with the situation at own pace; refer to *The Patient Manifesting Denial*, page 52, and *The Patient Experiencing Grief and Loss*, page 80.
- Teach relaxation techniques (e.g., deep breathing, visual imagery).

☐ EVALUATION CRITERIA/DESIRED OUTCOMES

The Patient
- Recognizes symptoms of anxiety and uses reduction techniques
- Overcomes shock/disbelief and seeks care of health care professionals
- Reports symptoms, problems, concerns
- Accepts and participates in treatment

NURSING DIAGNOSIS #2

Disturbance in self-concept: body image, self-esteem, role performance related to illness

Rationale: Serious illness and hospitalization may produce alterations in physical appearance that change the patient's perception of self. This situation also affects the family and the social roles the patient fulfills. These perceived negative changes decrease the patient's self-esteem.

☐ GOAL

The patient will achieve realistic perception of body changes; will resume customary role responsibilities at appropriate time; will regain self-confidence.

☐ IMPLEMENTATION

- Create a trusting nurse-patient relationship by showing interest, concern, and empathy for patient/family.
- Provide privacy and treat patient with respect at all times; know that patient needs to feel the positive regard of the care giver.
- Encourage expression of feelings about how patient views self, fears of changes produced by ill-

ness, and manner in which s/he and the family plan to cope.
- Provide information as indicated; know this may be required on a continuing basis.
- Assist to accept assistance from all members of the interdisciplinary team (e.g., physical therapist, occupational therapist, social worker); promote expectation that concentrated efforts can hasten recovery.
- Explore meaning of loss or change in body part or function; encourage sharing of feelings by patient and family members; expect shock, denial, anger, and frustration.
- Use role playing to assist patient/family to ventilate feelings of loss and grief.
- Discuss possible reconstruction or rehabilitation; encourage contact of outside support groups that may be helpful to patient/family.
- Assist to identify ways in which role strain can be minimized; changes in family responsibilities may be necessary with the sharing of parenting and other duties the patient normally performs with brothers, sisters, or friends.
- Involve as many support systems as possible to assist family so that stress on both patient and family is decreased and recovery facilitated.
- Promote involvement of both patient and family in plan of care; continue to allow as much control over activities of daily living (ADL) as possible.
- Focus on patient's strengths and strengths of family; assist to identify how these can be further developed.
- Accept ambivalent feelings of gratitude and resentment towards staff, family, friends if patient has lost independence and self-esteem as a result of illness and hospitalization.
- Provide continued support and encouragement for progress made; be positive and sincere in approach; praise both patient and family for adjustments made.
- Refer to *The Patient Experiencing a Threat to Self-Esteem*, page 127.

☐ EVALUATION CRITERIA/DESIRED OUTCOMES

The Patient
- Demonstrates acceptance of body changes
- Resumes role responsibilities gradually
- States realistic perceptions of self and abilities
- Demonstrates realistic planning for the future

NURSING DIAGNOSIS #3

Powerlessness relating to inability to control illness

Rationale: The patient who is hospitalized experiences a loss of control regarding his/her state of health. S/he feels helpless and may develop hope-lessness in the face of a poor or uncertain prog-nosis. This feeling of lack of control may produce anger, hostility, apathy, or depression.

☐ GOAL

The patient will discuss feelings and concerns about perceived lack of control of illness and state of health; will participate in planning for care.

☐ IMPLEMENTATION

- Demonstrate interest and concern; listen to requests and encourage as much patient and family participation as possible in planning for care; ask for feedback and maintain interest by using suggestions whenever possible.
- Assist in verbalizing feelings regarding lack of control; help to identify which situation can be changed and which cannot; encourage realistic expectations.
- Provide appropriate information so that indicated adjustments can be started; encourage communication between patient and family so perceptions regarding the illness are accurate.
- Accept expressions of hostility or anger which may be directed at care givers by realizing they are not meant personally; listen, reflect, and restate feelings in respectful and assertive manner.
- Be alert for signs of depression; refer to *The Patient Experiencing Depression*, page 57.
- Refer to *The Patient Experiencing Powerlessness*, page 115.

☐ EVALUATION CRITERIA/DESIRED OUTCOMES

The Patient
- Verbalizes feelings and concerns about perceived lack of control of illness and state of health
- Participates actively in planning and executing care plan

☐ GOAL

The patient will adapt to the sick role by coping effectively with necessary limitations, preserving existing abilities, and regaining maximum function in impaired areas.

☐ IMPLEMENTATION

- Determine patient and family goals, priorities, and preferences; offer support and information as needed.
- Work with patient to set realistic and acceptable goals; plan care based on patient's current level of functioning; advance patient participation as status tolerates.
- Discuss concerns regarding the letting go of usual family, work, or social roles and responsibilities; encourage patient to ask for help from spouse, family, and friends.
- Introduce appropriate self-help devices and assist patient to use.
- Encourage patient to ventilate feelings and concerns about illness, hospitalization, body functions, progress, prognosis; accept feelings and preoccupation with somatic concerns.
- Be consistent in encouragement and care giving; provide structure in environment to reduce stress.
- Encourage to do appropriate self-care; offer emotional support and praise; see *Behavior Modification*, page 250.
- Maintain a positive attitude despite frustration and anger that patient may show.

☐ EVALUATION CRITERIA/DESIRED OUTCOMES

The Patient
- Assumes increasing responsibility for self-care; states understanding of use of self-care devices
- Demonstrates knowledge of convalescent care plan
- Understands use of medications, treatments
- Convalesces and returns to highest level of health possible

---

NURSING DIAGNOSIS #4

Self-care deficit related to limitations resulting from illness

Rationale: The presence of physical limitations caused by illness results in decreased abilities to manage ADL. This is an acceptable situation in acute stages of illness and requires the care giver to assist the patient while encouraging progress toward regaining optimal performance.

NURSING DIAGNOSIS #5

Knowledge deficit regarding convalescence and rehabilitation

Rationale: The patient must gradually relinquish the sick role and begin to assume previous roles and gain independence. The patient and family will require information regarding postdischarge management of illness and teaching regarding medications, treatments, and care.

☐ GOAL

The patient will make transition from illness to convalescence by participation in and cooperation with convalescent treatment plan.

☐ IMPLEMENTATION

- Discuss progress and anticipate convalescence with patient/family.
- Assist patient to resume roles and responsibilities as appropriate; encourage to ask for help from staff, spouse, friends, family, co-workers.
- Using anticipatory guidance, assist patient to plan for discharge from hospital; problem solve and teach as needed to ensure patient/family understand discharge orders (e.g., medication, treatments, activity, rest, diet, when to call physician).
- Assist patient/family to explore community resources (e.g., Visiting Nurses Aassociation, Meals-on-Wheels, hospital equipment rental, homemaker service, Cancer Society, Colostomy Club, or other self-help groups).
- Ask open-ended questions (e.g., "How do you plan to manage . . .?" "What are your plans for . . .?").

☐ EVALUATION CRITERIA/DESIRED OUTCOMES

The Patient

- States understanding of convalescent treatment plan
- Identifies support groups and has made initial contact
- Demonstrates knowledge of course of illness and recovery
- Demonstrates increasingly independent assumption of ADL

Table 6
Characteristic Behaviors of the Patient Adapting to the Sick Role

Adaptive Behaviors	Maladaptive Behaviors
Stage I, Transition from Health to Illness	
Recognizes symptoms; may have some shock and disbelief	Does not recognize symptoms or completely denies symptoms
Seeks care of health care worker or doctor	Does not seek care of health care provider or doctor
Reports symptoms, problems, concerns	Makes no mention of symptoms, problems, concerns, or exaggerates and confuses them; quiet and hyperactive
Stage II, Actual Illness	
Participates with health care worker to plan treatment, set priorities	Refuses to participate in treatment plan
Complies with treatment plan	Does not comply with treatment plan; unresponsive or negative
Seeks relief from usual roles and responsibilities	Continues with usual roles and responsibilities inappropriately
Asks for aid from spouse, friends, family	Does not request aid; does everything or nothing
Asks for acceptance of illness and love in spite of illness	Defensive or aggressive, passive-aggressive behaviors; may be seductive toward staff
Talks about body functions and progress; is preoccupied with self and somatic concerns	Complains constantly and does not acknowledge progress; negative or denies concerns or problems
Shares feelings and concerns; is ambivalent with dependency, both grateful and resentful	Does not express or seem aware of own feelings
Asks for help appropriately from staff	Asks for care from others which s/he is capable of doing for self, or will not ask for help; demands, withdraws, complains constantly
Stage III, Convalescence	
Asks for guidance in resuming previous roles and responsibilities	Does not ask for guidance; assumes roles and responsibilities prematurely or not at all
Asks for help from spouse, friends, family, and co-workers in resuming previous tasks	Does not ask for help; does too much, too little for self; resents offers of help
Anticipates needs and asks for convalescent medication, treatment, activity, and rest orders	Does not think ahead and refuses to discuss treatment plan for convalescence
Convalesces and returns to previous state of health	Refuses to give up sick role; perceives self as sick when care givers perceive as convalescent or healthy

The Patient with a Substance Abuse: Alcohol

Definition/Discussion

Alcoholism is a physiologic dependence (addiction) on alcohol as a result of excessive use. The *DSM-III-R* classification is Substance Abuse Disorder.

Nursing Assessment

☐ **PERTINENT HISTORY**

Onset of acute symptoms, history of alcohol or other substance abuse, family history of alcohol/substance abuse

☐ **PHYSICAL FINDINGS**

Gastrointestinal disturbances (e.g., gastritis, chronic diarrhea); vitamin and nutritional deficiencies, disorders of neurologic and cardiac systems, biliary problems (e.g., pancreatitis, fatty liver, cirrhosis); hypoglycemia; withdrawal is a progressive process and includes 4 stages
- *stage I* (8 hours or more after cessation): mild tremors, nausea, nervousness, tachycardia, increased blood pressure, diaphoresis
- *stage II:* gross tremors, nervousness and hyperactivity, insomnia, anorexia, general weakness, disorientation, illusions, nightmares; auditory and visual hallucinations
- *stage III* (12-48 hours after cessation): all symptoms of stage I and stage II, as well as severe hallucinations and grand mal seizures; stages II and III are known as "delirium tremens"
- *stage IV* (3-5 days after cessation): initial and continuing delirium tremens characterized by confusion, severe psychomotor activity, agitation, sleeplessness, hallucinations, uncontrolled and unexplained tachycardia at onset

☐ **PSYCHOSOCIAL CONCERNS/ DEVELOPMENTAL FACTORS**

Denial; personality traits such as unease and dissatisfaction with life; tendency to excess in areas such as work, sex, recreation; difficulty tolerating anxiety or frustration, poor impulse control, dependence on others; poor ability to cope with stress; low self-esteem; strengths, abilities, interests, positive coping methods

☐ **PATIENT AND FAMILY KNOWLEDGE**

Prognosis, treatment plan, community resources; readiness and willingness to learn

Nursing Care

☐ **LONG-TERM GOAL**

The patient will recognize and accept addiction; the patient will develop situational supports and coping mechanisms that reflect adaptation to a life-style without alcohol.

NURSING DIAGNOSIS #1
a. **Fluid volume deficit** related to hypermetabolic state, not taking in liquids
b. **Potential for injury** related to complications of withdrawal from alcohol
c. **Hyperthermia** related to dehydration, increased metabolic rate

Rationale: The severity of withdrawal symptoms is the direct result of the increased level of acetaldehyde (breakdown product of alcohol) and decreased magnesium level in the blood. Untreated alcohol withdrawal can lead to life-threatening hypermetabolic state, fluid and electrolyte imbalance, delirium tremens, or convulsions.

☐ **GOAL**

The patient will withdraw from alcohol free from complications of dehydration, electrolyte or nutritional imbalance; will be free from injury related to delirium tremens.

☐ **IMPLEMENTATION**

- Know that the severity of withdrawal symptoms is related to the length and extent of drinking preceding the withdrawal period, complete cessation of use of alcohol is not necessary for the development of withdrawal symptoms; realize that diminished alcohol use in those who have developed a high tolerance and physical dependence may precipitate withdrawal symptoms.

- Observe for withdrawal symptoms as early as 8 hours after cessation of drinking; be aware that trauma victims (and others admitted to the hospital suddenly) must be observed for withdrawal symptoms.
- Chart behaviors and stage of withdrawal; report early hallucinations and delirium tremens or convulsions to physician; strive to identify and report stage I behaviors and control symptoms via PRN medication to avoid progressing to stage II or III; take vital signs every 2 hours and report any elevations; if patient's symptoms progress to stage III/IV, monitor temperature and heart rate at least hourly.
- Stay with patient if agitated, confused; ensure safety; reassure that current symptoms are only result of body's response to alcohol use, that they are temporary, and that control will return.
- Protect from injury; use restraints only if patient out of control and absolutely necessary.
- Deal with hallucinations by reinforcing reality; speak to patient slowly in a calm voice; provide a quiet environment; have someone stay with patient until the frightening symptoms have decreased.
- Monitor intake and output at least every 8 hours; ensure a daily fluid intake of at least 2,500 cc orally (unless contraindicated); offer favorite juices every 2 hours during waking hours; discuss IV hydration with physician if intake drops.
- Avoid providing patient with caffeine (e.g., coffee, tea, cola soft drinks, chocolate).
- Identify patient's food preferences; provide frequent small feedings or between-meal snacks of high-protein foods; involve patient in food planning if possible; give multivitamin and mineral supplements as ordered.
- Provide physical care advocated for any additional diseases/conditions.
- Ambulate patients in stage II withdrawal as much as possible; if necessary, walk with patient several times a day; help to bathroom, rather than providing bedpan or urinal; avoid ambulation/stimulation of patients in stages III and IV.

☐ EVALUATION CRITERIA/DESIRED OUTCOMES

The Patient
- Maintains fluid and electrolyte balance
- Has a normal temperature
- Remains free from injury

NURSING DIAGNOSIS #2
Ineffective individual coping related to dependence on alcohol

---

Rationale: Alcohol depresses higher cortical functions, has a disinhibitor and sedative effect, and serves to reduce anxiety rapidly; excessive drinking is often the way a person copes with anxiety. Alcohol addiction creates behavioral responses that are considered erratic, irresponsible, destructive. It may create a situation where the alcohol need is dominant and the purpose of living is to maintain alcohol intake.

☐ GOAL

The patient will discuss and develop the use of coping mechanisms other than alcohol to deal with the stress and strain of daily life; will discuss with others how they can help support patient to live without alcohol; will accept the support of others.

☐ IMPLEMENTATION

- Help to learn to tolerate psychologic stress, to do advance planning for anticipated painful events (e.g., surgery, separation from a loved one) and to reduce social isolation.
- Sit with patient at least twice daily; your presence will reinforce that patient is not being rejected for any undesirable behavior.
- Observe patient's behavior; discuss your observations with patient to help develop insight into behavior's relationship to alcohol intake.
- Discuss nonjudgmentally the relationship between alcohol and ineffective coping.
- Provide information as needed; refer to psychiatric nurse or mental health specialist if necessary.
- Recognize and share with patient that a life-style without alcohol is a major loss (refer to *The Patient Experiencing Grief and Loss,* page 80); anticipate what this may mean and help to plan adaptive ways to compensate for the loss (e.g., keep a glass of seltzer or iced tea in hand at social functions, replace drinking with a specified enjoyable activity).
- Do not punish or reprimand patient for failures or nonresponse to suggestions/interventions (punishment serves only to give patient fuel for continuing to deal with failure or rejection by drinking); praise any positive responses.
- Have patient participate in decisions about daily care in hospital; involve in some type of occupational therapy (may result in some measure of success to help increase self-confidence).
- Provide opportunities to decrease social isolation and to improve social skills with patient/recreation groups; encourage social interaction by insisting patient take meals in the dining room when possible; reinforce positive social behaviors (e.g., initiating friendly conversations); praise all efforts at participation in activities.
- Point out unacceptable behavior calmly and gently

(e.g., intellectualizing, making excuses, verbally abusing staff or others); let patient know this is not acceptable.

- Hold weekly health-team conferences to discuss aspects of alcoholism, to share feelings and responses to caring for an alcoholic patient, and to coordinate care; explain that it is normal for staff to feel frustrated, angry, guilty, rejecting, anxious when caring for alcoholic patients; staff often feel they have failed if a patient is readmitted in an alcoholic state after discharge; include a psychiatric nurse or other mental health specialist.
- Request inservice education programs (e.g., films, literature) on alcoholism.
- Invite a member of Alcoholics Anonymous (AA)/ AlAnon (family group of AA) to a staff conference to share their aims and approaches, or go to a meeting with a colleague.
- Provide opportunity for family to express their anger about patient; listen to and support them; put family in touch with a community group where consistent support and help are available (e.g., AlAnon).

☐ EVALUATION CRITERIA/DESIRED OUTCOMES

The Patient
- Demonstrates at least 2 positive coping mechanisms to deal with stress
- Develops plan for activities of daily living without alcohol
- Demonstrates appropriate social skills
- Has at least one plan to help decrease social isolation and strengthen new behaviors

---

NURSING DIAGNOSIS #3

Noncompliance related to difficulty in making major life changes

Rationale: Denial of alcohol problem and eventual life-threatening deterioration, as well as psychologic dependency, may lead to noncompliance. Research shows a lack of knowledge about disease and its treatment adversely affects compliance; however, patient knowledge of treatment does not necessarily increase compliance. The person needs to believe that the changes will be personally bene-

---

ficial and are worth the difficulty involved. Continued emotional support is needed to maintain an alcohol-free life-style.

☐ GOAL

The patient will perceive sobriety as a desirable goal; will follow the treatments as prescribed.

☐ IMPLEMENTATION

- Explain to patients on Antabuse therapy effects that develop with ingestion of alcohol (e.g., severe nausea and vomiting, flushed face, rapid pulse and respirations, drop in blood pressure).
- Arrange for patient/family to attend group counseling sessions, if available in hospital, to discuss feelings, problems, changing behaviors, pressures, sources of support (e.g., Al-Anon, community mental health agencies).
- Discuss AA with patient; offer to arrange for a member to visit and encourage patient to accept; provide information about other types of therapy available (e.g., local mental health clinics).
- Recognize that until patient is able to accept the fact a drinking problem exists, the patient will not be motivated to follow treatment, to attend AA, or to change behavior.
- Promote compliance by identifying the benefits of not drinking; realize that the patient must perceive that compliance will reduce discomfort with life and with self.
- Know that compliance is most difficult to achieve when personal habits must be broken; to stop drinking is an extremely difficult change to make under any circumstances.
- Teach about prescribed medications (e.g., rationale, schedule, side effects, how and where to get refills).

☐ EVALUATION CRITERIA/DESIRED OUTCOMES

The Patient
- Acknowledges alcohol problem and need for support to maintain alcohol-free life-style
- Has a contact with AA/other community mental health group
- States actions and side effects of current medications; has an adequate supply

The Patient with a Substance Abuse: Drugs

Definition/Discussion

A drug abuser is a person who repeatedly uses a chemical substance or substances in a way that is harmful to self and society.

- *Drug habituation:* psychologic dependence on a drug
- *Drug addiction:* psychologic and physical dependence on a drug with tolerance for increasing doses and development of withdrawal symptoms without drug
- *Drug dependence:* "Psychological/physical dependence on drug that is taken periodically or on a scheduled basis." (World Health Organization)

The *DSM-III-R* classification is Substance Abuse Disorder. Alcohol abuse is also considered substance abuse. For specific information on alcoholism, refer to *The Patient with a Substance Abuse: Alcohol, page 138*.

Nursing Assessment

☐ PERTINENT HISTORY

Drugs used, amount, frequency, length of time used; toxic effects or withdrawal symptoms; purposeful drug-seeking behavior; manipulation; acting out

☐ PHYSICAL FINDINGS

Physical problems related to poor nutrition status, fluid and electrolyte imbalance, dental caries, high blood pressure, infections from injections given under septic conditions, respiratory infections, alterations in level of consciousness (LOC), coma, seizures

☐ PSYCHOSOCIAL CONCERNS/ DEVELOPMENTAL FACTORS

Maladaptive coping with anxiety (difficulty tolerating anxiety or frustration; use of drugs to escape from tension and to obtain feelings of relief, oblivion, or euphoria), poor impulse control, passivity, inability to express anger and other intense feelings, dependency conflicts, problems with close relationships, family dynamics (dependency/independency conflict, presence of role models for drug/alcohol abuse, maladaptive coping with anxiety and stress); strengths, abilities, interests, adaptive coping measures, devel-opmental level, significance of peers, cognitive dysfunction, denial

☐ PATIENT AND FAMILY KNOWLEDGE

Available community resources, treatment plan, disease prognosis, readiness and willingness to learn

Nursing Care

☐ LONG-TERM GOAL

The patient will recognize and admit to drug addiction or dependence; the patient will develop situational supports and coping mechanisms that reflect adaptation to a lifestyle without drug use.

NURSING DIAGNOSIS #1

Potential for injury: trauma, poisoning related to drug overdose, withdrawal from drug(s)

Rationale: There is an increasing tendency for drug abusers to mix multiple drugs and to mix drugs with alcohol, resulting in dangerous potentiation of action and side effects. The patient needs protection from life-threatening complications of intoxication, overdose, and withdrawal (e.g., fluid and electrolyte imbalance, respiratory or renal failure, seizures, shock, toxic psychosis).

☐ GOAL

The patient will recover from the drug overdose or withdrawal period; will be free from complications such as fluid and electrolyte imbalance, respiratory failure, shock, and toxic psychosis.

☐ IMPLEMENTATION

- Treat patient symptomatically if abused substance is unknown (do not waste time playing detective).
- Avoid jumping to conclusions, moralizing, or making accusations, but do not accept what patient says at face value if clinical signs are contradictory.

141

- Assess and chart LOC and report changes to physician
  - *full consciousness*: alert, responsive; oriented to person, time, place; memory for recent events intact; verbalizes readily, coherently, and distinctly
  - *impaired consciousness*: drowsy, lethargic, loss of recent memory, slow thinking but still has appropriate responses
  - *confusion/delirium*: transient periods of disorientation, restlessness, uncooperativeness; dazed; easily agitated and irritable when disturbed; fearful; noisy; still responds to verbal stimuli and light tactile stimuli
  - *stupor*: responds only to repeated insistent verbal stimuli or continuous, painful tactile stimuli
  - *coma*: response to intense stimuli is either reflex or absent
- Check vital signs every 15 minutes until full consciousness returns; assess for patency of airway and adequacy of ventilation; observe closely for respiratory tract obstructions (e.g., mucus plugs, vomitus, tongue); turn head to side to prevent aspiration until patient is alert; have suction equipment available.
- Monitor for any abnormal respiratory patterns (e.g., wheezing, crowing, apnea, retraction) and report to physician STAT.
- Keep accurate intake and output; administer IV fluids as ordered; monitor effectiveness.
- Offer oral fluids and diet when permitted; consider patient's likes and dislikes as well as physical condition when offering choices.
- Administer drugs (e.g., sedatives, psychotropics) as ordered to treat withdrawal symptoms or to prevent/treat toxic psychosis; evaluate effectiveness.

☐ EVALUATION CRITERIA/DESIRED OUTCOMES

The Patient
- Shows no evidence of shock, toxic psychosis
- Maintains fluid and electrolyte balance
- Breathes easily, has adequate gas exchange

NURSING DIAGNOSIS #2

Ineffective individual coping related to dependence on drug(s)

Rationale: Taking drugs serves a purpose for the substance abuser. Drugs "do" things for the individual, such as relieve anxiety and uncomfortable feelings, increase pleasure, provide an escape from reality, express feelings or repress emotions. Abuse of drugs is an attempt to adapt to the stresses of life in a maladaptive manner.

☐ GOAL

The patient will discuss and demonstrate the use of coping mechanisms other than drugs to deal with stress of daily living; will decrease use of denial, manipulation, and purposeful drug seeking; will participate in self-care and problem solving.

☐ IMPLEMENTATION

- Hold weekly team conferences to discuss aspects of drug abuse; share feelings and responses to caring for the drug abuser (staff may feel angry, resentful, or as if they have failed if patient relapses—as a very high percentage do).
- Ensure that entire staff uses a consistent approach to patient's behavior.
- Set firm and consistent limits; be clear about definition of acceptable and unacceptable behavior.
- Involve patient in planning and doing self-care; give choices in activities of daily living (ADL), exercise, and leisure time.
- Keep focus on patient's responsibility for self and own choices; avoid intellectualizations about staff/society/family problems or faults.
- Discuss your observations of patient's behavior with patient; reinforce positive social behaviors (e.g., participation in unit activities, discussing problems related to drug use, initiating friendly conversation); calmly point out manipulative or acting-out behaviors (e.g., blaming society, intellectualizing, making excuses, verbally abusing staff or other patients, picking fights); let patient know that this is not acceptable.
- Recognize and share with patient that a life-style without drugs is a major change and a loss; refer to *The Patient Experiencing Grief and Loss*, page 80; discuss what this might mean and help patient to plan adaptive ways to compensate by utilizing strengths, interests, abilities, and developing adaptive coping strategies; refer to Table 1, *Stress Management*, page 24.
- Assist to identify most threatening aspect(s) of giving up drug (e.g., "friends," lack of responsibility); observe when patient has increased anxiety, reacts most intensely, acts out, or resumes denial; discuss these with patient.
- Do not support efforts at denial; listen to realistic thoughts and concerns (e.g., how to re-enter work force, what to do if peers apply pressure to use drugs); role play ways to deal with stressful situations; explore plans that seem unrealistic in order to identify the realities of the situation.
- Help patient express angry/sad/guilty feelings by using open-ended questions and by listening; spend time with patient identifying feelings and problems and problem solving.
- Teach to deal with anxiety and stress; refer to *The Patient Experiencing Anxiety*, page 22.
- Praise patient's efforts to care for self, to recognize reality of own behaviors, to participate in problem identification and problem solving.

EVALUATION CRITERIA/DESIRED OUTCOMES

The Patient

- Discusses/demonstrates coping mechanisms other than drugs
- Participates in self-care and problem solving in ADL
- Participates in planning life-style without drugs

NURSING DIAGNOSIS #3

Noncompliance related to difficulty in making major life changes to adapt to a life-style free of drugs

Rationale: Denial of drug problem, psychologic dependency/environmental reinforcers may lead to noncompliance with treatment plan. Feelings of powerlessness to learn healthy methods of coping with life's stresses and to break long-time habits can be a hindrance to compliance.

GOAL

The patient will demonstrate ability to cope with life without drugs; will accept treatment and will participate in plans for discharge.

IMPLEMENTATION

- Assess level of knowledge, ability and willingness to comply with treatment plan; recognize that until patient is able to accept the fact that a drug problem exists, the patient will not be motivated to follow treatment, to attend self-help groups, or to change behavior.
- Assist to identify behaviors related to stress and to develop strategies to cope effectively with stress and anxiety.
- Help patient to define support systems (e.g., family/friends); include them in discharge planning if possible.
- Arrange for patient/family/friends to attend group counseling sessions, if available in hospital, to discuss feelings, problems, changing behaviors, pressures, stress management, and sources of community support (e.g., community mental health agencies, Alcoholics Anonymous, AlAnon); know that narcotics-abuser groups led by former addicts seem to be the most effective method of treatment for drug abuse.
- Plan with patient ways to maintain self after discharge (e.g., hygiene, nutrition, finding friends and pastimes without drugs, recreation and work, school); help set personal goals and offer support for these.
- Plan for daily outlets for productive activity (e.g., occupational or industrial therapy); ask patient to set own activity goals; provide support to achieve them.
- Encourage verbalization and questions; ask patient to describe (in own words) treatment plan, follow-up care, symptoms to report to physician.
- Role play stressful situations; focus on realistic problems and solutions.

EVALUATION CRITERIA/DESIRED OUTCOMES

The Patient

- States willingness to accept drug treatment program
- Verbalizes plans to comply with treatment regimen
- Contacts a community support group (e.g., Narcotics Anonymous, self-help group, community mental health agency)

The Patient who is Suicidal

Definition/Discussion

Suicide may be defined as an act to voluntarily end one's own life; it may be the ultimate act of self-hatred, or an attempt to control the time and circumstances of death. Suicide is a method of communication, a cry for help, a visible sign that the person wishes to escape an intolerable situation and has run out of positive alternatives.

Attitudes of health care personnel have a critical effect on the suicidal patient. Many nursing care providers experience feelings of anger, frustration, unsympathetic attitudes, and fear of involvement while working with patients who have attempted suicide. Since they are actively involved in measures to preserve and prolong life, it is difficult to understand and accept patients who are trying to end theirs. Furthermore, attention-seeking behavior and demands for special treatment often seen in these patients tend to alienate staff. Perceived rejection of the patient by the staff increases the patient's feelings of self-deprecation, worthlessness, helplessness, and hopelessness. Changes in the patient's attitude toward self and the feeling of hope come primarily through therapeutic staff-patient relationships. It is, therefore, necessary for the health care providers to recognize their negative feelings, to share them with each other, and to receive counseling and encouragement from colleagues so that empathic understanding and a positive therapeutic attitude may prevail.

Suicides occur in hospitals at a much greater rate than in the general community: 3 1/2 times higher for medical and surgical patients and 30 times higher for neuropsychiatric patients. Jumping or hanging are the most frequently used methods. Legal implications necessitate clearly written hospital policies and guidelines for safeguarding suicidal patients. These policies should cover areas of lethality assessment, environmental precautions, safe care procedures, staff communications, attitudes and behavior, and record documentation. These guidelines provide staff with competent, community-based professional practices.

Nursing Assessment

☐ PERTINENT HISTORY

Prior suicidal attempts (when, how many, outcome); recent loss(es) (real or perceived), especially of a relationship, crisis situations; stresses (job, relationship); overt or covert actions or statements (giving away prized possessions); recent changes in behavior or activities of daily living (retirement); loss of job, home, abilities; changes in location or environment; changes in financial situation; cultural isolation; previous aggressive behaviors; recent physical illness(es); alcohol or substance abuse, recent withdrawal; anhedonia; hopelessness; previous or present mental illness (hospitalization, treatments, medications, psychoses, hallucinations, delusions, confusion, depression)

☐ PHYSICAL FINDINGS

Age, sex, race, outward manifestations of previous attempts, flat affect, lack of eye contact, somatic complaints, agitation and restlessness, apathy and withdrawal

☐ PSYCHOSOCIAL CONCERNS/ DEVELOPMENTAL FACTORS

Social network or lack of friends, developmental level, isolation, alienation, loneliness, prone to accidents, inability to cope, failure and poor performance pattern, frequent or severe stressors, patterns of communication, cultural influences, divorce(s), occupation (physicians, police, dentists at higher risk), disorganized life-style, personality styles (higher risk in dependent, manipulative, borderline, impulsive, and histrionic), poor impulse control, family dynamics, family history of suicide
Children: hyperactivity, with or without irritability; slow learning, boredom, phobias, mood and temper swings
Adolescents: family stress or disharmony, problem life-style, poor impulse control, dissolution of relationship (trigger event), truancy, delinquency, lack of parental acceptance, school problems, stress from developmental phases, fantasizing about death
Elderly: acute or chronic physical or mental illness, loss of loved one(s), social isolation, loneliness, retirement, poverty

☐ PATIENT AND FAMILY KNOWLEDGE

Indications of suicidal ideation (precipitating factors, conditions), lethality of methods, availability of means, use and availability of community or private organizations or support systems

Nursing Care

☐ LONG-TERM GOAL

The patient will be free from suicidal ideation, thoughts, and feelings; the patient will develop new alternatives to cope with the conditions that contributed to the suicidal state.

NURSING DIAGNOSIS #1

Potential for violence: self-directed related to suicidal ideation

Rationale: The first priority when a patient is actively suicidal is to protect the individual from harming self. This is the legal responsibility of the hospital staff. They have the opportunity to share their commitment to life, caring, and hope with the patient. This is necessary to cope with and decrease the wish to die.

☐ GOAL

The patient will not harm self; will establish a trusting relationship and rapport with at least one staff member.

☐ IMPLEMENTATION

- Assume responsibility for safety of patient; inspect unit for potentially hazardous situations; ensure windows are shatterproof; use first-floor facilities if available; remove sharp or dangerous objects (e.g., scissors, nail files, razor blades, medications, straps, cords, all potentially toxic agents) from patient's access.
- Restrict patient to observable areas; assign to room near nurses station and close to other patients' rooms.
- Follow hospital procedures for suicide precautions; ensure that all persons coming in contact with patient clearly understand restrictions.
- Explain reasons for one-to-one and tell patient what you are doing; observe sleeping and eating habits and attitude displayed; be an interested, active, supportive listener for the patient wishing to talk; accompany at all times, even to bathroom; know if it is permissible for family/friends to be in attendance.
- Assure patient s/he is safe from own self-destructive impulses; know that patients usually accept these safety precautions as an indication staff cares about them and takes their suicidal threats seriously.
- Know that patients will observe unit coverage and layout carefully to find opportunities to act; plan

staffing so that unit is always covered by experienced staff, especially at staff meal times, breaks, change of shift, and vacations; suicide occurs most often in hospital settings during change of shift, at mealtimes, or on weekends.
- Distinguish between rational and irrational communication; know that patients having visual or auditory hallucinations, delusions, or agitated depression are especially vulnerable to suicide.
- Assess for signs or statements that patient is hallucinating or describing a misperception of reality (e.g., "The voices are telling me I do not deserve to live."); intervene and reinforce reality before acting out occurs.
- Ascertain suicide plan and lethality (e.g., when, where, how, with what tools); take all suicide threats seriously; remember that plans are more lethal when they are specific (e.g., person has planned specific time and isolated place, or plans severe or self-mutilating act such as large amount of lethal medications); they are less lethal when plans are vague, involve a minor dose of medications or superficial cuts of the wrist in a place where they are likely to be discovered.
- Establish intensity of wish to die and determination of patient by paying careful attention to statements and affect.
- Monitor changes in affect; calmness or cheerfulness that is new to the patient's affect may signal that s/he has made up his/her mind to attempt to commit suicide and has formulated an effective plan to do so.
- Listen to patient who has previously attempted suicide for attitude about the attempt (is patient sorry attempt was not successful and threatening to try again? does s/he state behavior is regretted and agree to come for help if loss of control occurs again?).
- Ask patient to notify staff when suicidal feelings occur; attempt to obtain a suicide prevention contract in which the patient contracts to, for, and with self using the staff as facilitator and witness; encourage patient that most suicidal ideations are time limiting.
- Rally the support of caring family members and friends; the more friends a person has, the stronger the support system; allow them to ventilate own feelings regarding suicide and the patient so they can work more effectively with the patient in this situation; provide support and encouragement.
- Spend time with patient to observe behaviors and begin building a trusting relationship; combining a therapeutic relationship with staff and a safe, secure environment are 2 of the most important deterrents to suicide; the suicidal patient has an intense need to trust, to be accepted and have increased self-esteem; respect, caring, and concern are vitally important.
- Avoid judgmental attitude; show interest in the

patient and concern for present and future welfare.
- Evaluate behaviors carefully before discontinuing suicide precautions and before discharge, even if patient denies ideation.
- Use the interdisciplinary team approach for increased support for both the patient and staff (working with the suicidal patient requires mutual support and supervision to achieve maximum effectiveness in intervention).

☐ EVALUATION CRITERIA/DESIRED OUTCOMES

The Patient
- Seeks contact with staff when suicidal feelings occur
- Contracts to not attempt suicide
- Accepts necessity of temporarily restrictive environment of suicide precautions
- Accepts concern and support of staff and family
- Does not attempt suicide
- States fewer occurrences of suicidal ideation

NURSING DIAGNOSIS #2

Ineffective individual coping related to feelings of hopelessness, powerlessness

Rationale: The failure of regularly used coping mechanisms causes feelings of hopelessness and powerlessness leading the patient to consider suicide as the most desirable option.

☐ GOAL

The patient will identify causes of feelings of hopelessness and powerlessness; will develop effective ways to manage them.

☐ IMPLEMENTATION

- Encourage patient to discuss painful feelings that preceded suicidal thoughts; if causes of feelings can be identified, explore these to achieve some insight.
- Reflect your understanding of patient's perception of the situation so feelings of alienation will be decreased (e.g., "You must have felt as if there was no other alternative.").
- Monitor for increased anxiety and assist with management; refer to *The Patient Experiencing Anxiety*, page 22.
- Urge regular attendance at group therapy.
- Assist to determine how feelings of hopelessness and powerlessness can be alleviated and to identify ways control can be achieved by patient over own life; begin with small problems and their solutions and work up to those that are more diffi-

cult; refer to *The Patient Experiencing Powerlessness*, page 115.
- Ask how patient views the current situation and how this could be changed; assist to identify alternatives to suicide as a coping mechanism; refer to *Problem Solving*, page 248.
- Correct distorted perceptions (e.g., "It feels to you that nothing can change, but there might be some other possibilities you haven't considered. Let's talk more about it.").
- Teach art of requesting and accepting assistance when it is needed; work at the level of patient knowledge so that communication is clear and mutually understood.
- Allow to have as much control over life as is consistent with safety; set limits as needed for self-control and security.
- Evaluate current abilities to cope with stress; refer to Table 1, *Stress Management*, page 24.
- Work out a regular exercise or recreational program if physical condition permits; establish a pattern that can be adhered to after discharge.
- Focus on ambivalence patient has toward suicide (e.g., wants suffering to end but does not necessarily wish to die); help to find something to hope for in the future, to focus not on the past but on positive events that can now be created; the ability to be hopeful will be effective in preventing recurrence of suicidal ideation.
- Involve the interdisciplinary team for assistance in increasing effective management of all areas of functioning.

☐ EVALUATION CRITERIA/DESIRED OUTCOMES

The Patient
- Identifies factors precipitating feelings of hopelessness and powerlessness
- States how these feelings can be alleviated through changes in response
- Acknowledges alternative behaviors
- Participates regularly in exercise program and group therapy
- Participates in planning for care
- Expresses hopeful feelings in at least one area

NURSING DIAGNOSIS #3

Disturbance in self-concept: self-esteem related to maladaptive situational, maturational, or physiologic factors (specify)

Rationale: The individual with an impaired self-esteem experiences feelings of failure, unworthiness, lack of appreciation for own value, and alienation from others. This pattern of devaluing self and withdrawal may intensify as a result of internal or environmental factors and culminate in the percep-

tion that the taking of his/her own life is the only solution.

☐ GOAL

The patient will develop a feeling of increased self-worth and an ability to initiate and maintain social relationships.

☐ IMPLEMENTATION

- Establish a relationship that expresses respect, sensitivity, honesty, concern, and consistency.
- Spend time with patient and show positive regard.
- Sit in silence with the patient if necessary; if patient rejects you, state you will return at a specific time and then do so; continue to convey that you consider patient a valuable and worthwhile human being.
- Encourage patient to do as much self-care as possible; invite to participate in the treatment plan; allow input on favorite activities and provide opportunity for participation.
- Show recognition for all accomplishments; be sincere in praise.
- Ask patient to describe feelings of loneliness; identify if perceived rejection is a contributing factor and encourage realistic appraisal; role play initiations of social contacts until patient is comfortable in doing so.
- Urge regular attendance at group therapy to increase contact with others and provide opportunities to verbalize feelings.
- Respond to self-deprecating remarks in a positive way; do not allow patient to reinforce negative ideas about self; explain that when patient acknowledges feelings, it will be possible to begin to manage them.
- Structure time so patient is kept distracted and busy (productive activities produce a feeling of accomplishment); peer group activities are especially helpful for adolescents and the elderly.
- Work with patient to identify communication problems and assist in development of clear communication patterns.
- Set realistic goals with the patient (e.g., initiate 1 social interaction/day); increase as tolerated.
- Help to identify positive aspects of self and abilities and benefits of social interactions so that new and less isolated patterns of living can be instituted; refer to *The Patient Experiencing a Threat to Self-Esteem*, page 127.
- Work with patient on planning for increased individual and group contact after discharge; introduce to possible interest, support, or religious contacts prior to discharge so that follow-up will be facilitated.

☐ EVALUATION CRITERIA/DESIRED OUTCOMES

The Patient
- Expresses positive feelings about self
- Attends group therapy regularly and participates occasionally
- Initiates one social contact daily
- Identifies one enjoyable activity that is done well

NURSING DIAGNOSIS #4

Knowledge deficit regarding support services and constructive methods of life management

Rationale: *The patient can become a constructive member of society rather than elect to be self-destructive when provided with the opportunity to gain knowledge regarding effective ways to handle problems through the availability and utilization of individual and community support for crisis intervention and suicide.*

☐ GOAL

The patient will recognize and utilize individual or community assistance as needed; the family will recognize signs of impending suicide attempt; will identify resources available.

☐ IMPLEMENTATION

- Discuss discharge plans and evaluate patient's acceptance of the need for mental health counseling; point out that such follow-up will strengthen own coping strategies and independence.
- Determine what resources are most comfortable and appropriate for patient follow-up (e.g., a school counselor, social worker, clergy, marriage/family counselor, mental health specialist, psychologist, psychiatrist).
- Teach family/peers warning signs of suicide (e.g., change in affect/behaviors, sudden poor grades, withdrawal from usual activities, giving away favored possessions, fascination with death/dying).
- Involve family as much as possible, especially for adolescents and the elderly; family therapy can be of great value in working through feelings of guilt, frustration, or anger.
- Provide information regarding available community support groups, hot lines, suicide prevention and crisis intervention centers, and local mental health facilities that provide a variety of services; provide information regarding alternative sources of assistance in case emergency sources are not available.
- After consultation with physician/family/friends, initiate appropriate referrals; arrange first contact prior to discharge from hospital.
- Know that a directory listing all suicide preven-

tion and crisis intervention centers throughout the country is available from the American Association of Suicidology, 220 West 20th Avenue, San Mateo, CA 94403; arrange to obtain one for staff use.

☐ **EVALUATION CRITERIA/DESIRED OUTCOMES**

The Patient
- States no present suicidal ideation
- Identifies and has telephone numbers of private

and community support groups and health centers providing assistance for suicidal individuals
- Agrees to call a designated person before attempting suicide

The Family
- States knowledge of the clues or danger signals of suicidal ideation; indicates immediate professional help will be sought if/when these occur

The Patient Who is Violent

Definitions/Discussions

Violence is any physical behavior destructive to self, others, or property.

Acting out is any aggressive/angry behavior short of violence and includes verbal and nonverbal threats.

Aggression is a state of inner tension causing some discomfort to an individual and energizing her/him to overcome the environment, often using gross motor behavior.

Nursing Assessment

☐ **PERTINENT HISTORY**

Previous episodes of violent or acting-out behavior, history of abuse to self or others, alcohol or drug use, history of emotional difficulties in person or family

☐ **PHYSICAL FINDINGS**

Physiologic disease processes (e.g., trauma, brain tumor, temporal lobe epilepsy, hormonal imbalance, organic brain syndrome); toxic reaction to chemicals, prescribed or nonprescribed drugs

☐ **PSYCHOSOCIAL CONCERNS/ DEVELOPMENTAL FACTORS**

Perception of self as worthless, helpless, impotent, hopeless; perception of environment as frightening, hostile; delusions or hallucinations; dysfunctional family throughout developmental stages to adulthood; dysfunctional communication patterns, drug or alcohol use; flight of ideas, looseness of thoughts, suspiciousness or paranoid ideation; fear of loss of control; increase of stressors within a short period of time

☐ **PATIENT AND FAMILY KNOWLEDGE**

Ability to recognize behaviors of anxiety, fear or suspicion; identification of motor retardation or agitation; dysfunctional family coping patterns and patterns of communication; community pattern that uses violence as a way of coping

Nursing Care

☐ **LONG-TERM GOAL**

The patient will develop and use alternative adaptive coping mechanisms to deal with aggressive impulses; the patient will experience control of own behavior and will not harm self or others.

NURSING DIAGNOSIS #1

Potential for violence: self-directed or directed toward others related to inability to control behavior

Rationale: Violence is a response to feelings of impotence and helplessness in the face of a perceived threat. As anxiety and stress increase, cognitive abilities decrease and the individual responds more to isolated stimuli and less to the content of the situation. The loss of control that results from the decrease in cognitive abilities may lead the individual to harm self or others.

☒ **GOAL**

The patient will cease any violent behavior; will experience control of violent behavior, with staff assistance; and will demonstrate increased ability to control aggressive impulses.

☐ **IMPLEMENTATION** *approaches*

- Be honest, clear, and concise during all interactions.
- Allow patient to remain in present position; give space and keep some distance away.
- Observe patient while placing self between patient and door if possible; do not turn back to patient; move slowly and deliberately.
- Ask others to withdraw and leave area; speak in a calm, quiet tone.
- Identify feeling of anxiety: "You seem upset; I'm concerned you might hurt yourself or others here."

- Encourage verbalization rather than acting out: "What happened to make you so upset just now?"; offer alternatives: "I'll walk with you and we can talk about this." "Let's walk back to your room and discuss this." "Let's have a cup of coffee and talk about it." "I'll stay with you while you hit the punching bag."
- Provide reassurance or support and set limits: "I want to help you control your behavior right now so that you do not hurt yourself or someone else."
- Assess patient's ability to use self-control; if unable to control self, assemble equipment and staff; four staff members necessary to restrain average-sized patient; if time available, staff should remove glasses or pens or other potentially harmful articles from their person; a blanket or sheet and soft leather arm and leg restraints may be needed; prepare a private room that contains a bed with a metal frame to which restraints can be secured; clear this room of other potentially dangerous items; hallway to room should be cleared.
- Explain "We're concerned about this behavior and we're going to help you control it now so that you don't hurt yourself or others."
- Distract the patient with blanket or sheet as if you were about to wrap him totally with it; during this attempt to distract, each staff member should take an arm or leg, raise patient off feet and place face down on floor, removing base of support for physically assaultive behavior; use good body mechanics and be aware of patient's body alignment to prevent injuries to staff and patient.
- Transport patient to room (each limb still carried by a staff member, with the legs carried from above the knees); if necessary for control, carry face down; protect head; if necessary, one staff member can carry both legs.
- Follow facility procedure for application of restraints; care should be taken to ensure that the restraints do not impair circulation or cause pressure to underlying nerves; **a patient in restraints must be monitored at all times;** stay with and encourage patient to express thoughts and feelings about the incident; explore the situation that cause increased anxiety and loss of control.
- Remove all items from clothing, especially potentially dangerous, sharp items, and matches.
- Obtain physician's order for restraints prior to or immediately after emergency situation; a parenteral medication may be given either at site of loss of control or after transporting patient to room.
- Take blood pressure and pulse every 30 minutes and check extremities for signs of lack of circulation or pressure; offer snacks and fluids; give mouth care as needed.
- Remove restraints as soon as possible when acute agitation subsides.
- Allow others who may have observed restraining and transporting to ventilate their feelings and

concerns about patient or their own potential loss of control.
- Explore violent episode or loss of control with patient; identify why this act was done at this time (e.g., did this act have a "payoff" of decreased anxiety or relief of frustration?).
- Help to identify precipitating factors that led to anxiety and impulsive behaviors.
- Assess knowledge of own symptoms of increasing anxiety; teach as needed; explore alternative, appropriate ways to deal with anxiety.
- Explore attitudes about and teach appropriate expressions of resentment, anger, frustration, and other intense emotions; explore alternatives to overcontrol and withdrawal; use role playing and practice assertion techniques in group and individual settings.
- Assess for knowledge and behaviors of problem solving and stress management; refer to *Problem Solving*, page 248, and Table 1, *Stress Management*, page 24; teach as needed, using patient's strengths to help with weaknesses.
- Validate appropriate responses to frustration, resentment, anger, and anxiety.
- Make contract that patient will contact staff member when feeling symptoms of increasing anxiety and possible loss of control; plan for alternative behaviors to control aggressive impulses and express feelings in effective, nonviolent way.
- Work with family/spouse/partner so they may understand and work with patient to develop and support new coping.
- Establish measurable, time-limited short-term goals with the patient.
- Assist to establish long-term goals.
- Contract with patient to spend a specific amount of time together each day (e.g., 20 minutes twice/shift).
- Utilize behavior modification techniques; reward for positive behavior verbally or by spending extra time with patient.
- Function as a positive role model.
- Encourage verbalization of anger rather than physically acting out.

☑ EVALUATION CRITERIA/DESIRED OUTCOMES

The Patient

- Verbalizes chain of events that have usually preceded a violent episode
- Verbalizes feelings that have preceded a violent episode
- Has developed at least 1 new alternative for dealing with aggressive impulses
- Expresses feelings in an appropriate way that is not harmful to self, others, or environment

NURSING DIAGNOSIS #2

Potential for violence related to sensory-perceptual alteration

Rationale: The perception of objects or individuals in the environment as hostile, frightening, or threatening may increase the potential for violence since the individual is unable to evaluate the environment realistically. Such sensory-perceptual alteration may be manifested by paranoia, suspiciousness, or hallucinations.

☐ GOAL

The patient will have decreased sensory overload, fear, and contributing factors (e.g., medication, drugs, alcohol); will learn to define and test reality.

☐ IMPLEMENTATION

- Establish a positive relationship; demonstrate an accepting attitude.
- Use same personnel for care to promote trust; be honest at all times; provide short, clear statements and answers regarding hospital policy, routines, and procedures.
- Decrease environmental stimuli noise level and remove extra equipment.
- Limit number of people present in surroundings.
- Discuss current concerns and feelings; identify available support systems.
- Help to verbalize fears concerning hospitalization and loss of power.
- Encourage and listen to expression of feelings.
- Allow maximum autonomy and self-care.
- Monitor effectiveness of any prescribed medications every 15 minutes; notify physician of any serious side effects, toxic reaction.
- Discontinue use of medications causing toxic reaction until patient treated by physician.
- Assess patient's behavior frequently (every 15-30 minutes).
- Provide for safety (remove belts, ties, shoe laces, razors, and other sharp objects.
- Assess for suicide ideation and intent; assess for suicide lethality; provide constant monitoring for the suicidal individual by staff.
- Interpret reality for patient experiencing hallucinations, delusions, or ideas of reference by saying that you do not see, hear, or believe these things and that s/he must be feeling very anxious and fearful right now.
- Supply external controls with one-to-one support.
- Assess with patient/family possible causes of the sensory-perceptual alterations.
- Help identify situations, persons, and objects that increase anxiety or stress and discuss adaptive coping methods.

- Provide physical activity in accordance with patient's abilities.

☐ EVALUATION CRITERIA/DESIRED OUTCOMES

The Patient
- Identifies environmental stressors and demonstrates one adaptive method of coping
- Differentiates verbally between hallucination and reality

NURSING DIAGNOSIS #3

Knowledge deficit regarding treatment plan, medications, follow-up care, adaptive coping mechanisms, reportable symptoms, community resources

Rationale: Inadequate preparation for discharge may lead to noncompliance with treatment program and to reversion to previous maladaptive coping mechanisms.

☐ GOAL

The patient will maintain daily needs (e.g., grooming, hygiene, nutritional care); will continue positive interpersonal interactions and effective communication; will use adaptive coping mechanisms in dealing with negative feelings and in the control of aggressive impulses; the patient/family will discuss treatment plan and follow-up care, including medication schedule and side effects to watch for.

☐ IMPLEMENTATION

- Determine ability to comply with medication and treatment plan.
- Teach the importance of adhering to the medication schedule; give patient responsibility for requesting and taking own medications prior to discharge.
- Teach side/toxic effects of medications; provide name and telephone number of health care provider/clinic to contact if side/toxic effects occur.
- Discuss and role play adaptive methods of coping with stressful situations.
- Include family in discharge planning whenever possible.
- Discuss follow-up care schedule and develop a specific written plan of care with patient; provide written direction as needed.
- Plan ways patient will maintain self after discharge; help write out personal goals.
- Discuss available community resources and support groups and provide list of needed groups.

☐ EVALUATION CRITERIA/DESIRED OUTCOMES

The Patient

- Lists medications; verbalizes importance of taking them; verbalizes schedule and potential side effects; states how to obtain refills
- Has appointment for follow-up care; knows how to contact physician/therapist/clinic if needs help prior to appointment date
- Maintains self on a daily basis as evidenced by maintenance of personal grooming, hygiene, adequate diet and interaction with others
- Knows community resources and support groups

Geriatrics

The Patient with Alzheimer's Disease

Definition/Discussion

Alzheimer's disease is a progressive deterioration in intellectual functioning caused by cellular degeneration and formation of "senile plaques" in the cerebral cortex. It is the major cause of severe organic brain dysfunction in older people and accounts for 50% of senile dementias; it is a strong factor in an additional 24%. Onset is insidious and may begin at any time from age 30 to old age.

Nursing Assessment

☐ PERTINENT HISTORY

Onset of dysfunction, disturbed memory function, failure of perception, decline in intellectual function, medications used, eating pattern

☐ PHYSICAL FINDINGS

Decreased ability to care for self, deterioration in appearance and hygiene, changes in gait, increased activity and movement (pacing)

☐ PSYCHOSOCIAL CONCERNS/ DEVELOPMENTAL FACTORS

Regressed behaviors, altered ability to cope with fears, anger, confusion, fantasies; disturbed memory function, failure of perception, progressive decline in intellectual functioning and communication; availability of family

☐ PATIENT AND FAMILY KNOWLEDGE

Prognosis, progression of family through stages of loss of functioning of loved one, treatment, medications, community resources; family's level of knowledge, readiness and willingness to learn

Nursing Care

☐ LONG-TERM GOAL

The patient will be maintained for as long as possible in a state of biopsychosocial integrity in a comfortable and protected environment; the family will receive information and emotional support.

NURSING DIAGNOSIS #1

Self-care deficit: hygiene, nutrition, toileting related to forgetfulness, confusion, regressed behaviors

Rationale: Patients with Alzheimer's disease have a progressive deterioration of function. Prognosis is poor with eventual breakdown of intellect and personality until the person is totally dependent on others; bowel and bladder control diminishes and the patient becomes like an infant.

☐ GOAL

The patient will receive help to maintain personal hygiene; will drink a minimum of 1,500 ml/day; will ingest prescribed diet; will maintain mobility as much as possible; will take prescribed medications.

☐ IMPLEMENTATION

- Evaluate the extent of patient's ability to care for self; provide assistance as required.
- Urge to do as much for self as possible; reward all efforts and accomplishments.
- If patient does not want to do an activity, do not argue, but do talk calmly and try to distract patient; when patient is calm, try activity again.
- Keep self-care/personal items within easy reach.
- Provide food and fluid intake compatible with caloric needs; many of these patients walk and pace and require a high-calorie diet.
- If patient is bedridden, perform range-of-motion exercises following physician's instructions at least once daily.
- Assess medication ordered for drugs known to lower serum folate levels (e.g., barbiturates, phenytoin, primidone, phenylbutazone, nitrofurantoin, some analgesics, and possible phenothiazines [Mellaril, thorazine, Compazine, Phenergan]); these drugs are contraindicated for persons with Alzheimer's disease unless a folic acid supplement is taken; know that alcohol also lowers serum folate levels and should be used sparingly.

155

- Work with family to set realistic goals for self-care/patient care at home.
- For additional nursing actions refer to *The Patient with Chronic Organic Brain Syndrome*, page 158.

☐ EVALUATION CRITERIA/DESIRED OUTCOMES

The Patient
- Maintains personal hygiene with assistance
- Ambulates daily
- Takes daily medications
- Ingests daily allotment of food and fluids
- Maintains clear lungs and normal vital signs

NURSING DIAGNOSIS #2

Alteration in thought processes related to forgetfulness, confusion, inability to perceive realistically or interact appropriately with others

Rationale: Symptoms may include disturbed memory function, failure of perception, and decline in intellectual functioning. Patients seem unaware of any changes in mental functioning and cannot understand why others are concerned about them. Many elderly persons with Alzheimer's become like good children and are amiable and cooperative. Twenty percent have paranoid reactions; as they begin to lose ability for insight and self-evaluation, they lose the ability to perceive self and others realistically. Suspicion, hostility, and hallucinations may occur.

☐ GOAL

The patient will be oriented to time/place/person; will interact voluntarily with others and with environment in socially appropriate ways; will communicate effectively with others.

☐ IMPLEMENTATION

- Know that a stable environment with warm acceptance will help patient achieve optimal functioning with the limitations of the disease process.
- Interview family to identify usual schedule, preferences, and adaptive coping mechanisms previously used by patient; utilize these as much as possible.
- Use environmental manipulation to assist patient to cooperate with plan for activities of daily living (e.g., make dining room a warm and inviting place with plants, pets [such as birds or fish], soft music, art objects, bulletin boards, round tables with opportunity for socialization and conversation during meals).
- Allow use of toilet articles brought from home, play soft music or relaxation tapes at rest or bed-

time; put daily schedule and clock in each patient's room.
- Give positive reinforcement with praise, smiles, and rewarding experiences for cooperation in activities.
- Establish an effective communication pattern; depending on degree of deterioration, patient's words may be unintelligible or not make sense and you may need to depend on patient's body language to understand what s/he is trying to convey.
- Speak calmly, clearly, and slowly, one sentence at a time and repeat as necessary; use short, simple sentences.
- If patient is confrontive, yelling, or belligerent, do not argue or raise your voice; speak gently and calmly and patient will calm down.

☐ EVALUATION CRITERIA/DESIRED OUTCOMES

The Patient
- Is oriented to time, place, and person
- Interacts with others in socially appropriate ways
- Makes some decisions about activities and leisure time

NURSING DIAGNOSIS #3

a. **Grieving** related to loss of functioning and role
b. **Knowledge deficit** regarding prognosis, grief and mourning process, treatment, medications, community resources

Rationale: The patient with Alzheimer's may be maintained at home or in various community settings. Family members need support and guidance so that they can directly or indirectly provide adequate care and safeguard the patient's quality of life, as well as progress through the stages of loss of a healthy and functioning loved one who is gradually deteriorating emotionally and intellectually.

☐ GOAL

The family will receive emotional support and information about disease process and prognosis.

☐ IMPLEMENTATION

- Assess family for stage of loss; offer to spend time with them for the purpose of ventilation of feelings and concerns.
- Know that your presence is comforting as the family goes through the process of grief and mourning for their previously normal, mentally-intact loved one who must be cared for in special ways.
- Accept family feelings in their time of actual loss

when the patient is diagnosed, when plans are made for long-term care, and as they anticipate the gradual deterioration in intellectual functioning and finally, death; refer to *The Patient Experiencing Grief and Loss*, page 80.

- Assess family's knowledge of the disease process and prognosis; clarify information and teach as needed; help them to understand, accept and cope with patient's behavior.
- Problem solve with family to discover ways they can visit and support patient (e.g., spend time reading to patient, bring in photographs or family albums, and share appropriate hobbies or interests with patient).

☐ **EVALUATION CRITERIA/DESIRED OUTCOMES**

The Family
- Expresses understanding of disease process, prognosis, and the prescribed medical regimen
- Recognizes need for ongoing care in a comfortable and protected environment
- Expresses understanding of grief and mourning process; grieves for loved one
- Has name and telephone number of attending physician, available community resource groups, social worker for financial and insurance help, and a mental health counselor for crisis and coping with chronic illness situation

The Patient with Chronic Organic Brain Syndrome

Definition/Discussion

Organic brain syndrome (OBS), also known as organic mental disorder, confusional state, brain failure, senile dementia, or senility, is a mental dysfunction due to the response of the aging brain to disease or damage. Chronic organic brain syndrome is caused by Alzheimer's disease (see page 155), cerebrovascular disease (a multi-infarct dementia, formerly called cerebral arteriosclerotic disease), intracranial neoplasms and infections, normal pressure hydrocephalus, and exposure to toxic substances. Chronic alcoholics may develop Korsakoff's syndrome from prolonged thiamine deficiency causing permanent neurologic damage and chronic dysfunction. Acute organic brain syndrome may be caused by a wide range of conditions (e.g., cardiovascular or respiratory disease, metabolic disorders, infection, drug intoxication, dehydration, and electrolyte imbalance).

Nursing Assessment

☐ PERTINENT HISTORY

Onset of dysfunction, impaired memory for recent events, disorientation, poor judgment, emotional lability, regressed behavior, altered ability to comprehend accurately, medications used

☐ PHYSICAL FINDINGS

Pathophysiology, activity level, status of sensory modalities, decreased ability to care for self, deterioration in appearance and hygiene

☐ PSYCHOSOCIAL CONCERNS/ DEVELOPMENTAL FACTORS

Regressive behaviors, disturbed memory function and intellectual functioning, altered ability to cope with fears, fantasies, paranoid delusions or other strange ideas; confusion; strengths; previous hobbies and interests; living arrangements

☐ PATIENT AND FAMILY KNOWLEDGE

Prognosis, progression of family through stages of loss of functioning loved one, community support groups, treatment, rules and procedures in care facility, level of knowledge, readiness and willingness to learn

Nursing Care

☐ LONG-TERM GOAL

The patient will be maintained for as long as possible in a state of biopsychosocial integrity with as much independence and contact with reality as possible.

NURSING DIAGNOSIS #1

Self-care deficit: feeding, bathing/hygiene, dressing, grooming, toileting related to confusion, forgetfulness, regressed behaviors

Rationale: As mental and physical dysfunction increase, the individual has a decreased ability to coordinate and perform activities of daily living (ADL) and self-care. With assistance and support, the patient may be able to resume self-care activities within limitations of mental and physical deterioration.

☐ GOAL

The patient will perform some ADL with minimal necessary assistance; will drink a minimum of 1,500 cc/day; will attain and maintain desired weight; will participate in exercise and rest periods daily, ambulating with assistance as necessary.

☐ IMPLEMENTATION

• Have patient do as much self-care as possible for as long as able; be readily accessible and willing to

help with dressing, feeding, ambulation, and ADL as needed.
- Consider safety and patient capabilities when planning care, not just your own time, convenience, or workload.
- Keep nursing care plan and expectations realistic; explain this approach to family/friends to preserve consistency.
- Record vital signs and intake and output at least once daily and weight at least 2 times/week.
- Offer 6 small feedings daily of nutritionally-balanced foods and fluids to achieve goals for fluid intake and output; assist with feeding as needed.
- Arrange for patient to have eyeglasses, hearing aid, false teeth, and other assistive devices as needed.
- Assist with choice of clean wearing apparel appropriate to climate.
- Supervise medication consumption (kind, time, and amount); know side effects of drugs given and carefully observe and record patient responses to all medications and treatments.
- Provide physical activity as possible; if not mobile, provide range-of-motion exercises at least once daily.

☐ EVALUATION CRITERIA/DESIRED OUTCOMES

The Patient
- Performs some ADL with assistance
- Maintains desired weight and fluid and electrolyte balance
- Has adequate rest and sleep
- Exhibits normal bowel elimination

NURSING DIAGNOSIS #2

Alteration in thought processes (disorientation, forgetfulness, confusion) related to cerebral pathology

Rationale: Confusion is a state of mental disorder, derangement, and perplexion in which attention, comprehension, memory, and perceptions are disturbed or adversely affected. It may be temporary, but in only 10%-15% of OBS cases is the confusion potentially reversible.

☐ GOAL

The patient will be oriented to time/place/person; will interact voluntarily with others and with environment in socially appropriate ways; will make some decisions and choices related to own care and activities; will reminisce to integrate life experiences.

☐ IMPLEMENTATION

- Get patient's attention before speaking; say name, wait for eye contact, speak slowly, distinctly, and loud enough to be heard; turn off radio, television, and shut out other distractions.
- Use a voice tone that indicates sincerity, sensitivity, respect, and acceptance.
- Give patient choices when possible, but avoid meaningless, unnecessary changes (e.g., in roommate, decor, routines), which are often upsetting to OBS patients.
- Answer questions repeatedly as necessary, using short, simple sentences; reinforce verbal communication with gestures; build on the sensible statements of the patient to strengthen reality-based conversation.
- Provide orientation to time/place/person every hour; use clocks, calendars, signs, pictures, and written reminders; put patient's picture and name (in big letters) on the door to room and on bed.
- Use concrete symbols (photographs, tangible creations, and products) of patient's past to strengthen and reassure patient's sense of continuity of self (now threatened with brain deterioration).
- Encourage to review past in order to remember and savor happy events, friendships, trips, achievements, etc.; even if content of reminiscences produces sadness, resentment, or angry outbursts, there is value in ventilation and working through those feelings before changing subject to a more pleasant one.
- Celebrate special events in patient's life (e.g., birthdays, anniversaries, religious days); observe customary national holidays with parties, decorations, special refreshments, and entertainment.
- Utilize volunteers to visit or write letters for patient, to show films, hold concerts, or entertain, to take patients for outings of grounds or in neighborhood, etc.
- Arrange for some kind of meaningful occupational therapy (e.g., simple repetitive activities such as clipping coupons, packaging items, stuffing envelopes).

☐ EVALUATION CRITERIA/DESIRED OUTCOMES

The Patient
- Is oriented to time/place/person
- Interacts appropriately with others
- Participates in some decisions about ADL
- Reminisces about life experiences

NURSING DIAGNOSIS #3

Ineffective individual coping related to confused state and uncontrolled, intense feelings (e.g., fear, anxiety, anger, sadness, depression)

Rationale: The individual with acute or chronic OBS experiences labile (rapidly shifting) emotions, which interfere with the ability to cope with change and the stress of everyday life. Anxiety, fear, confusion, and frustration may increase as physiologic and mental functioning decrease; accumulated losses (e.g., death of loved ones; loss of function, roles, independence; changes in living arrangements) may overwhelm the individual with intense and uncontrollable feelings of grief.

☐ GOAL

The patient will communicate feelings and concerns; will utilize previous coping methods (e.g., laughing, crying, joking, hobbies, comfort measures); will utilize new coping measures (e.g., comfort measures, relaxation, stress-reduction measures).

☐ IMPLEMENTATION

- Observe, describe, and record patient's common behavior patterns; identify cues that trigger adverse reactions and plan to avoid/control these; note whether patient is agitated by certain persons, topics of conversation, or situations.
- Recognize that episodes of paranoia, aggression, temper tantrums, delusions, anxiety, despondency, rigid orderliness, fears, fantasies, apathy, stubbornness might occur from time to time.
- Know that medication (tranquilizers usually) can control much asocial, difficult-to-handle behavior and need to be considered for the safety and peace of mind of family; reduce medication dosages when sufficient numbers of skilled geriatric personnel are available to work with patient.
- Interview family and friends to identify successful coping mechanisms previously used by patient for anxiety, depression, stress; attempt to incorporate their usage with necessary modifications.
- Show you care by providing small gifts (e.g., a flower, a favorite food or drink, a picture of a special pet or friend, a coathanger mobile of greeting cards); use touch therapeutically if you feel comfortable in doing so.
- Respect the patient's privacy (i.e., space, time, possessions).
- Try carefully planned music as therapy for relaxation, mood lifting, sensory stimulation, or as a vehicle for communication and not just as a monotonous alternative to background noise.

☐ EVALUATION CRITERIA/DESIRED OUTCOMES

The Patient
- Demonstrates increased ability to communicate feelings
- Demonstrates decrease in uncontrolled mood swings

- Discusses concerns and feelings
- Accepts comfort measures
- Participates in relaxation and stress-reduction programs

NURSING DIAGNOSIS #4

Knowledge deficit regarding prognosis, treatment, medications, community resources

Rationale: The aged patient with chronic OBS may be maintained at home or in a variety of community or hospital settings; the family needs support, guidance, and information so they can directly or indirectly provide adequate care and safeguard the quality of life for the patient.

☐ GOAL

The patient/family will discuss treatment plan and follow-up care, including medication schedule and side effects to watch for; will develop a plan to maintain daily needs such as hygiene, grooming, diet, and interaction with others; will use community resources.

☐ IMPLEMENTATION

- Educate family and friends so they will not withdraw from the patient; help them to understand and accept the patient's behavior, to accept and work through their feelings of helplessness, anger, depression, love, and guilt.
- Help family prepare for the patient's return home (if applicable) by raising questions, considering solutions, exploring alternatives, and deciding on a goal and plan of action that meets their needs as well as the patient's.
- Assess level of knowledge and ability to comply with medication and treatment plan.
- Teach the importance of taking medications daily; discuss their desired effects and side effects.
- Discuss a follow-up care schedule; develop a plan of activities to strengthen patient's thought processes (i.e., continue with implementations per Nursing Diagnosis #2).
- Encourage verbalization and questions; ask patient/family to describe medication, treatment plan, follow-up care, and symptoms to report to physician.
- Discuss community resources (e.g., support groups, residential facilities, day-care centers), and how to access them.

☐ EVALUATION CRITERIA/DESIRED OUTCOMES

The Patient/Family
- Expresses understanding of chronic disability and the medical regimen prescribed

- Indicates a willingness to continue to keep patient oriented to reality, interacting with others
- Recognizes need for ongoing medical and nursing supervision and consultation
- Has name and phone number of attending physician, community health nurse, and available community resource groups (e.g., Meals-on-Wheels, homemaker services, senior citizen self-help groups)

The Patient Coping with the Problems of Aging

Definition/Discussion

Aging refers to that period of adult development that occurs in the later years of an individual's life cycle. Presently, age 60-70 (or retirement age) is used as a marker. There are specific developmental tasks of this age period as with all others. Illness, loss of significant others, retirement among others may threaten the individual's ability to complete tasks of the last period of life.

Nursing Assessment

☐ PERTINENT HISTORY

Losses of friends and family members and how resolved, past physical history, styles of coping, present living arrangements

☐ PHYSICAL FINDINGS

Any chronic diseases and level of disabilities; physical changes common to the aging process (e.g., loss of acuity of sensory modalities, gait changes); sexual, dietary and sleep habits; activity level; current medications and response to medications

☐ PSYCHOSOCIAL CONCERNS/ DEVELOPMENTAL FACTORS

Support system; significant others; progress in developmental tasks of aging: desire/plan for leaving a legacy; desire/method of sharing accumulated knowledge with the young; familiar objects (homes, pets, heirlooms, photos) to which individual is attached; hobbies; changing sense of time of immediacy (since less time is left) and significance (of treasured objects and people); experience of age and disability; amount of independence and dependence; usual pattern of activities of daily living (ADL) (e.g., bathing, elimination, sleeping routines)

☐ PATIENT AND FAMILY KNOWLEDGE

Developmental tasks; need for mutual understanding, respect, love, and intimacy; availability of emotional and spiritual counseling; community services of seniors for activities, meals, and transportation at no or reduced costs

Nursing Care

☐ LONG-TERM GOAL

The patient will accept physical, emotional, and behavioral changes that occur in the later adult years; the patient will accept support and assistance for maintenance of a sense of self-identity and self-esteem.

NURSING DIAGNOSIS #1

Social isolation related to fear of being unable to obtain warmth and companionship from others

Rationale: *The individual with social isolation experiences a need or desire for contact with others but is unable to make that contact. The isolation is perceived as imposed by others. It is not voluntary solitude but is experienced as loneliness. It is a common concern and common experience of the older person partially related to decreased mobility.*

☐ GOAL

The patient will discuss reasons for feelings of isolation and ways of increasing meaningful relationships and diversional activities.

☐ IMPLEMENTATION

- Provide frequent contacts (staff, other patients, visitors) that are expressions of interest, concern, and involvement; seek out other patients with similar interests.
- Involve patient in planning when and with whom activities will be scheduled.
- Have patient list interests; consider past hobbies and new activities that might be learned.
- Encourage discussion of feelings and the reasons that they exist.
- Help identify strategies to expand the world of meaningful relationships.
- Do not isolate patient; encourage involvement in

planned social groups (e.g., friendly club, sports fan club, resocialization and recreational groups).
- Refer to appropriate community services.

☐ EVALUATION CRITERIA/DESIRED OUTCOMES

The Patient
- Expresses feelings of loneliness
- Plans for interaction with others
- Seeks contact with and participates with others

NURSING DIAGNOSIS #2

Grieving related to actual or anticipated losses, situational events

Rationale: The older adult experiences many losses. As part of the grieving process the patient will experience the stages of grief. Events such as having to give up one's home, roles, and/or loss of significant others precipitate the grief response. This occurs in increasing degrees and frequency with the older adult. Many responses of grieving may be frightening to the individual (e.g., confusion, fatigue, depression, and somatic symptoms). The individual may be afraid that these symptoms herald serious illness and needs to learn that even though these responses are uncomfortable they are typical. Feelings of guilt are part of the grieving process. When reviewing one's life events, guilt may be a response of the individual who does not appreciate the value of past life's work. Unresolved guilt can impede the grieving process resulting in ineffective coping. Aggression sometimes is experienced; with the older adult it is often directed at the losses experienced and at the indignities, neglect and lack of respect for the older adult.

☐ GOAL

The patient will resolve the loss and will mobilize hope and interest outside self; will accept the process of grieving as normal; will express feelings of guilt and accept support of others to resolve; will express anger appropriately.

☐ IMPLEMENTATION

- Assess for insomnia, despair, lethargy, anorexia, loss of interest, somatic complaints, refusal to participate in ADL.
- Identify losses the patient is experiencing (e.g., loss of body part, function, previous life-style, independence, loved one).
- Permit patient to respond behaviorly to the loss in any nondestructive way; reassure that the sadness, anger, loneliness associated with the grief process is normal, expected, and generally temporary; when the grief runs its course, the person

will be able to look towards the future, make new friends, and make plans about how life will go on.
- Discuss how the stress of multiple losses can exacerbate chronic physical problems and that careful attention to good health practices is essential during the mourning process.
- Assess for appropriate grief behaviors and intervene appropriately.
- Refer to *The Patient Experiencing Grief and Loss*, page 80.
- Support attempts dealing with the guilt; do not give any reassurance about the blaming since this response often evokes anger in the person who feels the guilt.
- Communicate that you respect and do not blame patient for any shortcomings.
- Lend perspective regarding how the person did the best they could under the circumstances, and how it is easier in hindsight to see a better way.
- Encourage the patient to forgive themselves and accept the circumstances as part of the human condition.
- Allow patient to express angry feelings without reprimands.
- Deal with physically destructive aggression by use of limit-setting; praise constructive or verbally expressed feelings.
- Refer to *The Patient Manifesting Aggression*, page 10 and *The Patient Manifesting Anger*, page 13.
- Refer to *The Patient Experiencing Depression*, page 57.
- Refrain from pity, overconcern, and rewarding patient for clinging, whining, or self-preoccupation behaviors.
- Praise all efforts at participating in daily care, talking to others, etc.

☐ EVALUATION CRITERIA/DESIRED OUTCOMES

The Patient
- Demonstrates grief behaviors appropriate to the phases of grief and mourning
- Acknowledges that process of grieving is appropriate and necessary
- Participates in ADL, activities, and interacts with others
- Grieves appropriately
- Verbalizes acceptance and feelings of worth
- Expresses guilt
- Begins to develop new ways of coping with guilt
- Expresses anger appropriately
- Expresses other feelings of frustration, fears, and sorrows

---

NURSING DIAGNOSIS #3

Anxiety related to pathophysiologic, situational, or maturational events

Rationale: Anxiety is a state in which the individual experiences feelings of tension and activation of the autonomic nervous system in response to a vague, nonspecific threat. Anxiety in the older individual may be triggered by illness, rehabilitation, dependence on others for ADL, threats to self-concept, loss of significant others, change in environment, sensory or motor losses, and financial problems. Overemphasis on physical symptoms may occur when an individual is concerned about health and well-being and coping with the future.

☐ GOAL

The patient will experience an increase in psychologic and physiologic comfort; will use effective coping mechanisms in managing anxiety; will focus on activities and interactions with others; will describe accurately own health status.

☐ IMPLEMENTATION

- Refer to *The Patient Experiencing Anxiety,* page 22.
- Stay with the individual; speak slowly and clearly.
- Support coping mechanisms of walking, talking, crying.
- Make as few demands as possible.
- Utilize face-to-face contact and conversation, especially when the focus is patient concern.
- Manipulate sensory stimulation to optimal level; refer to *The Patient Experiencing a Sensory Alteration,* page 129.
- Provide physical activity (e.g., walking, needlepoint, knitting) as a tension outlet.
- Use music therapy and dancing for relaxation.
- Assist in devising a plan to deal with anxiety.
- Show a sincere interest and desire to assess accurately and realistically all complaints, but refrain from showing excessive sympathy or concern; give correct information when needed about individual's status, and point out discrepancy between beliefs and actual status.
- Do not acknowledge the same complaints over and over by giving your attention to them; rather, give attention for positive efforts (e.g., doing own ADL, participating in activities).
- Base your evaluation and intervention on observed behavior and objective signs rather than asking how patient feels; this minimizes overemphasizing physical complaints.
- Keep patient busily involved in purposeful social or occupational activities and conversation.

☐ EVALUATION CRITERIA/DESIRED OUTCOMES

The Patient
- Focuses on activity and is able to concentrate on topic at hand
- Expresses that anxiety level is lower

- Has a plan for coping with anxiety in the future

NURSING DIAGNOSIS #4
Powerlessness related to feelings of lack of control

Rationale: Powerlessness is a state in which an individual perceives a lack of personal control over events or situations. This feeling of lack of power and influence occurs in many older people and is more common in older, white, male adults who have previously held responsible positions in society. Powerless individuals may display apathy, anger, or depression.

☐ GOAL

The patient will maintain a sense of control by identifying factors that are within control; will make decisions regarding care, treatment, and future when possible; will increase self-care activities.

☐ IMPLEMENTATION

- Refer to *The Patient Experiencing Powerlessness,* page 115.
- Give patient as much control as possible over planning and carrying out own care; let patient make as many decisions as possible.
- Be sure patient understands procedures and rules, condition and treatments, results of tests, encourage questions and answer them completely.
- Find some useful, appropriate daily activity and responsibility for patient to assume (e.g., messenger service, dining room duties, help with other patient, janitorial chores); praise efforts and successes.
- Encourage communication that promotes individual integrity by involving patient in establishing routine and giving patient as much responsibility as possible.
- Promote a well role by encouraging wearing of clothes and shoes in the daytime, eating meals out of bed and in a common dining room when possible, exercising, and planning an activity each day.
- Make patient responsible for bathing, grooming, getting to meals, and sensory input (gentle reminders may be necessary); offer praise for patient's efforts.
- Address patient by name preferred; avoid names like "Moms," "Honey," "Sweetie."
- Encourage to keep favored mementos at bedside.
- Allow liberal visiting of significant others.

☐ EVALUATION CRITERIA/DESIRED OUTCOMES

The Patient
- Participates in establishing and carrying out the daily routine

- Remains active and expresses satisfaction over self-care activities
- Experiences control over some part of life
- Makes decisions as possible

NURSING DIAGNOSIS #5

Ineffective individual coping related to hoarding, anxiety, powerlessness, and decreasing cognitive skills

Rationale: As the individual experiences decreasing control over the environment and loss of personal effects, hoarding may result. Hoarding means saving food, string, sacks, envelopes, or other miscellaneous items. The individual hoards in an attempt to keep things meaningful to him/her (from a limited choice). It is an attempt to control those things in the patient's environment.

☐ **GOAL**

The patient will surround self with familiar items of sentimental and personal value; will meet environmentally safe, clean standards for daily living.

☐ **IMPLEMENTATION**

- Provide reasonable shelves, closet and drawer space for photos, clocks, plants, letters, books, and cosmetic articles.
- Explain and enforce (kindly and firmly) rules for securing money, expensive jewelry, other valuables; provide patient/family with detailed list of items taken.
- Clean unit and bedside stand with patient's permission and presence.
- Try to obtain patient/family cooperation regarding storage of perishable food, explaining that it attracts insects, rodents.
- Provide with time alone to sort, look through, repack various personal items, mementos, etc., into suitcase or private box; show patient where these will be kept.
- Have bulletin boards or spaces to hang greeting cards, grandchildren's art work, etc.

☐ **EVALUATION CRITERIA/DESIRED OUTCOMES**

The Patient
- Keeps mementos in designated place and spends time with them regularly
- Participates in cleaning out unit or bedside stand

NURSING DIAGNOSIS #6

a. **Sensory-perceptual alterations: visual, auditory, tactile** related to aging
b. **Alteration in thought process** related to cognitive, mental deterioration

---

Rationale: This is a state in which the individual experiences or is at risk of experiencing a change in amount, pattern (meaningfulness), or interpretation of incoming stimuli. Specific disruptions that cause sensory-perceptual alterations in the aging may be social isolation, losses (environmental, motor, sensory, object person), attitudes and responses of others, and results of pathophysiology. Diminished acuity of the senses is to be expected with the aging process, and affects the individual's ability to receive and interpret information about the environment. Thus the older individual is at risk for misinterpreting stimuli, or confusion, and for altered level of alertness. Evening is the time of most confusion in the elderly and has been linked to the decrease of stimuli confronting the patient at that time.

☐ **GOAL**

The patient will receive optimal level of stimulation; will demonstrate contact with reality.

☐ **IMPLEMENTATION**

- Assess level of alertness and confusion daily.
- Assess for history of onset and duration if confusion develops, when worse, and when better.
- Determine amount and type of stimuli desired and needed by patient in context of the usual lifestyle (e.g., desired reading material, TV, radio, level of activity, social activities, support systems).
- Assist to incorporate desired meaningful stimuli into daily routine, alternating stimuli as boredom or fatigue set in.
- Provide clocks, newspapers, pictures, and personal effects as a way of orienting patient to daily life.
- Limit numbers of staff caring for patient at risk.
- Increase stimuli consciously in the evening by way of lighting, TV, radio, and most important of all, social contacts.
- Use reality orientation with the confused patient.
- Teach about medical regimen, nursing care plan, unit routine, and other information that will increase knowledge (and therefore control) of the environment.
- Reduce unnecessary stimuli: noises, equipment, extraneous personnel.
- Encourage significant others to visit frequently; know that loved ones are the most powerful, meaningful stimuli available, and that their pictures at the bedside are important.
- Spend as much time with patient as possible; introduce to other staff, volunteers, and patients for social contacts.
- Provide periods for rest throughout the day and undisturbed sleep at night.

☐ EVALUATION CRITERIA/DESIRED OUTCOMES

The Patient

- Remains alert and oriented; is free from injury
- Expresses satisfaction with the level of stimulation received

The Patient Requiring
Reality Orientation

Definition/Discussion

Reality Orientation Therapy (ROT) is a group of psychosocial techniques that continually stimulate the brain to function in compensation for brain damage caused by disease, injury, senility, or disuse deterioration. ROT involves a program of total professional staff and visitor actions along with patient activities on a 24-hour, 7-day-a-week basis. The earlier therapy begins following the onset of confusion, the more effective it is likely to be. The key to success is consistency of expectations, attitudes, and approach on the part of staff, family, and friends.

Nursing Assessment

☐ PERTINENT HISTORY

Hobbies and interests during adolescence and adulthood, job and family history, health history

☐ PHYSICAL FINDINGS

Physical status and limitations, prognosis; energy level, cognitive status (confusion, forgetfulness, times of day that cognitive functioning is better/worse, precipitating factors); status of visual, auditory, tactile senses

☐ PSYCHOSOCIAL CONCERNS/ DEVELOPMENTAL FACTORS

Family/support system, likes and dislikes for activities and hobbies

☐ PATIENT AND FAMILY KNOWLEDGE

Caretakers, environmental structures and layout; facility routine, rules and regulations, patient prognosis

Nursing Care

☐ LONG-TERM GOAL

The patient will regain contact with reality, behaving with lessened confusion, disorientation, forgetfulness, and dependency.

NURSING DIAGNOSIS #1

Sensory-perceptual alterations related to monotony, distortion, overload

Rationale: At the present, the patient is not able to interpret presenting stimuli accurately as s/he may be experiencing deprivation, monotony, distortion or overload.

☐ GOAL

The patient will correctly perceive sensory stimuli; will interpret environment more accurately than before ROT; will appear more alert and responsive.

☐ IMPLEMENTATION

- Secure eye glasses, hearing aid, false teeth, and other assistive devices needed for activities of daily living (ADL).
- Place patient in upright position, preferably walking or sitting as often as feasible.
- Provide physical exercise in different settings (e.g., a walk, exercises while sitting).
- Call attention to sights, sounds, smells, taste, and interpretation of these stimuli.
- Increase sensory input with flower arrangements, new taste treats, use of spices (e.g., sucking on a clove, putting spices into jars and smelling to identify, using various flavorings in tea or desserts such as mint, almond, orange, or lemon, as alternatives to vanilla and chocolate).
- Use a variety of music (e.g., marches, polkas, lyrical, restful, jazz, sing-along) via tapes, radio, records; sing to patient while giving care; arrange for music groups from local schools to give concerts.
- Refer to *The Patient Experiencing a Sensory Alteration*, page 129, for additional information and suggestions.
- Observe and record behavioral changes; communicate changes to other staff members/family.

167

EVALUATION CRITERIA/DESIRED OUTCOMES

The Patient

- Uses aids to sensory modalities (e.g., hearing aid, glasses, teeth)
- Responds positively to incoming stimuli
- Demonstrates some awareness of items in the environment
- Interacts with environment

NURSING DIAGNOSIS #2

Alteration in thought processes related to short attention span, disinterest, apathy

Rationale: The patient is experiencing a decrease in ability to think and problem solve. S/he may demonstrate forgetfulness, short attention span, or disinterest in the environment.

GOAL

The patient will demonstrate an increase in attention span; will concentrate for longer periods of time; will correctly identify self in environment; will know time, day, and date with the help of usual reminders such as clocks and calendars.

IMPLEMENTATION

- Plan an individualized orientation session based upon patient's specific needs; do not expect too much; keep goals attainable, in small increments.
- Identify previous and present reinforcers (rewards) that bring pleasure to the specific patient; incorporate this information into the written care plan and utilize whenever patient behaves in an acceptable or desired manner or gives a correct response.
- Think twice about placing a confused patient next to a nurses station so s/he can be more closely watched, as this is sometimes perceived as humiliating to the family/friends.
- Help reduce patient's frustrations by keeping questions to the easy, familiar, simple level until s/he achieves successful responses; allow sufficient time for patient to formulate and produce an appropriate reply.
- Provide clocks, calendars, and pictures of friends, family, pets, or favorite objects and interests (e.g., sports, nature, children, antiques); refer to these several times daily.
- Always address patient by name; state name of hospital and day of the week; add date with month and year.
- Conserve patient's energy for normal cognitive processes by reducing causes of fatigue (e.g., allow short naps, alternate periods of rest/exercise/teaching).

- Present facts in a friendly, kind, firm, yet matter-of-fact, simple, and clear manner; repeat, using same or different words ad lib.
- Reinforce information with sensory aids (e.g., audio, visual, tactile, olfactory) prn; ensure that patient has eyeglasses and hearing aid prn.
- Enlist help of family/friends/housekeeping staff to correct patient's misconceptions gently and pleasantly without criticism.
- Allow family and visitors to remain with patient as much as possible.
- Provide slow, careful, detailed information regarding all tests, treatments, medications, and care activities; try to elicit a reaction, comment, opinion, preference; praise any appropriate attempts to respond.
- Help patient assimilate knowledge provided by asking questions (who? what? why? when? how?); be patient, wait calmly for reply; smile and compliment patient for repeating information accurately; if patient cannot provide a correct answer, give the answer and ask to repeat it.
- Encourage to ask questions of staff and to write down questions for physician; help print or write as needed.
- Ask to identify feelings and thoughts; reflect these, encouraging elaboration.
- Use TV quiz shows, radio talk shows to stimulate thought; do not have music playing while teaching, conversing, or trying to stimulate brain function.
- Know that while the adaptive value of reminiscing has not been conclusively demonstrated, it is nevertheless considered to be beneficial for patients who may be otherwise confused on current events and recent memories; know that having patient review own life can sometimes provide important clues about former friends and activities that brought pleasure and satisfaction, can provide opportunities to enhance self-concept and self-esteem, and can provide a useful means to resolve old griefs or stressful events, thereby achieving a better level of adaption to present circumstances.

EVALUATION CRITERIA/DESIRED OUTCOMES

The Patient

- Correctly identifies self
- Recognizes staff/family members
- Increases time of concentration
- Uses clocks and calendars
- Begins to interact more with environment
- Is oriented to place

NURSING DIAGNOSIS #3

Knowledge deficit regarding daily schedule, activities of daily living

> **Rationale:** *When thought processes are altered some things are forgotten and must be relearned; this differs with each person.*

☐ GOAL

The patient will make some decisions and choices with increased frequency; will carry out some of own daily hygiene with increasing willingness and independence.

☐ IMPLEMENTATION

- Give certain kinds of control/choices and help to exercise this control (e.g., time or type of bath, location of chair in dayroom or dining room, type of fruit juice or food.
- Promote self-care within known abilities and limitations; give help as needed but do not take over tasks because it is easier or more convenient; allow patient plenty of time; do not hurry or show impatience as it may increase patient's feelings of helplessness and irritation.
- Avoid IV fluids and tube feedings unless absolutely necessary.
- Try to follow a set routine and assign the same care personnel as much as possible, as consistency and comfort will reduce confusion.
- Explain or demonstrate each new procedure slowly and repeatedly, as you assist patient to participate actively.
- Observe, report, and reward appropriately even small changes toward more independent behavior.
- Refer to *The Patient with a Dependent Personality Disorder*, page 54.

☐ EVALUATION CRITERIA/DESIRED OUTCOMES

The Patient
- Continues to make an increasing number of decisions and choices
- Performs as many ADL as is possible
- Performs treatments to the degree possible

The Patient Requiring Remotivation and Resocialization

Definition/Discussion

Remotivation is a type of nursing therapy that continually stimulates the patient to engage in activities for the productive use of time, for creative use of energy, and for restoration of desire to enjoy life more fully. Resocialization stimulates the patient to interact effectively with other persons and with the social environment. Together they improve the aged person's quality of life. These programs incorporate, but are not limited to, therapeutically designed, individualized rehabilitation (occupational, social, vocational, educational, recreational and/or physical therapy). They are used for brain-damaged or severely handicapped persons, but are more commonly employed for the aged patient. To be effective, nurses also need a fundamental understanding of the aged patient. Meaningful activities are geared to stimulate interest and participation. People need to feel involved in personal, loving, caring, and understanding relationships.

Nursing Assessment

☐ **PERTINENT HISTORY**

Losses experienced and methods of coping; level of resolution of losses; past occupations, skills, hobbies, and interests; changes in living arrangements

☐ **PHYSICAL FINDINGS**

Level of cognitive functioning; physical disabilities or limitations; esthetic problems such as odors, incontinence, surgery

☐ **PSYCHOSOCIAL CONCERNS/ DEVELOPMENTAL FACTORS**

Support system available; significant others and relationship to them, causes of feelings of isolation or depression, what makes feelings of isolation better or worse

☐ **PATIENT AND FAMILY KNOWLEDGE**

Developmental tasks, need for social contacts, meaningful projects, usefulness, availability of emotional and spiritual counseling, community resources and support groups

Nursing Care

☐ **LONG-TERM GOAL**

The patient will actively engage in activities designed to further knowledge, physical and mental fitness, and service to self or society; the patient will spend time with friends and relatives, initiating conversation, and focusing on others rather than on self.

NURSING DIAGNOSIS #1

Diversional activity deficit related to monotony of confinement or change in life-style

Rationale: *In this state, the individual experiences an environment that lacks interesting activities or pastimes, resulting in boredom or depression. Taking responsibility for doing something about a boring situation is a way to decrease boredom and increase activity. Activities should be planned with the individual's premorbid preinsitutionalization personality, hobbies, interests, and life achievements in mind. At the same time new skills, new interests, and new ideas can be introduced.*

☐ **GOAL**

The patient will demonstrate an interest and desire to participate in meaningful learning or doing activities; the patient will express feelings of satisfaction, pleasure, and accomplishment upon conclusion of remotivation sessions and redirect energy towards interests that are personally fulfilling.

☐ IMPLEMENTATION

- Portray a positive, enthusiastic attitude when discussing tentative plan with patient/family; encourage them to express goals, interests, and feelings; work out with patient/family a simple plan to achieve realistic goals.
- Encourage participation in group setting; ensure that all members feel welcome, needed, and recognized for their participation; talk to the whole group, redirect questions, give feedback, and help members to share need for information with each other.
- Know that having a group-directed, relaxed, work, or study session does not mean that the nurse/therapist is unprepared or uninformed, or that the session is completely informal without a goal or a well outlined plan.
- Let patient choose from a list of specific topics after selecting a general interest area (e.g., health, safety, nutrition, art, music, politics, gardening).
- Encourage members of the group (when ready) as they gain knowledge, skill, and confidence, to select topics, provide supplies or visual aids, read or give presentations, demonstrate a skill, or help others to grow within the group.
- Utilize group games (e.g., Bingo, card games), herb or flower planting activities, preparation of holiday or birthday gifts and decorations, arts and crafts to develop muscle coordination, new skills, and opportunities for socialized learning.
- Encourage patient to use strengths to help self and others.
- For teaching suggestions, refer to *Guidelines for Teaching Patients and Families*, page 229.
- Evaluate and document progress or change in patient's knowledge, behavior, and attitudes; remember effects are often short term unless remotivation sessions are continually ongoing and constantly reinforced with new ideas as well as repetition of knowledge and skills already gained.

☐ EVALUATION CRITERIA/DESIRED OUTCOMES

The Patient
- Discusses feelings of boredom and ways to increase diversional activity
- Engages in diversional activities with voiced satisfaction
- Expresses awareness of need for purposeful activity

NURSING DIAGNOSIS #2

Social isolation related to lack of meaningful relationships, alteration in life-style

Rationale: *Social isolation can result from a variety of situational and health problems that result in a loss of established relationships or a failure to generate new relationships. Social isolation is not a voluntary solitude, but is perceived as being imposed upon the individual. A person does not have to be alone to feel isolated. Lonely people tend to shun others.*

☐ GOAL

The patient will seek out the company of at least 1 other person; will demonstrate an interest in those around and in the environment; will increase communication skills, initiating conversations or single comments more frequently than before; will indicate an increase in confidence and self-respect through appearance and remarks.

☐ IMPLEMENTATION

- Assess patient's health status, background, and past or present interests to select (or offer choices of) most desirable activities (e.g., a walk outdoors, a visit to another section of institution, a drive, a sport event, musical or dramatic production, group games, attendance at religious services, shopping expedition).
- Discuss with passive, compliant patient in a matter-of-fact way the proposed social interaction, situation, or person s/he is to be with (e.g., scheduled activity, type of clothes needed, length of time it will take, expected behavior).
- Elicit comments, expressed preferences, choices of activity or companion after planned social activity; reward any positive behaviors with enthusiasm, smiles, and warmth; try to elicit an expression of choice about further similar contacts.
- Exercise judgment to avoid excessive stimulation, fright, or discomfort caused by too many strangers or too many activities too quickly; observe and record patient's reactions and adjustment to each new situation.
- Introduce 1 new patient or staff member at a time and allow time for getting acquainted; after a number of persons have become acquainted, arrange for small groups to meet for a specific purpose or activity.
- Prepare arrangements of wallet-sized pictures of staff members and patients with names and titles underneath; use these charts with patients and ask them to name each person they have met (while covering name underneath); offer special privileges or recognition to patients who can name them all or have made the most progress in learning names.
- Change beds or room assignments to encourage friendships, associates with mutual interests or similar backgrounds.
- Provide special recognition and celebration of birthdays or other important events and anniver-

saries; have other patients join in preparation and planning of treats, surprises, gifts, decorations, entertainment, selection of music.

- Assist patient to express feelings and concerns about social isolation and help cope with feelings associated with loneliness.

☐ EVALUATION CRITERIA/DESIRED OUTCOMES

The Patient
- Identifies reasons for feelings of isolation
- Discusses ways of increasing meaningful relationships
- Has increasingly more social contacts

NURSING DIAGNOSIS #3

Disturbance in self-concept: self-esteem related to life changes

Rationale: Purposeful activity is necessary for healthy self-esteem, optimal cognitive and physical functioning. The patient must be made aware of this and must assume responsibility for establishing a plan of activity that facilitates maintaining a healthy self-concept.

☐ GOAL

The patient will express awareness of the need for purposeful activity; will become involved in establishing a plan to increase self-esteem.

☐ IMPLEMENTATION

- Discuss patient's past experiences to identify present (or potential) successful coping mechanisms and strengths.
- Encourage to identify own strengths (e.g., "Tell me something you did that made you proud."); to talk about happiest period of life; to express dissatisfactions (e.g., with the younger set, with present society/government/economy); to describe what made life most worthwhile; to discuss philosophy of life/death/God/man; to talk about family, holiday celebrations, favorite foods, entertainers, sports, and sports figures.
- Assist to use past interests to plan for present activities/pastimes and to seek out new interests.
- Examine content of reminiscing sessions to identify possible fears, weaknesses, losses, regrets that may have a bearing on present perceptions, attitudes, opinions, or behavior; do not probe for details or offer interpretations; reinforce positive aspects.
- Offer support calmly through presence and quiet attentiveness if patient expresses angry outbursts, disappointment, resentments, vindictive or paranoid statements; do not attempt to quell the tirade

or reassure prematurely, but allow the ventilation for its healing benefits; then redirect reminiscences to more positive topics.

- Encourage to talk about something funny that happened long ago; use humorous incidents to relax tensions and feelings of discomfort, to restore a sense of perspective, not to avoid discussing painful stories.
- Arrange for room or age-mates who can share memories of similar eras.
- Lead a discussion group that follows a sequence of life-cycle events.
- Use photographs, scrapbooks, old letters, and memorabilia to jog story-telling; play songs, lead a sing-a-long, cook or serve foods that patient has not had for a long time.
- Discuss reasons one needs to have purposeful activity (e.g., self-esteem, cognitive functioning, physical functioning; use language and examples patient can understand).

☐ EVALUATION CRITERIA/DESIRED OUTCOMES

The Patient
- Becomes involved in establishing a plan to increase self-esteem
- Uses past interests and present strengths to plan for activities

---

NURSING DIAGNOSIS #4

Impaired social interactions related to fear, shyness, or lack of experience with group process

Rationale: The older individual benefits from group experience in several ways. A social milieu is created by the group. In addition, the older individual gets feedback from others who are experiencing similar feelings and issues, thus decreasing feelings of isolation. The older individual may not be aware of these benefits and this knowledge deficit must be corrected.

☐ GOAL

The patient will participate in group, listening actively, responding appropriately, offering comments, and relating with the other members; will express enjoyment or pleasure in the group activity; will express regret or sadness when it is over or when s/he must miss it.

☐ IMPLEMENTATION

- Plan formal structured group sessions of 4 to 8 patients to perform a task, study a topic, develop interest, or cultivate a hobby (e.g., sing-a-longs, travel or geography groups, sports fans, gardening club, charades or dramatics).

- Schedule regular times for meetings of group; limit length to 30 or 35 minutes because of short attention spans, need for change of positions.
- Use a small room and keep group members close to each other.
- Serve refreshments and have patient dress up for group meetings.
- Have group leader prepare for meeting by taking time to establish a personal, trusting relationship with each member prior to inviting them to join a group; social bonding of leader to member helps patients overcome fear of rejection and fear of attachment with anticipatory loss that are often the basis of resistance to joining a group; know that patients may also reject a group leader whom they feel will be leaving them after they become attached (e.g., a student leader on temporary assignment).
- Know that if group leader lowers the defenses of its members (thereby making them vulnerable to the painful loss of relationships), s/he must help them develop capacity to sustain other relationships so they can reduce and offset the painful discomfort of losing their leader.
- Share own feelings of attachment and subsequent sadness with group when group experience is about to end; this will help members to share their feelings openly.
- Allow and encourage patients to facilitate participation by each member; reward each person's contribution; encourage members to interact with each other, not just with the leader whom they trust.
- Keep membership of the group stable so that trust, openness, and role identification can take place; encourage members to shake hands, hug or kiss, welcome each other, express concern over how member feels, etc.
- Form a reminiscing group wherein members share experiences, accomplishments, travels; as group leader, listen attentively, express appreciation to contributing members, reinforce the value and importance of life-review reminiscing; acknowledge feelings expressed; encourage both negative and positive feelings ("It's all right to feel that way."); teach family members the significance of reminiscing behavior and how to encourage its satisfying expression.
- Consider establishing an intergenerational sharing program with local preschools or elementary schools whereby mutual visits can occur and friendships can develop.
- Explore the feasibility of having community-based senior citizen groups meet at the health care facility for luncheons, cards, movies, concerts, or other reasons so that inpatients may attend and become involved with others in community.
- Know the therapeutic value of programs and facilities that allow pet-visiting privileges and in-house animal "mascots" or birds; explore feasibility of establishing pet-oriented project in your geriatric facility.
- Hold staff and family conferences about the patient's progress, needs, social relationships; involve patient in these conferences to contribute own perceptions, ideas, and choices.

☐ EVALUATION CRITERIA/DESIRED OUTCOMES

The Patient
- Participates in group experiences
- Expresses enjoyment or pleasure in social contacts and group activities

Children

The Child Experiencing Anxiety

Definition/Discussion

Anxiety is the uncomfortable feeling of tension or dread that is unconnected to a specific stimulus; it can be vague or intense. It occurs as a reaction to some unconscious threat to biologic integrity/self-concept. Anxiety can be assessed according to level.
- *Mild:* increased alertness and motivation; increased ability to cope with daily problems
- *Moderate:* decreased perception of the environment with selective inattention; decreased ability to think clearly
- *Severe:* drastically reduced perceptual field; able to focus on only one detail at a time
- *Panic:* inability to integrate environment with the self; cannot function; physical activity is disorganized; the child may be "frozen"

Anxiety can be used as a motivating rather than a destructive force if it is recognized and successful coping mechanisms developed.

Nursing Assessment

☐ PERTINENT HISTORY

Recent environmental/family/school/life-style changes, family/employment stability, losses, absence of supportive relationships, confusion of values/beliefs, previously experienced anxiety and coping methods, financial/health status, accident proneness, child abuse/neglect, chronic fatigue, change in appetite, grinding of teeth during sleep, pain

☐ PHYSICAL FINDINGS

Increased vital signs, muscle tension, sweating, headaches, dizziness, tremors, sweaty palms, flushing, fatigue, GI discomfort/dysfunction, hyperventilation, somnolence or insomnia, nightmares, crying, irritability, dry mouth, capillary dilation, inability to concentrate/understand explanations, shortened attention span for age, bed wetting, frequent urination, headache, stuttering

☐ PSYCHOSOCIAL CONCERNS/ DEVELOPMENTAL FACTORS

Developmental level, age-appropriate ability to express self, degree of perceived disruption, feelings/attitudes associated with the disruption, patterns of dependency, coping patterns of family, socialization pattern (e.g., values, belief systems, culture), habits/routines (e.g., play times, favorite games, sleep/naps, preferred foods), deterioration in school performance, emotional instability/tension, impulsive/regressive/neurotic/psychotic behaviors, sexual acting out, withdrawal from peer/social groups

☐ PATIENT AND FAMILY KNOWLEDGE

Identifiable cause(s), realization that both positive and negative stressors lead to anxiety, involvement of community agencies, level of knowledge, readiness and willingness to learn

Nursing Care

☐ LONG-TERM GOAL

The child will cope effectively with anxiety and use it as a motivation for change as appropriate.

NURSING DIAGNOSIS #1

Ineffective individual coping related to perception of situation

Rationale: Anxiety of more than a mild level will impair the individual's ability to cope.

☐ GOAL

The child will cope with the anxiety and reduce it at least one level.

☐ IMPLEMENTATION

- Use interventions appropriate to level of anxiety
  mild: does not require any intervention
  moderate
  - determine cause if possible
  - do not allow your own personal anxieties to be perceived by the child
  - spend 5-10 minutes with the child at least 3 times daily; show interest and support

- use age-appropriate techniques to discuss situation (e.g., drawing, telling a story, or situation completion ["There once was a little boy/girl who was upset over. . ."], throw bean bags at targets, play tag); refer to *The Child Requiring Play Therapy*, page 220
- allow child to cry
- do not make demands
- do not argue with/confront the child regarding unrealistic perceptions
- focus on the immediate problem; stay in the "here and now"
- explain all treatments/procedures to child in developmentally appropriate language
- do not give more information than child can handle
- be clear and concise in communication/explanations; repeat if needed
- attend to physical comforts and needs
- teach relaxation exercises; refer to Table 1, *Stress Reduction Activities*, page 24

severe
- use previously stated interventions as applicable
- stay with child until anxiety is lessened
- provide a calm, quiet environment
- have child take slow deep breaths if hyperventilating; ask to focus on how body feels on expiration; breathe with child to provide support
- use brief, simple communications
- structure activities into concrete tasks that do not require concentration
- attend to somatic complaints
- administer medication if ordered; evaluate effectiveness

panic
- use previously stated interventions as appropriate
- do not leave child alone
- demonstrate competence; remain calm; use firm, professional manner
- use a small room or separate area to provide privacy and security
- use physical touch judiciously; some children are comforted by touch and some are threatened by it
- reassure child that control will be maintained
- direct child's energy into repetitive motor activities
- observe closely

☐ EVALUATION CRITERIA/ DESIRED OUTCOMES

The Child
- States anxiety is decreased to a tolerable level
- Demonstrates behaviors indicating a decrease in anxiety
- Channels energy into goal-directed activity

NURSING DIAGNOSIS #2
Sleep pattern disturbance related to anxiety

Rationale: *Physiologic disturbances caused by anxiety may be reflected in a disturbance in sleep patterns.*

☐ GOAL
The child will achieve a sleep/rest pattern appropriate to age/developmental needs.

☐ IMPLEMENTATION
- Determine type of sleep disturbance child is experiencing.
- Ask what the child/parents perceive as the reasons for the disturbed sleep pattern.
- Provide measures appropriate to reduce insomnia
  - maintain a quiet, secure environment
  - use relaxation techniques (e.g. rocking to sleep, rubbing back, singing lullabies, night light)
  - decrease the number of distractions (e.g., temperature taking during night)
  - structure bedtime routine to match home routine (e.g., consistent time, bath, reading, warm drink, music, security blanket, amount of covers, type of bed clothing)
- Provide daytime stimulation; schedule time for physical activities; discourage napping and dozing (as age appropriate).

☐ EVALUATION CRITERIA/DESIRED OUTCOMES
The Child
- Falls asleep within 20 minutes
- Appears rested, has energy for daytime activities

NURSING DIAGNOSIS #3
Knowledge deficit regarding recognition and effective management of anxiety

Rationale: *Children/parents can cope effectively with anxiety if they learn to recognize it. New coping strategies can replace old ineffective coping skills.*

☐ GOAL
The child/parents will identify sources of anxiety; will employ effective measures to manage anxiety.

☐ IMPLEMENTATION
- Be aware of the impact of anxiety on ability to learn

- *mild*: learning can occur at this level
- *moderate*: learning can occur but it must be directed
- *severe*: inability to learn at this level
- *panic*: unable to learn
- Continue planned interactions with child.
- Teach parents to recognize that a change in school performance may indicate anxiety.
- Help identify those tensions and environmental factors that create a feeling of anxiety; attempt to identify precipitating factors/situations.
- Give careful, age-appropriate explanations; encourage questions and verbalization of any concerns that child may have.
- Stress the importance of patience since the child may not respond as before.
- Involve family in prevention/management of anxiety as much as possible; include in decisions about care.

- Teach the importance of regular physical activity.
- Provide positive reinforcement to parents who maintain an environment that allows an understanding of/control over the anxiety.
- Discuss alternatives to, advantages, and disadvantages of reducing stressors; explore ways to alter stressors.
- Provide information regarding available community support services.

☐ EVALUATION CRITERIA/DESIRED OUTCOMES

The Child/Parents
- List environmental factors that elicit anxiety
- Discuss ways of keeping anxiety at a mild or moderate level
- State willingness to learn new coping strategies
- Verbalize ways to cope with severe anxiety if it occurs

The Child with Autism

Definition/Discussion

Autism is a severe developmental disorder with neurologic, perceptual, physiologic, and behavioral dysfunction in the child under 30 months of age. The *DSM-III-R* classification is Pervasive Developmental Disorders. Previous diagnostic labels included symbiotic psychosis and infantile autism (for children age 30 months to 12 years, the term is Childhood-Onset Pervasive Developmental Disorder). There is a positive outlook for the child able to establish meaningful speech by age 5 years; if not, the child has a poor prognosis and will probably need institutionalization or eventual residential care.

Nursing Assessment

☐ PERTINENT HISTORY

Unstable sleeping and eating patterns, slow and unusual language development, disturbed perceptual-motor development, withdrawal from relationship with parent or caretaker, self-stimulatory behaviors (e.g., body rocking, head banging, twirling, staring at lights), self-absorption, self-mutilating (e.g., picking at skin, hitting/banging body or head with resulting bruises)

☐ PHYSICAL FINDINGS

Symptoms of present illness, associated health problems and handicaps, inadequate nutrition, poor hygiene, changes in vital signs

☐ PSYCHOSOCIAL CONCERNS/ DEVELOPMENTAL FACTORS

Refer to *Normal Growth and Development*, pages 231–245; motor skills: possible delays in motor skills and adaptive behavior, or may be age appropriate with good large-motor coordination; language skills: possible immature grammatical structure, echolalia (echoes words or phrases), confused word meanings, developmental aphasia (mute); visual/perceptive problems: avoidance of eye contact, lag in ability to separate figure from background; may prefer peripheral vision with moving objects recognized more easily than stationary ones; social/interpersonal skills: isolation or withdrawal from relationship with parent or care

giver, lack of emotional responsiveness, no cuddling into parent's body when being held, no reaching out to parent/care giver in anticipation of being picked up, no separation anxiety, restricted and isolated play, ignoring interactions with others, child's strengths and abilities, usual schedule of activities of daily living (ADL)

☐ PATIENT AND FAMILY KNOWLEDGE

Parent/family strengths and abilities, coping techniques for problem behaviors, knowledge of condition and treatment plan, prognosis, readiness and willingness to learn

Nursing Care

☐ LONG-TERM GOAL

The child will grow and develop at own pace, increasing adaptive behaviors and decreasing maladaptive behaviors; the child will maintain/improve physical, social, and emotional functioning to own optimal level; the parents/family will accept child and make plans for care at home or in residential setting.

NURSING DIAGNOSES #1
a. **Impaired communication: verbal** related to neurologic dysfunction
b. **Impaired social interaction** related to dysfunctional behavior
c. **Alteration in parenting** related to child's withdrawing behavior

Rationale: The autistic infant is quiet and self-absorbed; as the infant demands little contact, the parent/care giver tends to decrease contact, initiating mutual withdrawal. The lack of infant-parent attachment is manifested by the infant's lack of anticipation of being picked up by parent, failure to mold to body of parent, and absence of separation anxiety. This withdrawal from the parent/care giver has a profound influence on the infant's communication and interpersonal skills; the parent/care giver tends to feel inadequate, helpless, and avoid contact with the infant. This cycle of withdrawal and dysfunctional communication interferes with establishment of parenting and continues as the infant becomes a toddler and preschooler.

☐ GOAL

The child will demonstrate ability to tolerate an increasing amount of contact with staff/parents; the parents will demonstrate increased ability to relate to child.

☐ IMPLEMENTATION

- Approach in unhurried and calm manner; begin by sitting near child and greeting in quiet, friendly voice.
- Note what objects or activities child likes and use these to spend time interacting with child; establish eye contact using favorite toy, food, music, or doing child's favorite activity.
- Use favorite soft toys (e.g., stuffed animals, hand puppets, blankets) to touch and stroke child.
- Touch gently in ADL, feeding, and when talking and playing; teach child games that require touch (e.g., "this little piggy," "pat-a-cake").
- Do not give up if child withdraws or does not respond; continue touching and interacting on a regular basis, increasing time gradually as tolerated.
- Demonstrate these interaction techniques to family members and assist them to touch and interact with child on a regular basis.

☐ EVALUATION CRITERIA/DESIRED OUTCOMES

The Child
- Tolerates increased contact with staff/parents
- Responds in adaptive ways to contact (e.g., allows staff/family to touch, bathe, help with hygiene, read, sing, play with toys)
- Interacts using simple words and short sentences expressing own needs

The Parents/Family Members
- Demonstrate ability to contact and relate to child

NURSING DIAGNOSIS #2

Ineffective individual coping related to hospitalization, new environment, new care givers

Rationale: The child may react intensely to changes in environment (e.g., new care giver, change in schedule) with an emotional outburst or rage, crying, screaming, or unusual fearfulness. The child may insist on specific ritual in daily life (for sense of sameness and control).

☐ GOAL

The child/parents will express feelings and concerns about hospitalization; the child will adjust to hospital environment; will accept care from staff and parents.

☐ IMPLEMENTATION

- Assess child's/parents' level of understanding and acceptance of hospitalization and health status; allow time for child/parents to express feelings and concerns in their own way.
- Accept feelings in nonjudgmental way; allow parents to be the experts on the child and ask for their assistance to interpret child's communication and behavior.
- Assess strengths and abilities of child/parents, usual schedule of ADL, level of functioning, preferences, and rituals; include these in nursing care plan.
- Assign same staff member to child as much as possible; provide sameness and consistency in nursing care (autistic child will not respond well to change).
- Permit toys or blankets from home to stay with child; provide toys appropriate to age and level of functioning.
- Know that these children tend to withdraw from contact with others; schedule regular time to be with child each shift; utilize ADL to interact with child and to build trusting relationship.

☐ EVALUATION CRITERIA/DESIRED OUTCOMES

The Child
- Expresses feelings and concerns about hospitalization and hospital routines as possible
- Accepts care from staff and parents

NURSING DIAGNOSIS #3

Potential for injury related to developmental delays

Rationale: Developmental delays in speech with difficulty in communicating pain, discomfort, and other needs; disturbed perceptual-motor development with lack of understanding of safety rules and/or lack of impulse control; a tendency to increase self-stimulation; and self-mutilating behaviors when fatigued or adjusting to changes all increase the autistic child's potential for injury.

☐ GOAL

The child will experience minimum pain and discomfort; will be safe from preventable accident or injury.

☐ IMPLEMENTATION

- Observe for restlessness, agitation, or changes in vital signs that might indicate pain, fever, infection, or other complications.
- Remember that these children may not use words to communicate needs so that ongoing observation and assessment is essential.
- Observe for fatigue and provide for daily naps and rest periods.
- Identify situations that precipitate head-banging or picking behaviors; protect child by using helmet or other protective devices.
- Encourage child to express needs and feelings in acceptable ways (e.g., gestures, words, sounds, toys).
- Check frequently that safety rails remain up and seat belts are in place; if restraints are necessary, check underlying skin frequently.
- Offer comfort measures (e.g., blankets, toys, pillows) to comfort and divert; know that touch or holding may not be comforting to an autistic child.
- Refer to individual nursing care plans for specific disease entities.

☐ EVALUATION CRITERIA/DESIRED OUTCOMES

The Child
- Experiences comfort and relief from pain
- Is free from self-inflicted injury and discomfort
- Experiences no accident or injury

NURSING DIAGNOSES #4

a. **Self-care deficit: feeding, hygiene, dressing, toileting** related to perceptual impairment
b. **Knowledge deficit (parental)** regarding behavior modification techniques, treatment plan, procedures to be carried out after discharge (e.g., dressings, medications, assessment for complications, reporting complications); follow-up care

Rationale: The autistic child has problems learning self-care related to perceptual-motor dysfunction, poor communication skills, and social withdrawal. Parents may need to learn behavior modification techniques as well as preparation for discharge.

☐ GOAL

The child will develop and maintain as much independence as possible in ADL; will ingest adequate food and fluid to meet body needs; will maintain skin integrity; will increase adaptive behaviors; the parents will learn and demonstrate behavior modification techniques in ADL; will demonstrate technical

skills/procedures to be carried out after discharge; will discuss follow-up care and community support resources.

☐ IMPLEMENTATION

- Identify problem areas in ADL (e.g., toilet training, dressing, bathing, eating).
- Allow child to do as much of usual ADL as is possible considering health status and hospitalization; encourage parents to interact and assist child as needed with ADL.
- Work out a positive reinforcement program and include it in the nursing care plan; review program with parents to ensure their understanding and compliance; ensure that they utilize behavior modification consistently with their child.
- Use child's need for ritual and sameness to assist with developing health hygiene and eating habits.
- Use child's own words or teach simple words and concepts; break concepts and procedures into small components and allow child to practice and talk about each component, giving positive reinforcement and constructive feedback with each practice.
- Use passive and active range-of-motion exercises as tolerated; encourage as much ambulation as tolerated.
- Ensure adequate intake of food and fluid; use supplements when necessary and allow choices of food when possible.
- Measure and record intake and output; note frequency and consistency of bowel movements.
- Remain with child during mealtime and until medications are safely swallowed; observe for mouthing of nonfood items.
- Preserve skin integrity by massage, bathing, use of lotions, sheepskins, water mattress; if incontinent, maintain cleanliness of child and bed with a matter-of-fact attitude.
- Teach parents essential nursing care and required skills (e.g., dressings) as needed.
- Offer verbal encouragement and support to parents; offer hope that this child will learn healthy habits and adaptive behaviors as each task is broken down into small behaviors and each desired behavior is consistently rewarded.
- Inform parents that child will learn healthy habits of ADL at own pace and that parents can learn techniques to cope effectively with behavior problems.
- Discuss treatment plan for discharge including medications, side effects, symptoms to report to physicians, procedures, and community resources.

☐ EVALUATION CRITERIA/DESIRED OUTCOMES

The Child
- Demonstrates self-care in eating, dressing, bathing, toileting

- Ingests adequate food and fluid to meet needs for growth and development
- Maintains skin integrity

The Child/Parents
- Are increasingly able to cope with ADL
- Demonstrate technical skills or procedures to be carried out after discharge and have an adequate amount of supplies

- Have a written list of medications, dosages, and schedules; state actions, possible side effects, and action to be taken
- Have an appointment for follow-up with physician/clinic and a referral to a community support agency (for language training, advice and counseling regarding appropriate preschools, schools, institutions, parent support groups)

The Child Experiencing a Body-Image Disturbance

Definition/Discussion

Body image is a person's image or concept of his/her own body. It is formed from internal development as well as from environmental experiences including input from others, societal views, cultural practices, and previous experience with persons whose bodies have changed.

Although the term "body image" is rarely used in conjunction with very young children, the child's sense of body is critical to early development. During the toddler phase of development, autonomy is the goal as the child strives for some body control. The child becomes aware of his/her body and its totality. The disappearance/removal of any body part threatens the child's existence (e.g., during toilet training, ritualistic activities may be necessary before the child will flush or allow the toilet to be flushed).

The preschool child begins to see self in relation to the rest of the world. However, thinking is not consistent with adult realities; magical thinking is the rule and the child views the world in relation to those things that are familiar (e.g., compares own body to a balloon—if there is a hole, all the air inside will leak out; a preschooler with a cut finger will not be consoled until a Band-Aid is placed on the cut to keep everything inside from leaking out). Children of this age also take things/words literally (e.g., on hearing "Jake will cut off his nose to spite his face," the child will picture Jake without his nose).

School-age children begin to look at the world in a more rational manner; at the same time, peers begin to play a significant role in the child's life. The child compares self to same-sex peer group (e.g., being the tallest boy or girl in the class may be very exciting or upsetting to the child). There is some evidence suggesting that children become weight conscious during the middle school-age years. Adolescents are very body conscious; the onset of puberty creates a great deal of confusion and body changes are magnified. The adolescent has a need to be the same as peers and deviations are not acceptable.

A body-image disturbance reflects the inability of an individual to perceive/adapt to an alteration in structure, function, or appearance of a part of or the entire body.

Nursing Assessment

☐ **PERTINENT HISTORY**

Surgeries, illness, trauma causing change in body form; rapidity of change; permanent or temporary refusal to participate in care; denial of change(s)

☐ **PHYSICAL FINDINGS**

Loss of body part or its function; neurologic, metabolic, or toxic disorders; anorexia/obesity; progressively deforming disorders; acute dismemberment; disability or handicap; visibility of change; withdrawal, apathy, crying, agitation

☐ **PSYCHOSOCIAL CONCERNS/ DEVELOPMENTAL FACTORS**

Cognitive/social/emotional/developmental level, academic achievement, peer relationships, previous experience with someone with altered physical appearance, cultural practices, coping patterns, personality style, dependency patterns, depression, shame, physical/sexual abuse, habits (e.g., what comforts child, eating/bedtime routines, favored objects)

☐ **PATIENT AND FAMILY KNOWLEDGE**

Possibility of rehabilitation or repair, degree of change in life-style and functional significance, value placed on alteration, perception of what change means, available community agencies, level of knowledge, readiness and willingness to learn

Nursing Care

☐ **LONG-TERM GOAL**

The child will acknowledge and integrate body change(s) into adaptive and realistic management of own life.

NURSING DIAGNOSIS #1
Disturbance in self-concept: body image related to altered body structure or function

Rationale: A real or perceived change in body image results in a need to modify one's self-concept. Certain areas of the body have greater value and meaning to an individual; threats to these areas cause more disruption and require more adjustment.

☐ GOAL

The child will acknowledge and begin to accept body change(s).

☐ IMPLEMENTATION

- Provide openings to enable child to express feelings by validating your observations and feelings (e.g., "You look down in the dumps. How are things going for you today?" or "You seem upset/sad. Are you?" Show child pictures and have him/her describe how the child in the picture is feeling and why); recognize that acting out behavior may be the child's way of expressing frustration; refer to *The Child Requiring Play Therapy,* page 220).
- Be a good listener and accept what child verbalizes; remember not to take anger or hostility personally (this may be the only way possible for the child to handle these feelings).
- Focus on the child's feelings and deal with the presenting behavior (e.g., do not challenge child's denial that a body change has actually occurred).
- Determine what the body-image change means to the child and what effect the child thinks it will have on life; do not challenge perceptions you think are unrealistic, but continue to provide opportunities for child to share these perceptions and feelings with you.
- Be accepting of child's body changes; if child is repulsed or ashamed of physical changes, s/he will be watching the faces of others for negative signs; assist the family to accept changes also and to avoid reinforcement of the child's negative feelings.
- Provide basic needs for child; dependent behaviors/regression in developmental achievements may be exhibited at this time.
- Assist child to normalize the change; use developmentally appropriate strategies (e.g., develop rituals, provide rational explanations, use make-up/adaptive devices to appear just like everyone else).
- Let the child know that the feelings and concerns that are being experienced are normal and that you are there to listen as well as to help cope with the changes.

☐ EVALUATION CRITERIA/DESIRED OUTCOMES

The Child
- States that a change in the body has occurred
- Begins verbalization of feelings regarding the change

- Exhibits fewer negative reactions to staff and environment
- Shows occasional interest in self-care

NURSING DIAGNOSIS #2

Grieving related to loss or alteration in body form, function

Rationale: Resolution of a loss through successful management of the grief process will allow the child to progress effectively toward adjustment to changes in body structure and function.

☐ GOAL

The child will acknowledge, express, and resolve grief related to change(s) in body form or function.

☐ IMPLEMENTATION

- Recognize individual responses to grief; these are determined by ego strengths, perception and meaning of loss, previous experiences, and present support systems; refer to *The Parent Experiencing Grief and Loss,* page 211, for review of the grief process.
- Know that the nurse's personal feelings toward loss must be recognized before the nurse can accept those of others.
- Be empathic and understanding; educate child/family regarding normal grief reactions to permit more realistic expectations.
- Encourage verbalization of feelings toward the loss of the body part or function (e.g., the pleasures provided and the needs it fulfilled in the past) in order to promote acceptance and to lessen denial.
- Allow child to cry.
- Be alert for signs of depression (e.g., isolation or withdrawal, inability to grieve, fatigue, anorexia).
- Do not encourage fantasizing or false hopes regarding reversal of change in body form or function.
- Know that resolution of loss is accomplished a little at a time; be realistic about time required to achieve resolution.

☐ EVALUATION CRITERIA/DESIRED OUTCOMES

The Child
- Verbalizes/demonstrates, through play, sadness and feelings of loss
- States what the body change means
- Shows evidence of adapting to body change

NURSING DIAGNOSIS #3
Knowledge deficit regarding adaptation to alteration in body image

Rationale: When body changes occur, new coping mechanisms and changes in life-style may be required for successful adjustment.

☐ **GOAL**

The child/family will accept the alteration in body and successfully adapt to required changes in lifestyle.

☐ **IMPLEMENTATION**

- Give positive reinforcement for efforts to adapt; child/family behavior will indicate when acceptance of body alterations has begun (e.g., may ask questions; will start to look at the incision, dressings, etc.).
- Accept, but do not support, expressions of denial.
- Assist child in choice of prosthesis (if one is to be used) by providing information and arranging for a visit by a member of an ostomy club, or other appropriate group; let child/family determine time of visit as appropriate, but try to arrange it as soon as possible.
- Involve child/family in child-care activities; begin slowly and add new activities one at a time; reinforce any efforts to participate.
- Assist adjustment to awareness of the extent of the loss since there is frequently a lag between initial alteration and realistic perception.
- Tell family how they can help by listening, supporting reality, allowing expressions of anger, denial, and not challenging them, permitting child to cry and giving positive reinforcement for all efforts to cope/adapt; praise the family for participation in efforts to assist.
- Hold a team conference, including family if you wish, and share information on grief and loss (see page 211) and crisis intervention (see page 191) with each other; discuss what parts of these concepts apply at this time; revise the care plan as necessary.
- Refer for continued contact with community support group, home health nurse, and appropriate community agencies.

☐ **EVALUATION CRITERIA/DESIRED OUTCOMES**
The Child
- Accepts continued support and positive input from family
- Utilizes community resources such as ostomy club, therapy, to provide ongoing support, reassurance, and assistance in recovery
- Resumes predisturbance activities
The Family
- Supports the child and provides positive input

The Child/Family Adapting to Chronic Illness

Definition/Discussion

Chronic illness refers to a physical disorder with a protracted course (usually longer than 3 months) that can be progressive and fatal, or associated with a relatively normal life span despite impaired functioning. Such an illness frequently has acute exacerbations requiring intensive medical attention, followed by a long period of supervision, observation, and care at home; usually it is the child and family who must manage the illness on a day-to-day basis. The most common chronic illnesses are asthma, cardiac conditions, and diabetes mellitus. It is estimated that 7%–10% of children are affected with a serious chronic illness.

Nursing Assessment

☐ PERTINENT HISTORY

Course of illness (e.g., time since diagnosis, characteristics of acute exacerbations requiring hospitalization, number of days in hospital and absent from school during past year); treatment strategies (e.g., medical management, teacher or school nurse management); academic achievement; use of community and social support systems

☐ PHYSICAL FINDINGS

Physical growth; physical limitation from the illness itself, or from prescribed treatments; pain or discomfort; other handicapping conditions (e.g., mental retardation, cerebral palsy); physical/behavioral symptoms indicating episodic illness or acute exacerbation of the chronic condition

☐ PSYCHOSOCIAL CONCERNS/ DEVELOPMENTAL FACTORS

Cognitive/social/emotional/developmental level of functioning including academic achievement and peer relationships; coping mechanisms, including use of support systems, daily routine at home; impact of hospitalization(s) and school absence(s); changes in child's development as a result of illness/treatment; parental attitudes towards the child's illness; impact of treatment regimen on the child/family

☐ PATIENT AND FAMILY KNOWLEDGE

Previous educational efforts; need for compliance with therapeutic regimen; knowledge of treatment plan, ability to perform plan and give medications, as well as readiness (emotionally and financially) to manage the child's health at home; level of knowledge, readiness and willingness to learn

Nursing Care

☐ LONG-TERM GOAL

The parents will manage and will help the child manage the complex treatment procedures at home; the parents will work to prevent the illness from disrupting normal family functioning or the family's involvement in the community; the child will cope with the realities of the illness while continuing to attend school and participating in age-appropriate activities as much as possible; the family will encourage achievement of age-appropriate developmental tasks by the child.

NURSING DIAGNOSIS #1

Alteration in health maintenance related to chronic disease process with its remissions and exacerbations, need for a lifelong period of medical treatment

Rationale: A chronic illness is usually treatable but not curable, and requires a lifelong commitment to complex, expensive, and sometimes painful procedures for managing the illness and maintaining optimal level of health. Treatment regimen may be beyond the child's cognitive capabilities, or it may be too time consuming for parents to supervise the child's daily illness-related tasks.

☐ GOAL

The child/parents will perform the necessary home treatments and procedures to manage the illness and maintain the child at home; the child will perform necessary treatment procedures under parental supervision as age and condition permit.

☐ **IMPLEMENTATION**

- Recognize the primary role of the parents as care givers.
- Discuss which aspects of the management of the illness should be the child's responsibility, which the parents', and how the physician, nurse, and other health professionals will remain involved.
- Plan discussions at regular intervals as the illness changes over time and as the child becomes capable of greater responsibilities.
- Encourage the child's involvement in age-appropriate health promotion and illness management tasks (at home and in the hospital).
- Provide educational sessions and materials that will enable the child/parents to learn day-to-day illness management tasks.
- Identify community health providers who can reinforce health teaching/procedures and assist with health maintenance activities at home; encourage parents to communicate with these providers (including school nurse) to describe ongoing treatments, report observations and the results of daily tests relevant to the child's condition.
- Evaluate roles of all family members (especially the child) in the management of the child's health on a regular basis.

☐ **EVALUATION CRITERIA/DESIRED OUTCOMES**

The Child
- Is maintained at home
- Participates in illness-management tasks as able

The Child/Parents
- Establish an efficient daily routine for ongoing home treatments.
- Perform home treatments and procedures appropriately

NURSING DIAGNOSIS #2

Family coping: potential for growth related to impact of the child's disease on the family's functioning

Rationale: A family with a chronically ill child must exert a great deal of effort to effectively manage the child's disease while encouraging normal development in the child. Preventing the illness from disrupting normal family functioning is an important goal to work toward.

☐ **GOAL**

The family will cope with and master the stress of the illness; will increase sharing, support, and heighten self-esteem.

☐ **IMPLEMENTATION**

- Support parents with reassurance, realism, and repetition, as family members come to grips with the reality of the child's illness and treatment.
- Help parents develop strategies to adjust to the crisis of chronic illness.
- Encourage parents to expect age-appropriate behavior and set realistic limits for their child.
- Analyze support systems and use of community resources (medical, financial, social) that help in the process of long-term adjustment to chronic illness.
- Recognize the need for additional supports and refer for services in the community.
- Coordinate services and help family and health care team to communicate effectively with one another.

☐ **EVALUATION CRITERIA/DESIRED OUTCOMES**

The Family
- Communicates effectively with one another and with other family members to function as a stable family system
- Establishes and maintains healthy relationships with friends and effective relationships with community resources
- Assists all members of the family unit to achieve developmental tasks

---

NURSING DIAGNOSIS #3

Disturbance in self-concept: body image, self-esteem, role performance, personal identity related to impact of specific illness characteristics (e.g., visibility, prognosis, treatment requirements, functional capabilities)

Rationale: In some cases, the severity of the illness and the child's generally poor health may limit functioning so that the child is deprived of critical experiences resulting in poor social skills, lowered self-esteem, and greater dependence on parents than is developmentally appropriate.

☐ **GOAL**

The child will participate in school programs, family and peer activities; will be as independent from parents as developmentally appropriate.

☐ **IMPLEMENTATION**

- Assess the child's attitude toward the illness and treatment.
- Encourage compliance with treatment regimen.
- Encourage school attendance (educational continuity is of vital concern).
- Communicate regularly with teachers and com-

munity health providers when homebound/hospital teaching is needed.

- Help parents to think of creative ways to revise/adapt treatment routines allowing for play time with peers and other normalizing experiences in the community.
- Recommend participation in discussion, activity, or support groups (counseling) that can provide peer support and decrease social isolation.
- Teach the child to perform developmentally appropriate self-care activities and illness management tasks; counsel parents to encourage the child's independence in these areas.

☐ EVALUATION CRITERIA/DESIRED OUTCOMES

The Child
- Performs developmentally appropriate self-care activities
- Participates in age-appropriate recreation with peers
- Expresses feelings

NURSING DIAGNOSIS #4

Social isolation related to the parents' gradual withdrawal from friends and community resources after diagnosis of chronic illness in their child

Rationale: Decreased energy, decreased financial resources, embarrassment or shame about their child's condition, and anger that others were spared the pain of a chronically ill child can lead to self-imposed social isolation.

☐ GOAL

The parents will develop and maintain social relationships with family members, friends, and neighbors; the family will utilize community resources appropriately.

☐ IMPLEMENTATION

- Assist parents in the identification of possible activities that promote enjoyable family and community interactions.
- Involve family in parent/sibling/family support groups, or in social/recreational activities sponsored by disease-related foundations or organizations.
- Promote the child's participation in school and after-school social activities.

☐ EVALUATION CRITERIA/DESIRED OUTCOMES

The Family
- Participates regularly in social activities

NURSING DIAGNOSIS #5

Anxiety related to unpleasant treatments, prognosis, loss of control, and the variable course of the illness

Rationale: The child/parents experience anxiety when faced with learning and carrying out complex, often painful treatments; children and parents worry about what the future holds for them; parents' anxieties about their child's health may influence child-rearing patterns.

☐ GOAL

The child/parents will be supported while adjusting to the diagnosis of chronic illness; will express feelings and concerns to health care professionals; the parents will be motivated and comfortable in the daily care and decision making regarding their child.

☐ IMPLEMENTATION

- Assess child, parents, and sibling(s) for behaviors reflecting anxiety.
- Listen and give emotional support; refer for counseling if indicated or requested.
- Encourage child/family to learn about the illness and treatment.
- Prepare child for procedures or consequences of the illness in an age-appropriate manner.
- Give parents positive reinforcement for cooperation with treatment plan, learning new skills, and realistic child-rearing practices.
- Maintain sensitivity towards families who are battling with feelings of anxiety and may be angry with health care providers; consider mental health referral if appropriate.

☐ EVALUATION CRITERIA/DESIRED OUTCOMES

The Child/Parents
- Express feelings to the health care team
- Respond positively to the support and encouragement of team members
- Carry out treatments at home while maintaining positive family functioning
- Identify community resources that provide emotional support or services during the variable course of the child's illness

---

NURSING DIAGNOSIS #6

Activity intolerance related to illness and exacerbation of symptoms or treatment complications, with accompanying loss of functioning

---

> **Rationale:** A chronic illness, with its up-and-down course, affects the child's physical functioning and energy level. The child may experience pain or discomfort and resist involvement in physical activities.

> **Rationale:** If knowledge deficit exists, the family cannot appropriately maintain the child's optimal level of functioning or prevent complications and deformities related to the illness.

☐ GOAL

The child will engage in daily care activities to the fullest extent possible as well as participate in developmentally appropriate recreation/social activities.

☐ IMPLEMENTATION

- Encourage the child to do as much daily personal care as the chronic illness will allow.
- Teach parents behavioral management techniques to reinforce the child's participation at home.
- Set up a schedule with consultation from health care team (physician, occupational and physical therapists) for participation in recreation activities and exercise programs; give praise and attention for the child's progress with the program.
- Assist the child to acquire and use self-help devices as well as adaptive equipment if recommended by health care team.
- Communicate the child's functional potential and recommended activity level (including rest periods if necessary) to school personnel; reassess functional potential periodically and communicate results to parents and school.

☐ EVALUATION CRITERIA/DESIRED OUTCOMES

The Child
- Performs developmentally appropriate activities of daily living within limits of disability
- Participates in exercise program and/or recreational activities with peers on a regular basis

The Parents
- Communicate regularly with health care team regarding child's functional potential and activity level

---

NURSING DIAGNOSIS #7

Knowledge deficit regarding measures to promote maintenance of independent functioning, prevent complications, exacerbation of symptoms, deformities

---

☐ GOAL

The child/parents will verbalize an understanding of the chronic illness, treatment plan, use of medications, home care responsibilities, and available support services.

☐ IMPLEMENTATION

- Instruct in technical skills/procedures to be carried out at home; help parents decide what aspects of the management of the disease should be the child's responsibility (according to developmental/cognitive abilities).
- Teach how and when to communicate with the physician between clinic appointments, to describe ongoing management behaviors, personal observations, and the results of daily tests relevant to the child's condition.
- Refer to community health nurse to provide reinforcement of health teaching at home; help parents to communicate relevant information with school nurse.
- Teach about maintenance of medical or adaptive equipment to be used at home or school.
- Teach signs and symptoms of illness complications, including crisis situations and how to obtain emergency care.
- Reinforce importance of regular communication and follow-up appointments with health care team, community health nurse, and school nurse.
- Provide written information (if available) published by disease-specific foundations or associations, including educational programs sponsored by these organizations.

☐ EVALUATION CRITERIA/DESIRED OUTCOMES

The Child/Parents
- Describe the chronic illness and prescribed treatment program
- Demonstrate home management skills and use of medical or adaptive equipment
- Communicate concerns and information with health care providers at appropriate times
- Keep follow-up appointments
- Use community support services

The Family Requiring Crisis Intervention

Definition/Discussion

Crisis intervention refers to those approaches used to restore someone to a state of emotional equilibrium, from one of disequilibrium (the crisis state).

Nursing Assessment

☐ **PERTINENT HISTORY**

Recent illness or loss; stresses of the past year; transitions; trauma, catastrophic illness or accident; job, family stability; decreased ability to carry out activities of daily living (ADL); current threatening event

☐ **PHYSICAL FINDINGS**

Altered vital signs, anxiety (e.g., moderate, severe, panic), decreased concentration, somatic complaints, agitation, tension, neglect in self-care

☐ **PSYCHOSOCIAL CONCERNS/ DEVELOPMENTAL FACTORS**

Developmental level, normal coping methods, supportive or dysfunctional family history, ego strengths, dependency patterns, apathy, distorted perceptions, regression to lower levels of functioning, habits/routines at home

☐ **PATIENT AND FAMILY KNOWLEDGE**

Previous experiences; perception of the problem, severity of disruption; internal and outside support or agencies; ability to decrease anxiety; socialization, interpersonal, and communication skills; level of knowledge, readiness and willingness to learn

Nursing Care

☐ **LONG-TERM GOAL**

The child/family will achieve adaptive resolution of the crisis; the child/family will return to usual roles with a realistic perception of what has occurred and with adequate coping mechanisms.

NURSING DIAGNOSIS #1

Ineffective individual/family coping related to perceived inability to deal with problem, distorted perception of the problem

Rationale: *Usual coping mechanisms may not prevent increased stress when a threatening event occurs. The child/family may have a distorted perception of the problem and may feel unable to deal with it. The inability to manage the stress situation results in disequilibrium.*

☐ **GOAL**

The child/family will state perception of stressful situation and develop coping mechanisms effective in the crisis state.

☐ **IMPLEMENTATION**

- Assess feelings regarding the stressful event and what the perception of the problem is; remember child's/family's perception is what is important and may differ from yours.
- Allow to respond at length and in detail to your questions; do not challenge any statements; try to determine exactly what is most threatening; listen and encourage child/family to keep talking.
- Determine the real/anticipated loss(es) involved; assess behavior in light of the grief and mourning process.
- Determine usual coping strategies and how successful these methods are.
- Encourage verbalization about supportive individuals or agencies and whether or not they would be of value in the present situation.
- Ask what you could do to make child/family feel better right now; if at all possible, provide it.
- Provide basic needs; if child becomes very dependent in ADL, allow this dependency to occur for the immediate time.
- Help child to gradually increase independence in ADL; involve in self-care, slowly at first, then gradually add more activities.

- Provide opportunities for child/family to make decisions about daily care; give some control over own situation; praise them for making decisions, for coping with current stress, for helping self/selves to feel better.
- Ask for child's/family's ideas on what can be done next to improve the situation; incorporate your ideas with theirs to give a sense of control.
- Support and reinforce reality when behavior indicates that child/family is beginning to adapt or cope (e.g., asking questions, focusing on reality); share with them how you see it; ask them to clarify or validate your perceptions.
- Incorporate into the nursing care plan suggestions for new methods of coping with the crisis state; enlist the cooperation of staff in assisting the child/family with these.

☐ EVALUATION CRITERIA/DESIRED OUTCOMES

The Child/Family
- Appraises situation realistically
- Verbalizes feelings regarding the threatening event
- Identifies usual methods of coping with problems
- States need for new ways to handle the disequilibrium
- Identifies at least 2 effective strategies

NURSING DIAGNOSIS #2

Anxiety related to feelings of being overwhelmed by threatening event

Rationale: *Situations perceived as threatening produce increased anxiety that can result in inability to manage situation, which leads to feeling overwhelmed.*

☐ GOAL

The child/family will identify causes of threat; will achieve skill in managing the anxiety.

☐ IMPLEMENTATION

- Refer to *The Child/Family Experiencing Anxiety*, page 177.
- Ask what the child/family is feeling at this time (e.g., scared, anxious, panicky) and what occurred to cause these feelings (e.g., new diagnosis, new roommate, new equipment).
- Encourage verbalization of all feelings of anxiety and discern those that are the most threatening; listen actively and with empathy.
- Make any environmental changes that are possible to decrease the impact of the threat (e.g., change room, allow family to stay for additional support).
- Share information regarding tests, procedures,

etc.; tell what to expect and how orders are carried out.
- Enlist the help of other personnel in planning for care that will decrease anxiety; share your perceptions and information with them.
- Teach simple relaxation techniques (e.g., deep breathing) to use whenever needed to keep anxiety from increasing.
- When leaving room, tell when you will be back; return at the appointed time.

☐ EVALUATION CRITERIA/DESIRED OUTCOMES

The Child/Family
- Identifies causes of threat and describes threatening event
- Makes realistic requests to keep anxiety manageable
- Uses relaxation techniques
- Requests staff assistance appropriately

NURSING DIAGNOSIS #3

Grieving related to an actual or perceived loss

Rationale: *An individual's grief is affected by many factors, including personality, previous losses, intimacy of relationship, and personal resources. Unresolved grief is a pathologic response of prolonged denial of the loss or a profound psychotic response that leads to problems in coping. Dysfunctional grieving is evidenced by loss of self-esteem, depression, excessively strong dependency needs, and ambivalent feelings for the lost person or object. Such unresolved grief leaves the individual susceptible to further psychologic trauma that can in turn lead to crisis, depression, and suicide.*

☐ GOAL

The child/family will describe loss and the meaning of the loss; will express and share grief with others; will resolve the loss in an adaptive manner.

☐ IMPLEMENTATION

- Refer to *The Parent Experiencing Grief and Loss*, page 211, for review of the grief process.
- Assess for any contributing/causative factors that may delay the grief work.
- Listen and encourage expression of feelings (e.g., fear, despair, anger, sadness).
- Develop a relationship of trust through one-to-one interactions.
- Give support and reassurance by accepting feelings and experiences.
- Explore, if indicated, what it is that makes child feel hopeless, worthless, that life is not worth living.

- Provide support by discussing feelings and coping mechanisms.
- Encourage to share grief and provide support for each other.
- Discuss new coping mechanisms; encourage to practice them.
- Involve in the decision-making process.

☐ EVALUATION CRITERIA/DESIRED OUTCOMES

The Child/Family
- Expresses feelings
- Shares feelings and concerns with family members
- Participates in decision making for the future

NURSING DIAGNOSIS #4

Alteration in family process related to situational or pathophysiologic stressor

Rationale: When the normally supportive and adaptively functioning family experiences a stressor, the family's previously effective functioning ability may be challenged. Common factors that contribute to an alteration in family process include illness of a family member, trauma, loss of a family member or valued object, gain of a new family member, disaster, economic crisis, change in family roles, conflict, psychiatric illness, and social deviance. When the child's/family's usual problem-solving methods are inadequate to resolve the situation, a crisis may occur. In response to crisis, the child/family will either return to precrisis functioning, develop a higher level of functioning, or develop an ineffective (lower) form of functioning.

☐ GOAL

The family will return to the precrisis level of functioning; will verbalize feelings to nurse and to each other on a regular basis; will maintain a functional system of mutual support for each other.

☐ IMPLEMENTATION

- Help identify feelings of stress, past and current methods of coping, strengths and weaknesses.
- Encourage to share thoughts and feelings with each other, to interact and communicate daily.
- Encourage recognition and verbalization of feelings including guilt, anger, hostility, and blame.
- Help to make realistic appraisal of the situation.
- Urge to list choices, available resources.
- Assist to reorganize roles as needed at home and to set priorities to maintain family integrity and to reduce stress.

☐ EVALUATION CRITERIA/DESIRED OUTCOMES

The Family
- Shares feelings and concerns
- Sets priorities and implements adaptive coping strategies
- Reorganizes home roles as needed
- Maintains or returns to precrisis level of functioning

NURSING DIAGNOSIS #5

Knowledge deficit regarding utilization of support systems, problem-solving techniques needed to avert a crisis state

Rationale: A crisis will not develop if situational supports are sufficient, perception of the problem is realistic, and effective coping solutions are available.

☐ GOAL

The child/family will identify available support; will develop alternative coping to solve current problem.

☐ IMPLEMENTATION

- Give information as needed (e.g., hospitalization, treatment therapy); ask for feedback to ensure understanding.
- Teach to brainstorm alternate solutions to current problem, to look at the pros and cons of each one; do not tell them what to do, but ask if one of the solutions could possibly work; role play alternative solutions.
- Check the effectiveness of new coping options by asking what actions they would take if confronted with a situation similar to the one just experienced; reinforce positive adaptation and coping; teach as necessary.
- Help to identify support systems available.
- Refer to outside support or agency to correct family or individual dysfunction once crisis is resolved.

☐ EVALUATION CRITERIA/DESIRED OUTCOMES

The Child/Family
- Has a realistic perception of what occurred
- Fosters situational supports in the form of family, friends, job
- States at least 3 options available to use to cope with stress
- Lists community resources to go to if another threatening situation occurs

The Child Experiencing Depression

Definition/Discussion

Depression is a reaction to one's inability to adapt to change/loss/separation. Depression in children is a constellation of factors characterized by sadness, low self-esteem, and internalization of anger/aggression, which interfere with the child's day-to-day activities. Manifestations vary according to the developmental level of the child, risk factors, and family interactions; however, symptoms of depression may include boredom, restlessness, fatigue, difficulty concentrating, behavioral changes/problems, "acting out," accident proneness, sighing, somatic complaints, sleep disturbance.

Nursing Assessment

☐ **PERTINENT HISTORY**

Duration and characteristics of symptoms; incidence of situational or maturational loss, chronic or terminal illness, trauma, physical/sexual abuse; alcohol/chemical dependency

☐ **PHYSICAL FINDINGS**

General appearance, sleep patterns, elimination, nutrition, activity patterns

☐ **PSYCHOSOCIAL CONCERNS/ DEVELOPMENTAL FACTORS**

Interactional patterns, developmental level, expression of affect, school functioning, peer/family relations, level of thought disruption; habits (e.g., what comforts child, eating/bedtime routines, favored objects)

☐ **PATIENT AND FAMILY KNOWLEDGE**

Child's self-evaluation, parental perception of child's behavior; awareness of existence of a problem and willingness to work toward a solution

Nursing Care

☐ **LONG-TERM GOAL**

The child will express feelings of increased self-esteem and hope; will demonstrate increased positive social interactions.

NURSING DIAGNOSIS #1
a. **Hopelessness** related to inability to feel positive about present life situation
b. **Powerlessness** related to feeling overwhelmed by events or emotions
c. **Ineffective individual coping** related to life events
d. **Altered growth and development** related to depressed mood

Rationale: *Hopelessness and powerlessness characterize depression and may result in passivity and despondency. This is debilitating to a child striving to achieve age-appropriate developmental tasks. Depression may be a response to traumatic life events (e.g., natural disasters, unexpected deaths, rape, physical/sexual abuse). A severely depressed child may experience reality disorientation, or an inability to problem solve even the simplest of motor tasks, speak cohesively and intelligibly, or comprehend conversation.*

☐ **GOAL**

The child will express feelings in age-appropriate ways; will perform age-appropriate developmental tasks.

☐ **IMPLEMENTATION**

- Ask child how s/he sees things, whether anything helps him/her feel better, and what might help improve situation.
- Use play therapy/role playing to assist the child in gaining mastery over the event; refer to *The Child Requiring Play Therapy*, page 220.
- Support disclosure of painful memories.
- Praise ability to share feelings whether it be through play therapy or verbalization.
- Administer prescribed antidepressants as ordered; note effectiveness.
- Assist child to engage in small structured social encounters.
- Praise child's efforts to participate.
- Familiarize self with age-appropriate developmen-

194

tal tasks; refer to *Normal Growth and Development*, pages 231–245.

- Engage child in activities that match or are slightly below developmental level; provide opportunities for success; avoid activities that set the child up for failure.
- Advance to increasingly higher-level tasks; praise and reinforce accomplishments.
- Allow child to make decisions concerning care (e.g., when to brush teeth) if appropriate; keep decisions simple; restrict choices so as not to overwhelm child.

☐ EVALUATION CRITERIA/DESIRED OUTCOMES

The Child
- Expresses fears, concerns
- Demonstrates age-appropriate developmental tasks
- Makes simple decisions regarding care
- Participates in play therapy

NURSING DIAGNOSIS #2

a. **Self-care deficit: hygiene/grooming** related to inability to make decisions, feelings of hopelessness/worthlessness
b. **Disturbance in self-concept: body image/self-esteem** related to distorted perception
c. **Alteration in bowel elimination: constipation/encopresis** related to lack of exercise, poor-quality intake, withholding
d. **Alteration in nutrition: more than body requirements** related to perceived comfort value of food
e. **Alteration in nutrition: less than body requirements** related to perceived negative connotations of food

Rationale: The depressed child may be immobilized to the point of not bathing, brushing teeth, combing hair, eating, sleeping, or dressing appropriately (e.g., too warm for hot days or vice versa, or not changing clothes, wearing unkempt clothing). This contributes increasingly to depression, distorted body image, and decreased self-esteem. Children may experience depressive symptoms as a result of internalized anger. This often presents itself psychologically as withholding attention and affection. It may further progress to the physical withholding of stool as the child attempts to gain control over these feelings. Lack of exercise and poor nutritional intake because of depression may also result in constipation. Regressive behavior (e.g., wetting during the day) may be seen. Children may use food as a comfort mechanism or avoid food altogether.

☐ GOAL

The child will take an active role in self-care; will resume a normal elimination pattern; will ingest a diet appropriate for nutritional needs.

☐ IMPLEMENTATION

- Assist child with hygiene and grooming; praise positive aspects of child's appearance.
- Praise and reinforce independent attempts at completing even small daily tasks.
- Reinforce (e.g., visually with star chart) efforts to participate in self-care, play/school work.
- Assist child in planning new, more effective skills for coping; practice mastery of coping skills via play therapy/role playing.
- Provide appropriate diet with increased roughage (e.g., fresh fruit, vegetables, high-fiber cereals).
- Encourage and reinforce participation in exercise.
- Administer stool softener, mineral oil as ordered; monitor for effectiveness.
- Set aside consistent toilet-time (e.g., after meals, before bedtime); praise and reinforce toilet use.

☐ EVALUATION CRITERIA/DESIRED OUTCOMES

The Child
- Participates successfully in self-care, play activities, and school
- Eats an appropriate diet
- Stays dry during the day if age appropriate
- Passes soft stool at least every 2 days

NURSING DIAGNOSIS #3

a. **Sleep pattern disturbance** related to fears, anxiety, inactivity or sleeping during the day
b. **Diversional activity deficit** related to inactivity

Rationale: The depressed child may be restless, have nightmares, or be fearful of being left alone. The child who withdraws from activity during the day or who is allowed to sleep for prolonged periods in the day may not be able to sleep at night.

☐ GOAL

The child will maintain/regain a normal sleep pattern; will actively participate in games, conversation, helping others.

☐ IMPLEMENTATION

- Explore child's fears and anxieties related to nighttime, being alone, sleeping through play therapy or conversation.

- Follow a consistent bedtime routine (e.g., drink of water, trip to bathroom, bedtime story, hug and a kiss).
- Provide a nightlight.
- Sit at child's doorway if necessary to keep child in room and as reassurance until child falls asleep.
- Choose activities, games, and possible playmates that are developmentally appropriate.
- Elicit activities/interests from child; encourage and praise the child's participation.
- Encourage physical activity from the child (e.g., running, tag, jump rope).
- Monitor the child's social interactional patterns.
- Assist the withdrawn child to tolerate brief periods of contact with another child (e.g., sit with child); increase gradually the group size as tolerated by the child.
- Structure activities with another higher functioning child to serve as a role model and help the withdrawn child participate.

☐ EVALUATION CRITERIA/DESIRED OUTCOMES

The Child
- Sleeps restfully without waking through the night
- Participates in bedtime routine
- Interacts appropriately with peers

NURSING DIAGNOSIS #4

Potential for injury related to self-abusive behavior, accidents

Rationale: The depressed child may engage in self-abusive behaviors (e.g., biting, hitting, scratching, head-banging), or appear very clumsy and accident prone (e.g., falling while climbing, running out into the street, touching a hot oven, falling down during play).

☐ GOAL

The child will redirect energies toward developmentally appropriate and safe behavior and play activities.

☐ IMPLEMENTATION

- Identify child's abusive/accidental tendencies.
- Prevent child physically from completing abusive/accident-potential behavior.
- Engage child in an activity that distracts the child so that abusive/accidental behavior cannot be continued when the new activity is begun.

- Praise child's participation in the new safe behavior.
- Stress your desire to keep child safe.
- Reinforce safe behavior (e.g., with star chart, hugs, praise, pats).

☐ EVALUATION CRITERIA/DESIRED OUTCOMES

The Child
- Engages in no self-abuse
- Verbalizes a safe behavior versus an unsafe behavior
- Does not participate in any unsafe behaviors

NURSING DIAGNOSIS #5

a. **Ineffective family coping** related to failure to comprehend severity of depression (meanings of behavioral changes)
b. **Alteration in family processes** related to inability to cope with a child member experiencing depression
c. **Knowledge deficit** regarding childhood depression

Rationale: Parents and others may underestimate the importance of behavioral symptoms, or may deny that the behavioral change exists. The normal supportive environment of the family is challenged when the child experiences depression. The family must be allowed to verbalize their feelings and receive external support when needed.

☐ GOAL

The family will recognize and effectively manage depressive changes in the child's behavior; will return to its functionally supportive state; will increase communication and understanding regarding the child's experience with depression.

☐ IMPLEMENTATION

- Assess family's understanding of the child's status.
- Assess level of disruption in family functioning.
- Point out changes in behavior (subtle or blatant) as they relate to depressive symptoms (e.g., withdrawal, increased motor activity, decreased appetite, increased appetite, decreased attentiveness, increased aggression); demonstrate and role play with family ways to manage these behaviors.
- Encourage family to express their feelings regarding the changes in the child.

- Encourage and allow family members to verbalize feelings to nurse and to one another.
- Assist family members in maintaining mutual support of one another.
- Encourage family to seek professional help when needed.

☐ EVALUATION CRITERIA/DESIRED OUTCOMES

The Family
- Demonstrates recognition of a symptom and effective management techniques by role playing
- Is mutually supportive of one another and of the child

The Child with a Developmental Disability

Definition/Discussion

Developmental disability, also known as mental retardation, refers to a subaverage general intellectual functioning that originates during the developmental period and is associated with impairment in adaptive behavior. Children with developmental disabilities need the same basic services that other human beings need for normal development, including education, vocational preparation, health services, and recreational opportunities. In addition, many moderately, severely, and profoundly retarded children need specialized services such as diagnostic evaluation centers, early intervention programs, special education services, and residential living.

Nursing Assessment

☐ **PERTINENT HISTORY**

Present complaints, course of illness or accidental injury (e.g., length, characteristics); home treatment for illness or injury; presence of chronic health impairments; number/length of prior hospitalizations; physical setting in which the child resides (e.g., home, residential, institutional); special services/procedures required by the child's developmental disability; previous level of function

☐ **PHYSICAL FINDINGS**

Vital signs; level of consciousness; weight; presence of other handicaps such as cerebral palsy, epilepsy, blindness, or deafness; presence of physical/behavioral symptoms indicating pain/discomfort; functional capabilities

☐ **PSYCHOSOCIAL CONCERNS/ DEVELOPMENTAL FACTORS**

Level of intellectual functioning; adaptive behavioral skills; overall developmental level; coping mechanisms/habits of child and family; impact of normal routine on child/family; stressors/concerns of family; support systems available

☐ **PATIENT AND FAMILY KNOWLEDGE**

Developmental program needs of child, adaptation/ acceptance of child's level of functioning/prognosis; level of knowledge, ability, readiness and willingness to learn

Nursing Care

☐ **LONG-TERM GOAL**

The developmentally disabled child will learn, develop, and grow at own rate to become a productive participant in society.

NURSING DIAGNOSIS #1
Self-care deficit: feeding, bathing/hygiene, dressing/grooming, toileting related to physical/mental deficit

Rationale: *The child with a developmental deficit may be unable to perform/communicate basic needs; therefore, parents, nurses, and other care providers may have to assist the child and be responsible for ensuring that basic needs are met.*

☐ **GOAL**

The child will ingest adequate food/fluids to meet body's needs; will have a normal bowel pattern.

☐ **IMPLEMENTATION**

- Maintain consistency and establish a routine; schedule meals, naps, medications, and treatments at the same time every day.
- Follow the child's normal routine as closely as possible.
- Assist the child in development of a communication system to express needs (e.g., make felt board with specific pictures [toilet, cup, wheelchair] and have child point to what is desired; teach sign language).
- Ensure adequate intake of food and fluid; use supplements when necessary and allow choice of food when possible; if child uses special feeding utensils, ensure they are present in advance.
- Attend to activities promoting good hygiene/oral

care; brush teeth after meals and upon rising; keep child clean; establish a routine bathing pattern; preserve skin integrity (e.g., massage, lotions, sheepskins, water mattress); support the child's efforts to perform self-care activities.
- Provide experiences that promote self-sufficiency in self-care skills; allow as much independence as Possible in activities of daily living.
- Ambulate as much as possible; use active and passive range-of-motion as appropriate.
- Monitor normal pattern of bowel/bladder elimination; clean perianal area of stool/urine immediately.

☐ EVALUATION CRITERIA/DESIRED OUTCOMES

The Child
- Maintains/regains admission weight and level of hydration
- Maintains good skin condition
- Maintains adequate level of personal hygiene

NURSING DIAGNOSIS #2

Anxiety related to hospitalization, separation from family, disruption of daily routines

Rationale: Developmentally delayed children have intellectual/emotional limitations that increase difficulties in adapting to hospitalization, or changes in caregivers and routines; in understanding the reason for hospitalization and related restrictions; and in communicating feelings of anxiety. Children with a developmental disability frequently are less anxious and more cooperative when schedules and time frames are exact.

☐ GOAL

The child will adjust to the hospital/altered environment; will exhibit behavioral indicators of trust and security; will maintain relationship with family.

☐ IMPLEMENTATION

- Encourage and allow time for child to express feelings/understanding in own way.
- Accept expressed feelings with nonjudgmental words and actions.
- Provide consistency in nursing care; assign one nurse per shift to do all care.
- Adjust hospital procedures to child's usual routine as much as possible.
- Follow through on promises made to child (e.g., if you say you will return at a specific time, do so).
- Provide diversions (e.g., toys, games) that are appropriate to level of functioning; tell family to

bring in favorite toys and to stay with child if possible.
- Encourage interaction with child's peers, family members, or care providers so child maintains significant relationships; ask for assistance in correctly interpreting communication and behavior; allow them to provide care when possible.
- Allow child to participate as much as possible in decision making regarding care.

☐ EVALUATION CRITERIA/DESIRED OUTCOMES

The Child
- Maintains admission level of functioning within limits imposed by physical illness

---

NURSING DIAGNOSIS #3

Altered growth and development related to mental/emotional/cognitive deficit

Rationale: Developmental disabilities are associated with impairments in adaptive behaviors; adaptive behavior refers to the child's adjustment to everyday life; children with developmental disabilities learn more slowly than others and reach a lower overall level of functioning.

☐ GOAL

The child will function at a level consistent with his/her cognitive skills and adaptive abilities.

☐ IMPLEMENTATION

- Discuss and promote the concept of "normalizing" experiences to promote self-sufficiency, adjustment, and mental growth (e.g., eating meals with others, music therapy in groups).
- Permit the child to express feelings, but at the same time do not allow unacceptable behavior (e.g., temper tantrums); reinforce appropriate behavior.
- Provide toys, games, equipment, educational supplies, and teaching that will enable the child to increase cognitive, social, motor skills.
- Communicate and interact with the child in an age-appropriate fashion; maintain dignity in all interactions with the child.
- Allow and encourage family members, siblings, and nondisabled peers to visit and interact with the child.
- Foster self-worth; provide personal space so child's belongings are accessible; encourage child to care for the physical environment if appropriate.

☐ EVALUATION CRITERIA/DESIRED OUTCOMES

The Child
- Maintains/improves level of function
- Participates in "normalizing" experiences, with family, siblings, nondisabled peers

---

NURSING DIAGNOSIS #4

Potential for injury related to developmental disability

Rationale: Cognitive and physical limitations associated with developmental disability may preclude the child's understanding of dangers, use of safeguards, and requesting help appropriately in dangerous situations. Because the child adapts slowly to new activities/situations/environments (e.g., the hospital), the developmentally delayed child is at risk for injury.

☐ GOAL

The child will cooperate with hospital rules and regulations regarding safety as able; will be free from preventable accident or injury.

☐ IMPLEMENTATION

- Institute safety precautions as appropriate (e.g., check safety rails frequently; restrain only if necessary; stay with anxious child; make frequent checks; do not underestimate child's strength).
- Plan for mobility aids as needed (e.g., wheelchair, walker, other special equipment).
- Observe for mouthing of nonfood items.
- Do not wait for call light; plan regular checks so child expects you.
- Remain with child until medications are swallowed safely; be alert to medication side effects that interfere with function/safety.
- Explain/demonstrate procedures and equipment (e.g., suctioning, gavaging) in advance so when used, will not cause fear or be removed by child.

☐ EVALUATION CRITERIA/DESIRED OUTCOMES

The Child
- Is free from accidents
- Complies with hospital rules
- Does not swallow toxic/nonedible items

NURSING DIAGNOSIS #5

a. **Family coping: potential for growth** related to having a child with a permanent disability
b. **Ineffective family coping** related to having a child with a permanent disability
c. **Alteration in family process** related to having a child with a permanent disability

---

Rationale: The developmentally disabled child's inability to perform age-appropriate tasks and need for specialized training, as well as "normalizing" experiences, forces the family into an adjustment process that includes developing alliances with professionals. The family struggles with adapting to life with a handicapped child in a world of nondisabled persons.

☐ GOAL

The parents will express an understanding of developmental disabilities; will facilitate the child's development; family members will express their feelings/concerns; will interact positively with the child.

☐ IMPLEMENTATION

- Provide opportunities for parents/family members to discuss feelings (e.g., anger, guilt, hostility); accept these expressions in a nonjudgmental manner by both words and actions.
- Provide information about changes in child's level of function, strengths and weaknesses.
- Include child/parents/family members in planning individual programs and routines for the child.
- Support families through the times when they are separated from the child.
- Provide opportunities for families of children in residential programs to discuss their feelings about home visits; assist them in planning for visits to prevent/avoid problems.
- Provide opportunities for families to interact with other families with developmentally delayed children, to share experiences and information.
- Be alert to indications of ineffective coping such as abuse or neglect of child and refer to counseling/appropriate agencies as necessary; refer to *The Child with Nonaccidental Trauma,* page 213.

☐ EVALUATION CRITERIA/DESIRED OUTCOMES

The Family Members
- Express feelings about the child's disabilities and level of function
- Develop an alliance with care givers who are seen as supportive and helpful
- Participate in decision making about child's program

NURSING DIAGNOSIS #6

Knowledge deficit regarding deficit, treatment, skills necessary to care for child at home/other setting

Rationale: If knowledge deficit exists, the child's health problems/behaviors cannot be appropriately

managed, nor can individualized educational/social/recreational experiences be planned to meet the child's special needs.

☐ GOAL

The child will maintain/improve current levels of function; family members will verbalize an understanding of the child's specific needs.

☐ IMPLEMENTATION

- Allow the child to participate as much as possible in the decision making process.
- Assist the family members to learn technical skills as well as behavioral techniques that are necessary in caring for the child (e.g., scheduling, routines, and equipment).
- Correct any misunderstandings and provide health teaching; refer to the appropriate nursing care planning guide for current medical diagnosis.
- Teach skills that may need to be employed after discharge (e.g., dressing changes).
- Review/teach about medications (e.g., dosage, time, method of administration, side effects).
- Visit the home or other transfer site to assess needs (e.g., additional equipment, supplies), or consult with home health nurse prior to discharge.
- Provide time for child/family members to practice necessary home care (e.g., dressing changes, soaks).
- Provide information regarding community agencies/resources; provide telephone numbers of physician, clinic, day treatment/residential programs.
- Ensure that family realizes that options (e.g., home care, residential care) may change as the child's/family's situation changes.

☐ EVALUATION CRITERIA/DESIRED OUTCOMES

The Child
- Maintains/improves functioning

The Family Members
- Describe child's care needs accurately
- Demonstrate skills/procedures to be carried out after discharge
- Schedule follow-up appointments with physician/clinic/program
- List community support services available

The Child who is Dying/Terminal

Definition/Discussion

Societal and cultural values influence both children and adults in their acceptance of death. Understanding those values influences the perceptions of/reactions to the knowledge that a child is dying. Previous experiences with death (e.g., pet, family member, friend, peer) will influence the child's perception of/reaction to death. Children convey their feelings and understanding of impending death through symbols and behaviors.

The age of the child must be considered in relation to his/her level of understanding regarding death and dying. Young children may equate death with separation, going into a grave, or sleep. The apparent lack of understanding on the child's part about what is happening does not mean the child has no anxiety about death and dying. Children perceive alterations in staff and family behavior around them and may adjust their own reaction to death based on adult behavior.

The development of a concept of death takes place in stages related to the child's maturing cognitive abilities, rather than the child's chronologic age. Factors such as cultural background, religious socialization, and real-life experiences with death and dying processes influence the concept formation. Children learn to cope with death mainly through observing parents, other family members, and friends. Emotional support and teaching of the family promote adaptive coping with death in both children and parents. Exposure to death in a matter-of-fact, non-frightening manner and at a developmentally appropriate level tends to be less fearful. This results in more adaptive coping compared to those who have not had this developmentally appropriate presentation.

Nursing Assessment

☐ PERTINENT HISTORY

Course of illness (e.g., length, characteristics), social and cultural values of family, previous experiences with death (e.g., relative, friend, pet), home measures to maintain child's comfort and to relieve anxiety

☐ PHYSICAL FINDINGS

Level of consciousness, vital signs, level of hydration, amount of pain/discomfort, energy available for self-care and diversional activities

☐ PSYCHOSOCIAL CONCERNS/ DEVELOPMENTAL FACTORS

Age and developmental level, coping mechanisms of child/family, support systems and resources available, behavior of parents and siblings around the child, expectations of child/family, habits/rituals of child at home

☐ PATIENT AND FAMILY KNOWLEDGE

Causes, options, level of knowledge, readiness and willingness to learn

Nursing Care

☐ LONG-TERM GOAL

The child will maintain physiologic/emotional functioning with comfort and reduced anxiety during the terminal process; the family will move toward acceptance and resolution of the terminal process so they can assist in providing comfort and support to the dying child.

NURSING DIAGNOSIS #1

Alteration in comfort: pain related to disease process

Rationale: Throughout the course of the illness and in particular close to the time of death, the pain the child experiences becomes the parent's pain, and the apprehension that the parents have is transferred to the child, increasing discomfort.

☐ GOAL

The child will experience minimal pain and discomfort, thus easing the parent's pain as well

☐ IMPLEMENTATION

- Refer to *The Child Experiencing Pain*, page 217.
- Prepare the parents in advance for the pain the child may be experiencing.
- Assure the family that care givers are monitoring the child, and prepared to help.

202

- Make sure the family knows how often the pain medication can be given and the time that it is due.
- Assess pain and provide medication PRN; use oral medications whenever possible; attempt to reserve heavy doses of any narcotics/shots until late in illness.
- Position the child to relieve pain.
- Give analgesic 30 minutes before painful procedures.
- Use gentle touch, soothing voice, distraction techniques (e.g., imagery, music) as appropriate.

☐ EVALUATION CRITERIA/DESIRED OUTCOMES

The Child
- Exhibits behaviors indicating comfort
- Denies pain verbally
- Sleeps comfortably

NURSING DIAGNOSIS #2

Anticipatory grieving related to probability of death

Rationale: As the child's illness progresses, emotional changes take place in the child and family reflecting stages of awareness and understanding of the terminal process. This grieving also occurs in care givers.

☐ GOAL

The child/family will express feelings, fears, anxieties and guilt; will verbalize their understanding of the child's physical health status and the terminal process.

☐ IMPLEMENTATION

- See Table 7—The Child's Conception of Death.
- Assess acceptance of the physical-health status; tell child/family that others in the same situation experience many kinds of feelings; ask what it is like for them.
- Allow and encourage parents to express feelings without the child being present.
- Provide opportunities for the child to share feelings without the parents.
- Accept feelings and expressions in a nonjudgmental manner.
- Permit expressions of anger and hostility, but do not allow unacceptable behavior; the child may perceive this as hopelessness and abandonment.
- Provide age-appropriate tools (e.g., toys, pens, pencils) that will enable the child to have normal experiences and symbolically express level of understanding about death; refer to *The Child Requiring Play Therapy*, page 220.

- Avoid false cheerfulness and evasiveness that may prevent the child from trusting/expressing true feelings.
- Allow discussion of the physical manifestations of the illness, the diagnosis, and possible outcomes; use language that can be understood by all.
- Give information to the child and family about changes that are occurring in the body.
- Encourage family members, friends, peers, to continue interaction with the child; be available to them if the child withdraws from their attempt to comfort.
- Allow the child to make decisions regarding physical care (e.g., setting the time for procedures and participating in daily activities whenever possible).
- Allow the family to assist with care, or if that is not feasible, to assist with the care of other children on the unit (if the child/family desire and accept this).
- Keep the family informed on the daily medical and nursing regimen so they can be kept abreast of the child's physical and emotional functioning.
- Assess the parents' coping behavior so that when they need support, or are unable to be with the child and need to be alone, feelings of guilt will be avoided; seek consultation from a psychiatric/mental health nurse if necessary.
- Assess the strengths of the parents; utilize those strengths in planning the management of the child.
- Provide opportunities for staff discussion of home care options.
- Explain the decision for home care is not irreversible if the family cannot cope.

☐ EVALUATION CRITERIA/DESIRED OUTCOMES

The Child/Parents
- Identify feelings
- Express understanding of prognosis
- List resources available for support

NURSING DIAGNOSIS #3

Self-care deficit: feeding, bathing/hygiene, dressing/grooming, toileting related to debilitated state

Rationale: As the terminal illness progresses, the child becomes weaker and less able to meet physical needs, and physiologic demands of illness manifest in fever, bleeding, drainage, and incontinence that increase physical care demands.

☐ GOAL

The child will maintain as much independence as possible in activities of daily living (ADL); will maintain physiologic functioning with comfort for as long as possible; the family will participate in the child's physical care.

☐ IMPLEMENTATION

- Encourage the child's participation in ADL as long as the child's energy levels are not depleted.
- Use passive/active range-of-motion exercises as tolerated; encourage as much ambulation as possible.
- Ensure adequate intake of fluid and food; use supplements when necessary; allow child choice of food when possible.
- Preserve skin integrity (e.g., massage, bathe, use lotions, sheepskins, water mattress); reposition every 2 hours and as necessary.
- Maintain a pleasing physical environment (e.g., allowing adequate ventilation of the room, use of room deodorants when necessary, permitting toys/material objects of importance to the child to be present).
- Allow the child to wear own clothing when possible.

☐ EVALUATION CRITERIA/DESIRED OUTCOMES

The Child
- Remains clean and dry
- Is positioned comfortably every 2 hours

The Parents
- Demonstrate moving and hygiene techniques

NURSING DIAGNOSIS #4
a. **Diversional activity deficit** related to immobility, lack of energy, isolation from friends
b. **Social isolation** related to separation from family, friends

Rationale: A child with a terminal illness may lack the physical stamina to engage in previous accustomed play activities. The child may withdraw from friends in preparing for death, friends may stay away because they are uncomfortable, friends/parents may prohibit visiting ill child so as to protect healthy child (physically/emotionally).

☐ GOAL

The child will not be bored; will accomplish age-appropriate activities as stamina permits.

☐ IMPLEMENTATION

- Talk with child to assess wants/desires regarding play, favorite activities.
- Provide age-appropriate play activities (e.g., playing jacks, baking cookies, making paper dolls, col-

oring, finger painting, clay modeling, reading, watching favorite movies/TV, listening to music, caring for pets, walking outside, riding in wagon).
- Include child in family activities as much as possible; if at home, suggest child be placed in central area where family gathers.

☐ EVALUATION CRITERIA/DESIRED OUTCOMES

The Child
- Shows no listlessness/irritability from lack of activity
- Does not complain, demonstrate behaviors of boredom

NURSING DIAGNOSIS #5
Knowledge deficit regarding preparation for transfer of child to home or nonacute setting

Rationale: Given the right set of circumstances and supportive help for the family, a death at home (or in a more home-like setting) can be more comfortable and more personal for both the child and the family. Training the parents to become the primary care givers can often help the family to overcome the feelings of helplessness and loss of control that accompany a death in the hospital setting.

☐ GOAL

The child will maintain current level of functioning in new setting; the child/family will perceive that home/nonacute hospital care is a viable alternative; the family will demonstrate understanding of the child's care; will state potential complications, and list community resources.

☐ IMPLEMENTATION

- Assist family members to learn the skills necessary to care for the child's physical needs at home (e.g., administration of medications, positioning, range-of-motion exercises, bathing, skin care, use of equipment, bedside commodes, suctioning devices).
- Assist to recognize need for pain medications and the amount necessary to maintain comfort.
- Make home visit to assist family in setting up the home for the child prior to discharge.
- Refer to appropriate agencies (e.g., VNA, health department, home health agency, hospice) for additional professional assistance.
- Assist the family in anticipating funeral arrangements; arrange for social service agencies and resource persons (e.g., clergy) to be available.
- Refer to self-help groups in their community; keep a list available at your nursing unit for convenient use; refer to the American Cancer Society or Com-

munity Mental Health Center for additional resources.
- Give family list of names/phone numbers to call in case of questions/emergency.

- Acknowledges the decision for home care is not irreversible if the family cannot cope
- Understands arrangements for the use of community resources including support/self-help group and clergy

☐ EVALUATION CRITERIA/DESIRED OUTCOMES

The Child/Family
- Demonstrates technical skills needed to care for self/child at home

Table 7
The Child's Conception of Death

Concepts	Nursing Implications
Infant (0–14 months) • Elementary sense of the meaning of separation. • Until about 5 months, the loss means the deprivation of the basic needs for food, comfort, and security. • Separation anxiety develops beginning with stranger anxiety about 7–8 months and then the concept of object permanence around 9 months. • Child is sensitive to parental reactions (e.g., anxiety, anger, sadness, crying).	• Note behaviors indicative of response to separation (e.g., excessive crying, irritability, apathy, listlessness, feeding disorders, weight loss, developmental delays). • Assist parents to deal with feelings about loss and death, which will allow the build-up of emotional reserves to meet the needs of the infant. • Provide visual, auditory, and tactile stimulation (e.g., talk to, play with, hold infant). • Provide age-appropriate play activities (e.g., peek-a-boo, "all-gone").
Toddler (15 months–2½ years) • Comprehension of loss remains limited in scope, but child can extend concept beyond the maternal figure to people and objects in the world around him. • Separation anxiety reaches its peak around 2 years. • Learns through repeated separations that reunions are an inevitable outcome; therefore, death is temporary.	• Note behaviors indicative of response to separation (e.g., anger, tantrums, depression, withdrawal, inappropriate attachment). • Listen attentively and be matter of fact and honest: "Grandpa can't come to dinner because he's dead and in (heaven, cemetery, or other explanation)." Use correct terms "death," "died," "buried," to prevent confusion; do not use "sleep" to describe death as toddler will be afraid to sleep. • Know that toddlers are adept at sensing inconsistencies between verbal and nonverbal messages; withholding real feelings will make toddler anxious. Say, "Crying makes me feel better when I'm sad," or "Grownups need to cry and be sad, too." • Provide appropriate play activities (e.g., hide and seek, peek-a-boo, jack-in-the-box).
Preschooler (2½–6 years) • Death does not imply cessation of life but an altered state of living (e.g., sleep, immobility). • Attributes life and consciousness to the dead. • Egocentric thinking results in the notion that dead people can be fed or given medicine to bring them back to life, because these kinds of things make the child feel better. Television and cartoons reinforce that death is not final. • Does not understand intent or reasons behind events; attributes magical or supernatural causes to what is seen and cannot be understood; may perceive death as a punishment or retribution for wrongdoing.	• Note behaviors that indicate a response to the death: ritualistic or superstitious behaviors (e.g., continuing to set a place at the table; may lie awake at night to ward off monsters; has repeated questions, may continue to ask when the deceased is coming home, or when will be the next time to see the person, why did the person die). • Utilize familiar situations to talk about death (e.g., talk about dead birds, bugs, autumn leaves, or dead flowers; read age-appropriate books and let child draw pictures). • Allow child to have funeral ritual for deceased pets (curious child may dig up the remains to see if still in ground). • Give concise and frequent explanations as requested by child regarding the death. • Explain death in terms child can understand (e.g., "Dead people [animals] cannot eat or run or play or be sad or happy"). • Explain that people cannot be "wished away"; inform child that everyone has these wishes sometimes and that thoughts and wishes cannot hurt others.

Table 7—*Continued*
The Child's Conception of Death, Cont.

Concepts	Nursing Implications
	• Know that preschoolers accept literal meaning of words; listen to thoughts and feelings and clarify understanding of death; familiarize yourself with words or phrases that connote death to the preschooler, and use them when referring to the deceased. Do not use them in association with the preschooler. For example, if child says pet is "sleeping," do not put child to bed stating "It is time to go to sleep." Use child's terms of "nite-nite," "bedtime," "tuck me in time."
	• Accept expressed feelings; give support until child feels safe enough and has enough self-control to grieve and begin to resolve loss.
	• Hold and comfort the child. Say "It's OK to cry or be angry"; let child know that s/he was not at fault or responsible for death.
School-age (6–12 years)	• Note behaviors that indicate a response to death: anxiety about changes in routine; creation of rituals or setting routines as magical or protective; nailbiting, thumbsucking; hyperactivity; mood swings; inappropriate gaiety.
• By 9 years, equates death with the cessation of life; is more reality oriented and logical in thought.	• Assess understanding and clarify meanings of statements and questions; ask "What do you think makes people (animals) die?" This age group responds well to logical explanation.
• Increased cognitive abilities facilitate an understanding of time and transformation of states.	• Listen to religious orientation and beliefs; allow child to talk about feelings; provide aggressive outlets through play, as well as opportunities to draw, write, read and tell stories. Use physical contact and bedtime rituals to encourage conversation about the happenings of the day, joys, fears, concerns, questions.
• Considers death as something that happens to someone else until about 9 years old, then death becomes universal.	• Allow child to attend or discuss funeral and burial services; tell what to expect in matter-of-fact way; arrange for friend or family member to sit with child and take child out of service if child wants to leave. Take child to burial site to visit grave if child desires. Answer questions about postdeath activities (e.g., mortuary, autopsy, or funerals).
• May feel varying degrees of responsibility; can still interpret death as punishment.	• Know that support given to parents about their concerns and feelings about death will help child. Allow child to laugh and play during periods of bereavement; play is the work of child and will facilitate grief work.
• Has pronounced fears of mutilation.	• Acknowledge child's concerns and fears about parents' possible death; let child know that they are not dying and who would care for the child if they did.
	• Provide appropriate play activities; reassure that child is not responsible for the death, that child did nothing wrong to cause the death. Reinforce that no physical harm will come to child because of the death.

Table 7—Continued
The Child's Conception of Death, Cont.

Concepts	Nursing Implications
Adolescent (13–18 years) • Understands death is universal, including self, but still does not accept it as believed reality (practices denial); anxiously avoids thought of death; directs energies at obtaining a sense of self and one's place in the world.	• Note behaviors that may indicate a response to the death: defiance, drug/ETOH abuse, reckless driving; tachycardia, tachypnea, flushed skin tone, diaphoresis; restlessness, pacing; mood swings; may ask many questions; will fear and resent any intrusion on independence; may regress in behavior and become demanding of help with the simplest tasks. • Listen to thoughts and feelings about death; answer questions honestly; discuss movies, television, and books with theme of death. • Treat with respect and as an individual who needs guidance and support and needs to retain independence, control, and decision-making power; facilitate peer-group contact. • Accept expressed feelings of anger or resentment; assist family to regard unpredictable outburst or projection of anger toward staff or parents as normal response to grief and mourning; observe for misconceptions and leftover "magical thinking" or responsibility/guilt for death. Focus on normalcy of experimentation with independence, sexuality, and aggression so that adolescent will release inappropriate guilt. Listen and give support to parents so they can support adolescent and believe in his/her growing process as mature person. • Discuss plans for future. Reinforce the need to be responsible for personal safety and have adolescent problem solve way to provide this. • See *Strategies for Counseling Adolescents*, page 000.

The Child with Failure to Thrive (Nonorganic)

Definition/Discussion

Failure to thrive (FTT) is the deviation of an infant's or child's growth rate below a normal standard. The weight may persist below the third percentile for age or may decrease to become less than 80% of ideal weight for age. The deceleration or persistence at a low weight may be the result of organic or nonorganic (psychosocial) etiologies.

- *organic:* physiologic cause is known to contribute to growth failure such as defects in digestion (e.g., cystic fibrosis) or absorption (e.g., gastroenteritis), failure to metabolize (e.g., inborn errors), disruption in utilization (e.g., infection, malignancy, cardiac disease), neurologic disorders (e.g., diencephalic syndrome)
- *nonorganic:* dysfunctional patterns of interaction between primary caretaker (usually mother) and infant/child; caretaker appears to be "out of touch" with the child

Nursing Assessment

☐ PERTINENT HISTORY

Prenatal history; birth and neonatal course (e.g., birth weight, discharge weight); past medical problems; height and weight of other family members; illnesses; nutritional intake; method and type of feeding; food preparation; behaviors during feeding; developmental milestones

☐ PHYSICAL FINDINGS

Weight, height, head circumference, vital signs, hydration status, presence of vomiting, characteristics of stool, cardiac/respiratory/gastrointestinal/genitourinary/neurologic status; observed behavior of child and parents during feeding

☐ PSYCHOSOCIAL CONCERNS/ DEVELOPMENTAL FACTORS

Family social history (e.g., father/mother employment, availability at home, relationship between parents, known/suspected child abuse, ability of family income to meet basic needs), age when major developmental milestones were achieved, comparison of child's development with any siblings or parental expectations, availability of support systems

☐ PATIENT AND FAMILY KNOWLEDGE

Appropriate interactional patterns, willingness to change and to accept support from outside the family, level of knowledge, readiness and willingness to learn

Nursing Care

☐ LONG-TERM GOAL

The infant/child will attain normal growth rate and establish functional patterns of interaction with caretaker.

NURSING DIAGNOSIS #1

Alteration in nutrition: less than body requirements related to insufficient caloric intake, difficulties in feeding

Rationale: The growing body has specific caloric intake requirements related to stages of growth and development. Insufficient intake of calories results in a growth deficit. Protein is necessary for tissue healing and fluid balance. Hypoproteinemia may lead to edema, which interferes with cellular nutrition. Anemia reduces oxygen-carrying capacity of the blood and may result in tissue hypoxia. Vitamins and minerals are necessary for many aspects of cell membrane formation and stability. Dehydration leads to decreased tissue perfusion. Infants and children with FTT can be frustrating to feed; they may turn away, refuse the nipple, fall asleep, vomit, spit, or fight feeding. Prior feeding experiences may have been unpleasant.

☐ GOAL

The child will ingest an adequate diet for age; will eat without resistance.

☐ IMPLEMENTATION

- Monitor and record intake and output accurately.
- Provide adequate caloric intake (may need 150–200 cal/kg/day); focus on protein intake.
- Offer small amounts of high-protein food and fluids at frequent intervals; consult dietician as needed.
- Weigh child daily on same scale, in same clothes, at same time.
- Include primary caretaker as much as possible in feeding care; observe interaction patterns.
- Demonstrate nurturing by holding, cuddling, and talking to child during feeding; teach parents to nurture during feeding.
- Provide feeding times that are conflict free.
- Encourage and praise child/parents for any behaviors that are conducive to successful feeding.
- Teach parents regarding the current developmental level of child; explain that child is not purposefully refusing to eat in order to frustrate them.

☐ EVALUATION CRITERIA/DESIRED OUTCOMES

The Child
- Gains weight
- Resumes normal growth pattern for developmental level
- Eats without resistance

The Parents
- Participate in feeding
- Describe child's current developmental level
- State realistic expectations for child's feeding behavior

The Child/Parents
- Interact appropriately with each other

NURSING DIAGNOSIS #2

Alteration in parenting related to low self-esteem

Rationale: Parents who have low self-esteem are not confident in their roles and may be depressed. These feelings disrupt healthy parent-child interaction and reduce chances for effective parenting.

☐ GOAL

The parents will express positive feelings and demonstrate adequacy in the parenting role.

☐ IMPLEMENTATION

- Provide time for parents to express feelings/concerns/doubts about parenting roles.

- Encourage parents to participate as much as possible in all aspects of child care.
- Praise even the smallest parental attempts to participate in care giving and nurturing.
- Show parents developmentally appropriate child care techniques.
- Role model positive parenting behaviors (e.g., talk soothingly to child, praise child for appropriate behavior, use distraction as appropriate to stop undesirable behavior in child instead of verbally belittling or physically handling child).
- Identify parental support groups (e.g., Parents Anonymous) available in the community.

☐ EVALUATION CRITERIA/DESIRED OUTCOMES

The Parents
- Care for child appropriately
- Verbalize positive feelings about parenting
- Demonstrate realistic, developmentally appropriate expectations for their child

---

NURSING DIAGNOSIS #3

Impairment of skin integrity related to decreased nutritional intake

Rationale: Children who fail to thrive often are emaciated and dehydrated as a result of insufficient nutritional intake. Any interference with cellular nutrition will disrupt skin integrity.

☐ GOAL

The patient will maintain intact skin surfaces while undergoing nutritional therapy.

☐ IMPLEMENTATION

- Bathe daily with mild soap and rinse completely; leave no residue on skin to contribute to breakdown.
- Clean diaper area quickly and gently after soiling.
- Use lubricating cream on entire body to prevent drying of surface.
- Reposition child every 1–2 hours.

☐ EVALUATION CRITERIA/DESIRED OUTCOMES

The Child
- Has no drying, cracking, peeling skin
- Maintains perineal skin integrity

NURSING DIAGNOSIS #4

Alteration in health maintenance related to impaired family dynamics, lack of resources

Rationale: Families of children who fail to thrive characteristically are isolated from the mainstream of society. They often have no extended family in the vicinity or a dysfunctional extended family. Mothers may withdraw from the family; fathers may be unable/unwilling to help or are not present. These families may demonstrate ineffective or non-existent use of medical and community resources. They may either not know about available resources or reject outside help.

☐ **GOAL**

The family will identify existing medical and community services; will accept assistance.

☐ **IMPLEMENTATION**

- Establish a trusting relationship with the family; use nonjudgmental listening techniques; acknowledge their concerns.
- Give family a list of community services available.
- Alert interdisciplinary team of need for social work involvement.
- Use relationship with the family to introduce the outside support; introduce social worker to family.
- Assist with scheduling of appointments for follow-up care prior to discharge (this will let family know they are not alone).

☐ **EVALUATION CRITERIA/DESIRED OUTCOMES**

The Family
- Allows nurse to interact with them
- Accepts outside assistance/support
- Establishes and keeps follow-up appointments

NURSING DIAGNOSIS #5

Knowledge deficit regarding normal child growth and development

Rationale: Parents who lack knowledge of normal growth and development will have unrealistic expectations for child behavior as each new developmental stage approaches. Expecting behavior beyond the child's capabilities, or labeling a child's normal behavior as spiteful, reduces the effectiveness of parenting.

☐ **GOAL**

Parents will understand normal behaviors in the next stage of child's development.

☐ **IMPLEMENTATION**

- Refer to *Normal Growth and Development*, pages 231–245, and *Guidelines for Teaching Patients and Families*, page 229.
- Teach parents about normal childhood growth and development; give them written material or suggest references to reinforce teaching.
- Praise parents for increased knowledge about their child.
- Identify resources available to assist with continued learning.

☐ **EVALUATION CRITERIA/DESIRED OUTCOMES**

The Parents
- Participate in teaching sessions
- List normal behaviors in the next stage of child's development
- Verbalize positive feelings regarding new knowledge

The Parent Experiencing Grief and Loss

Definition/Discussion

Grief is the set of normal responses a person goes through following the death of a loved one, or the loss of an idealized perfect child because of birth defects or prematurity. Mourning is the psychologic process that results from a loss. The grief and mourning process is the process of coping with and adapting to the loss. According to Engel (1965), the grief and mourning process involves three states: 1) shock and disbelief, 2) developing awareness of the loss, and 3) restitution. Full restitution may take a year or more and some people never completely recover. Each stage has its own adaptive responses and time frame.

Nursing Assessment

- [ ] **PERTINENT HISTORY**

    Medical history of child, length/type of illness, nature/cause of condition (e.g., hereditary, accidental, self-destructive)

- [ ] **PHYSICAL FINDINGS**

    General level of wellness/illness, ability to sleep, appetite

- [ ] **PSYCHOSOCIAL CONCERNS/ DEVELOPMENTAL FACTORS**

    Developmental stage and tasks; expectations for the outcome of the illness; meaning of the loss; past experiences with loss: what previous losses have occurred, rate of progression through the grief process, what helped them cope; support system; normal expression of emotions, communication patterns; degree of success in completing previous stages of development; habits/rituals (e.g., sleeping, eating, playing)

- [ ] **PATIENT AND FAMILY KNOWLEDGE**

    Stages of grief, what to expect in each stage; community resources; level of knowledge, readiness and willingness to learn

Nursing Care

- [ ] **LONG-TERM GOAL**

    The parents will cope with the loss by completing each stage of the grief and mourning process.

NURSING DIAGNOSIS #1

Grieving related to the death of a child, birth of an infant with major defects

Rationale: Grief is the expected and normal response to the death of a child or loss of the idealized perfect infant.

- [ ] **GOAL**

    The parents will go through the stages of grief in their own manner and reach resolution.

- [ ] **IMPLEMENTATION**

    - Help parents to talk about their feelings (e.g., "Would you like to talk about what has happened?" "What is it like for you just now?").
    - Expect a variety of grief reactions; know that all are adaptive and should be supported except suicidal ideation, destructive reactions; anger and hostility may be projected; know that it is not meant for you personally; do not reject the parents but rather give support (e.g., "You must be feeling very angry right now," or "I feel that you are really hurting inside"); continue to spend time with them.
    - Provide empathic listening (probably the most helpful intervention); do not challenge statements, but encourage more expressions of feelings.
    - Recognize individual responses to grief, which are determined by ego strengths, perception and meaning of loss, previous experience, and present support systems.
    - Avoid platitudes (e.g., "You're healthy, you'll be able to have another child").
    - Ask the parents if they wish to see the baby/child;

ask if they have seen a dead person before if the child is dead and they wish to view the body; assess expectations and provide information accordingly; wrap/cover the body in a blanket; handle it tenderly and carefully.

- Discuss the positive and negative aspects about seeing the body if parents are ambivalent; know that some view this as helpful to shorten the period of shock and disbelief.
- Adjust visiting hours if necessary to allow family/friends to visit and provide needed support.
- Be prepared to discuss such things as signing of autopsy or death certificate, disposing of child's clothes, possible future surgery and hospitalization for living baby.
- Have the same nurse each shift sit and talk with parents twice/shift if possible; allow family or friend to remain at bedside.
- Explain to the parents that the next stage of adaptive resolution involves behaviors of: asking questions (e.g., about the cause of death or deformity, what can be done for the living child); making outbursts (e.g., crying, anger, hostility); and feeling overwhelmed, interspersed with reality.
- Continue to support the grieving process; reinforce positive, adaptive grieving.
- Share the importance of allowing self to grieve openly rather than suppressing it; stress that both parents need to grieve and may not be able to support each other.
- Discuss with parents/family how they expect to cope at home; assess the need for ongoing support (e.g., public health or home health nurse, referral to a mental health clinic or a private mental health worker).
- Provide referrals and follow-up as needed; work with family so they can continue to give the parents support after discharge.

☐ EVALUATION CRITERIA/DESIRED OUTCOMES

The Parents
- Talk about the child and about feelings of loss
- Move through the stage of shock, disbelief, anger, and progress to developing an awareness of the reality of the loss
- Verbalize an understanding of the time span needed to complete the grief process

---

NURSING DIAGNOSIS #2
Knowledge deficit regarding the process of grief

Rationale: The experience of grief makes it difficult for the parents to take in and retain information. The parents may be experiencing a major loss for the first time.

☐ GOAL

The parents will verbalize where to obtain information and support for grieving.

☐ IMPLEMENTATION

- Discuss responses to grief, point out how responses are common and necessary, that others experiencing a loss have many of the same responses.
- Tell what to expect next in the grieving process.
- Explain that restitution will eventually occur and that frightening feelings/responses will diminish over time.
- Provide follow-up as necessary and when possible; tell parents they can call hospital staff for further support.
- Provide a written list of books on grief and community support services.

☐ EVALUATION CRITERIA/DESIRED OUTCOMES

The Parents
- State expectations for the future
- Explain that responses to grief are limited in time
- Identify resources available for information, support, and referral

The Child with Nonaccidental Trauma

Definition/Discussion

Child abuse is the nonaccidental injury or neglect inflicted upon children by their caretakers. It includes physical and emotional neglect, physical battering, psychologic attack, and sexual abuse. The presence of one physical or behavioral indicator (see Assessment) need not necessarily be viewed with alarm, but repeated "accidents" or multiple signs are a cause for suspicion and precautionary reporting. High-risk situations include presence of a child with a chronic illness, or family situations in which the parent has poor or nonexistent support systems.

In some cases, the abuse is unintended (e.g., the trauma is inflicted by someone who cannot cope or who has unrealistic expectations for the child). For others, the process of abuse may have to do with the sense of power it bestows upon the abuser. The aggressor may not be able to get these feelings of power from the peer/work environment, and so takes it out on the child who is dependent on the abuser for existence. Whether the abuse is intended or not, the consequences for the child are still the same.

Nursing Assessment

☐ PERTINENT HISTORY

Accident report of person(s) accompanying child, child's description of injuries, degree of agreement between accounts; person responsible for child's care at time of incident; probability that incident being described is feasible for the child's age/developmental stage; history of similar incidents for this child/sibling; history of abuse in extended family

☐ PHYSICAL FINDINGS

Vital signs; consciousness and orientation; general appearance (e.g., clean, dirty, clothing); bruises, locations and stages of healing; weight/height in relation to normal growth curve; untreated infections; dental hygiene; lumps on scalp; retinal hemorrhages, scars, lacerations, fractures (locations and quantity); multiple fractures, especially in children under age 2; burns (particularly from cigars or cigarettes) on soles of feet, palms of hands, buttocks, or genitalia; im-

mersion or scalding burns of hands, feet and buttocks with line of demarcation and few splash marks, degree of tissue damage; human bite marks, dental injuries, or cuts around mouth or eyes; areas of hair loss, location and description; trauma to genital area

☐ PSYCHOSOCIAL CONCERNS/ DEVELOPMENTAL FACTORS

Child's developmental/cognitive level; actual support systems; social interactions, behavior pattern (e.g., unresponsive, shy, fearful at approach or touch of an adult, passive while being examined, apprehensive when hearing other children cry, ignores friendly overtures, performs self-stimulating activities, seeks attention with asocial or deliquent acts, misses school frequently or falls asleep in class); verbal expectations of punishment for minor, childish accidents (e.g., spilling milk, wetting bed)

☐ PATIENT AND FAMILY KNOWLEDGE

Feelings toward the child, understanding of child's cognitive abilities, reactions to the incident, interactions, readiness and willingness to seek appropriate medical and mental health follow-up

Nursing Care

☐ LONG-TERM GOAL

The child will be free from pain, injury, fear, and neglect. The parents/caretakers will limit the potential for abuse of the child. The parents will implement new coping mechanisms, will seek appropriate help, and will not abuse the child.

NURSING DIAGNOSIS #1
a. **Potential for injury** related to abuse, neglect
b. **Alteration in comfort** related to physical injuries from abuse

Rationale: The array of physical injuries that a child may experience are varied. The trauma/neglect is usually severe enough to cause the child physical discomfort. Psychologically, the older

child may be suicidal or put him-/herself in a position to be harmed (e.g., drug/alcohol abuse, sexual promiscuity).

☐ GOAL

The child will be free from injury, self-abusive behavior; will be free from pain.

☐ IMPLEMENTATION

- Suspect abuse in children with unexplained injuries, injuries with several explanations, spiral fractures or head injuries in children under 2, repeated accidents, or cases in which siblings have had similar accidents.
- Conduct a complete nursing assessment.
- Restrict visitors if necessary.
- Explain all actions to child/parents.
- Follow hospital/state policies regarding the reporting of suspected child abuse; call a child abuse hotline.
- Confront self-abusive behavior; inform child that you will protect him/her from injuring self.
- Assess for behaviors indicating pain (e.g., guarding of an extremity, not letting anyone touch a particular area).
- Refer to *The Child Experiencing Pain,* page 217.
- Position child for comfort.
- Administer analgesics as ordered; assess and document effectiveness.
- Refer to Nursing Care Planning Guide specific to injuries (e.g., head injury, burns).

☐ EVALUATION CRITERIA/DESIRED OUTCOMES

The Child
- Is safe
- Is free from injury
- Does not engage in self-abusive behavior
- Verbalizes/demonstrates behaviors indicating comfort

NURSING DIAGNOSIS #2

Alteration in nutrition: less than body requirements related to neglect

Rationale: *Child abuse may take the form of willful neglect (e.g., withhold needed nutritional nourishment) or unintentional neglect (e.g., lack of knowledge). The child may be underweight for height, or have failure to thrive or signs of starvation.*

☐ GOAL

The child will gain weight according to the normal growth curve.

☐ IMPLEMENTATION

- Calculate caloric requirements appropriate for age; provide diet to meet these requirements.
- Weigh every other day, on same scale, in same clothes, at same time.
- Determine typical family activities associated with mealtime.
- Demonstrate appropriate mealtime behaviors; make mealtimes fun by socializing/eating with the child; have child eat with other children.
- Encourage regular mealtime intake as well as nutritious snacks.
- Provide positive reinforcement for appropriate mealtime behaviors.
- Refer to *The Child with Failure to Thrive,* page 208.

☐ EVALUATION CRITERIA/DESIRED OUTCOMES

The Child
- Gains weight according to normal growth chart
- Associates pleasure, enjoyment, and satiation with mealtimes

---

NURSING DIAGNOSIS #3

a. **Anxiety** related to a betrayal of trust by caretaker regarding safety and protection
b. **Fear** related to potential for repeat physical injury, abandonment

Rationale: *Children need to love and be loved. Once the child's trust has been betrayed, the child is likely to experience feelings of uneasiness. The child may fear that the abuser (particularly if it is a parent) will leave, or the school-age child may believe that the abuse is somehow deserved (i.e., punishment for some wrongdoing). Uneasy feelings about the abuser are generalized to all adults (e.g., hospital staff).*

☐ GOAL

The child will be protected from continued abuse; will realize that the responsibility for the abuse lies with the abuser; will verbalize feelings of safety/security.

☐ IMPLEMENTATION

- Observe and describe suspicious behavioral characteristics (e.g., flinching and ducking when anyone reaches out to touch; withdrawn, continual scanning of environment; searching for potential danger).
- Reassure child of safety while in your care.
- Offer to hold, rock, hug child; note child's reactions to/tolerance of this physical closeness; do not try to force physical closeness; carry infant in front carrier as much as possible.

- Determine what activities comfort child; establish a routine and stick to it as much as possible.
- Encourage verbal child to talk about feelings; be a concerned, quiet, nonjudgmental listener.
- Provide play materials; refer to *The Child Requiring Play Therapy*, page 220.

☐ EVALUATION CRITERIA/DESIRED OUTCOMES

The Child
- Discusses/plays out feelings
- Indicates comfort with staff verbally or through behaviors

NURSING DIAGNOSIS #4
a. **Disturbance in self-concept: self-esteem** related to parental abuse
b. **Ineffective individual coping** related to being unprotected and emotionally betrayed

Rationale: The basic relationship between child and parent is that of trust—to be protected, nourished, and loved. Children who are abused experience both physical and emotional traumas leading to a sense of worthlessness and feeling bad about oneself. In turn, the child may engage in self-deprecating statements and self-defeating behavior. Children are limited in their repertoire of coping mechanisms and trust their parents to keep them from harm. Abuse/neglect scars this trust and often pushes the child past the point of adaptive coping skills.

☐ GOAL

The child will begin to appreciate positive traits/aspects; will develop/implement adaptive coping skills.

☐ IMPLEMENTATION

- Observe for withdrawn behavior, and "setting self up" to get into trouble.
- Give positive reinforcement concerning appearance, participation in activities, abilities to complete projects; praise appropriately, not indiscriminately.
- Set appropriate limits; develop important task for child to do.
- Schedule time each day just for child; discuss perceived strengths/weaknesses; validate and reinforce strengths; assist to develop way to resolve weaknesses.
- Reinforce current adaptive coping skills; assist to develop new coping skills.
- Role play new coping skills with child to reinforce them.

☐ EVALUATION CRITERIA/DESIRED OUTCOMES

The Child
- Makes positive statements about self
- Accepts praise
- Role plays use of new coping skills
- Uses old adaptive and new coping skills in daily interactions

---

NURSING DIAGNOSIS #5
a. **Alterations in parenting** related to inappropriate limit setting/expectations for child's developmental/cognitive level
b. **Knowledge deficit** regarding presence of abuse, reasons for it, normal growth and development

Rationale: The family may deny the abuse, may be unaware that the child's injuries are a result of abuse, or may feel a need to "protect" the abuser for financial reasons or out of fear of abuse themselves. Few abusive parents really want to hurt their child and afterwards feel guilty, embarrassed, and a failure as a "good parent." Inappropriate expectations of age-appropriate skills can also potentiate an abusive situation.

☐ GOAL

The family will acknowledge abusive activities; the parents will understand normal child growth and development; will relate to their child on an appropriate developmental/cognitive level.

☐ IMPLEMENTATION

- Listen; be aware of your own nonverbal messages and feelings; maintain composure and compassion.
- Communicate support; refrain from criticism or rejection.
- Discuss abuse as a family problem; reinforce that everyone has a responsibility to protect the child.
- Explore alternative financial support/resources; connect with resources in community.
- Teach parents regarding their child's current developmental level; refer to *Normal Growth and Development*, pages 231–245.
- Give anticipatory guidance on the next level of development and appropriate expectations for that level; provide a list of resources for information about future developmental tasks; encourage follow-up to reinforce this learning.
- Role play with parents to help them internalize concepts of growth and development; allow them to identify with current cognitve level of child.
- Teach parents how to fulfill their wish to be good parents and "to do the right thing"; teach them to

enjoy their child, pointing out lovable attributes and features.

- Ask parents to join you and child in playing; role model for parent how to praise child; praise parent for participation; see *The Child Requiring Play Therapy*, page 220, and *Guidelines for Teaching Patients and Families*, page 229.
- Demonstrate how limits can be set and enforced; discuss how discipline can be given with consistency, fairness, and without physical force or uncontrolled anger; reinforce with praise and encouragement any parental attempts to nurture, comfort, cuddle, or express affection to the child.
- Help parents explore feelings; assist in defining stressors and help develop alternative methods of managing them.
- Assist parents to recognize behaviors that indicate increasing frustration/lack of coping; discuss actions to take to avoid abusing child.
- Explain that a child whose only emotional contact with parents is via abuse may provoke the parent deliberately in order to gain attention.

- Teach that the child will respond more positively and be better controlled if productive, emotionally satisfying activities are done together.
- Reassure parents that they have rights and needs also; provide them with names of organizations (e.g., Parents Anonymous) that assist parents who have abused their child; encourage involvement in follow-up visits.

☐ EVALUATION CRITERIA/DESIRED OUTCOMES

The Parents

- Recognize abuse, own high-risk behaviors
- Describe how they will protect the child(ren)
- Manage future stressful situations without resorting to abuse
- State appropriate developmental tasks, behaviors to expect of child
- Set appropriate limits on child's behavior
- Role play actions to take when high-risk behaviors/situations occur
- Contact community support groups

The Child Experiencing Pain

Definition/Discussion

Pain is a sensation of discomfort, distress, or agony resulting from a single stimulus or a class of stimuli. Emotions of anxiety, anger, depression, fear, loneliness, feelings of abandonment, and fear of body intrusion can alter perception and expression of pain. Research indicates that children experience as much pain as adults yet clinical studies show that physicians and nurses underestimate pain in children and tend not to offer pain medication or teach skills to cope with pain.

Nonverbal communication and changes in physiologic measures are present before verbal expression of pain in children; children may deny pain to be "good" or to avoid a "shot" or may fake pain to avoid school or unpleasant procedures, so observation of nonverbal and physiologic changes becomes important in differential diagnosis. Behavioral reactions to pain correlate with the age of the child. Pain reactions are subjective and individual, depending on individual life experience, maturity, and culture as well as type of pain, location, and stimuli.

Nursing Assessment

☐ PERTINENT HISTORY

Duration of pain; noxious stimuli: mechanical (trauma, friction), chemical (microorganisms, toxins, drugs), thermal (heat, cold), electrical; prior painful experiences and responses to them; use of pain medication (type, amount, time)

☐ PHYSICAL FINDINGS

Flushed skin; increased pulse, respirations, blood pressure; dilated pupils; vomiting; loss of appetite; favoring/guarding body part, location of pain; nature of pain (e.g., superficial, deep, referred), if able to differentiate; *newborn:* total body movement with brief, loud crying; *infant and toddler:* rolling head from side to side, pulling on ear for pain in ear or head, tense body postures, widely opened eyes, flexing knees for abdominal pain, refusing to move body part; *preschool/school-age child:* clenching teeth and fist, rigid posturing; *adolescent:* psychosomatic complaints

☐ PSYCHOSOCIAL CONCERNS/ DEVELOPMENTAL FACTORS

Cultural differences in expressing pain; ability to localize; words used to describe pain ("hurt," "owie," "boo-boo"); emotions, mood, affect; activity level; usual response to pain, coping mechanisms; *infants:* no memory of painful experience prior to 6 months, association of environment with painful experience; *toddlers:* fear of body intrusion; *preschooler:* magical thinking or fantasies (e.g., something they did/ thought caused the pain experience), increased verbal skills to communicate pain, poorly developed concept of body integrity, no understanding of temporal relationship, faking symptoms, *school-age child:* fear of body injury, exaggeration; *adolescent:* importance of body image, overconfidence compensating for fear

☐ PATIENT AND FAMILY KNOWLEDGE

Causes of pain, techniques for coping; level of knowledge, readiness and willingness to learn

Nursing Care

☐ LONG-TERM GOAL

The child will have pain recognized and treated; the child will be free from any pain that impairs day-to-day functioning or interferes with the attainment of life goals.

NURSING DIAGNOSIS #1

Alteration in comfort: pain related to condition

Rationale: Pain affects children's ability to cope with illness/hospitalization, interfering with their ability to reach their developmental potential.

☐ GOAL

The child will verbalize (or exhibit behaviors that indicate) a decrease in pain; will be free from pain-related immobility; will demonstrate an increased ability to cope with pain and discomfort; the parents/child will discuss feelings and concerns about pain and measures to relieve them.

☐ **IMPLEMENTATION**

- Help child talk (if able) about pain and relief measures.
- Discuss child's discomfort with parents; encourage them to carry out selected nursing care; ask to express their concern to you; explain rationale for comfort measures and pain medication.
- Administer analgesics as ordered; monitor frequently for effectiveness; report to physician if child's pain is not effectively relieved.

Infant/toddler
- Touch, comfort, hold; use soft voice or music.
- Observe for physiologic changes; monitor vital signs; examine part of body child pulls, rocks, or favors.
- Utilize distraction; rock, sing, carry, play peek-a-boo or other games that child enjoys.
- Maintain parent/child contact and do procedures as quickly as possible if distraction does not help; hold if restraints are needed; protect from injury (e.g., falling, breaking off the injection needle).
- Pay attention to toddler's complaints (can communicate verbally, localize their pain [e.g., "owie on my knee"], rarely fake pain).
- Ask parent what words, behaviors, and methods precipitate a response of intense physical resistance and emotional upset, and which methods of coping with pain are likely to be helpful.
- Listen to parents' feelings and concerns; include pertinent information from parents in care plan.
- Avoid intrusive procedures (e.g., rectal temperature, injections) as much as possible as these are threatening whether painless or painful; ask physician for oral medications, axillary temperature, or other alternatives.
- Accept regression (e.g., becoming incontinent even if toilet trained); give permission to cry.
- Have comfort objects available (e.g., bottle, blanket).
- Offer pain medication in forms that toddler will take (e.g., crush and put in gelatin or ice cream).

Older toddler/preschooler
- Monitor for self-imposed limitation of activity.
- Avoid use of heat, cathartics, or laxatives when abdominal pain is present.
- Report change of pain to physician.
- Do not take verbal attacks personally; understand that child is afraid; allow parent to do as much as possible for child.
- Tell child "It's OK to cry;" offer comfort; listen to child's concerns and feelings.
- Cover injection sites, abrasions, cuts with Band-Aids to give security that body injury is "fixed" and body integrity maintained; use progressively smaller dressings as size of dressing will be interpreted as progress in healing.

- Know that child may have exaggerated fears about body injury (e.g., worries about bleeding, insides falling out, needle punctures, mutilation, and castration); use term "fixed" rather than "removed."
- Measure axillary or oral rather than rectal temperature if child is able to cooperate.
- Use therapeutic play to prepare child for procedures and to discuss pain as part of illness/accident; use dolls, puppets, stuffed animals to demonstrate a procedure or to encourage a child to talk about an experience; refer to *The Child Requiring Play Therapy*, page 220.
- Clarify that child is not to blame for pain; magical thinking leads to guilt, shame, and idea that pain is punishment for wrongdoing.
- Desensitize to threatening equipment (e.g., needles, oxygen mask) by introducing it in pleasant, familiar surroundings, using play (e.g., dress a stuffed bear with an OR mask, cast, or give the bear a "shot"); if child shows fear, move equipment far away in room and reintroduce with play at a later time; allow child to touch and play with the equipment under supervision.
- Have child rate pain with a range of happy to sad faces or utilize colors to demonstrate discomfort; ask child to color or place an "x" in location of pain on a picture of child's body; give choice of comfort measures.
- Encourage child to draw pictures or use toys or dolls to tell stories about pain and hospitalization experience; allow child to project feelings onto dolls to learn child's perceptions and concerns.

School-age child
- Teach relaxation using imagery
  - "take deep breath and blow out slowly; let arms and legs be as limp as a wet noodle"
  - "breathe into painful area; let your breath blow out the pain; slowly breathe out and imagine pain is blowing away with the breath"
  - "put your hand or pillow over the 'hurt' and softly breathe into that area; as you breathe out, imagine that the tightness is melting away and that the hurt feels better"
- Observe nonverbal cues of fear or pain and offer support; know that crying or losing control may cause embarrassment; reassure as necessary.
- Limit procrastination and bargaining as delaying a dreaded event often increases anxiety.
- Ask preference as to presence of parents; discuss choice with parents.
- Tell child about available pain medications; explain that the sting of an injection or bad taste of medicine only lasts a moment, but will help take away some of pain for longer period of time.
- Allow child to plan and problem solve within reasonable limits for situation and condition, utilizing present cognitive skills.
- Use humor to distract or teach (e.g., comic books,

funny songs, stories) if child likes humor, jokes, and puns.
- Be extremely sensitive when examining genital area as touching the school-age child's genital area is very threatening.

Adolescent
- Approach with respect; ask what helps with pain/ discomfort and use these coping methods (e.g., pillow, hot tea, earphones with music, icepacks); offer privacy.
- Avoid authoritarian attitude; do not try to be "hip" or use adolescent jargon.
- Assess learning needs and offer information on techniques to distract or decrease pain; give something positive to do as well as to restore feelings of control (e.g., relaxation with imagery or cutaneous stimulation [e.g., rub skin in rhythmic pattern with lotion, powder, menthol, or cream; use pressure, heat, cold, electric vibrator set at moderate intensity]).
- Listen to and accept adolescent's concerns and feelings; use open-ended questions and be nonjudgmental.
- Assess knowledge and offer small amounts of information about pain, medications, and pain management as adolescent shows interest.
- Work with adolescent to find effective methods of coping with pain.
- Assess effectiveness of pain medications and techniques to distract or decrease pain.

☐ EVALUATION CRITERIA/DESIRED OUTCOMES

The Child
- Is relieved of pain
- Displays no physical behaviors indicating presence of pain
- Has no complaints of pain when asked (if verbal)

- Expresses feelings about pain and its relief at age-appropriate level
- Uses effective pain-relief measures at age-appropriate level

---

NURSING DIAGNOSIS #2
Knowledge deficit regarding cause of pain and pain management

Rationale: *If knowledge deficit exists child/parent cannot appropriately manage treatment of pain. A lack of understanding increases anxiety and tension, further increasing pain.*

☐ GOAL
The child/parents will adhere to pain management treatment at home and verbalize its importance.

☐ IMPLEMENTATION
- Answer questions using nonthreatening, brief, and honest information at child's level of understanding.
- Give child/parents verbal and written instructions regarding list of medications, dosages, schedule, possible side effects and when to report them to physician/clinic; where and how to obtain refills.
- Have child/parents demonstrate techniques to distract from or decrease pain.
- Make appointment for follow-up care.

☐ EVALUATION CRITERIA/DESIRED OUTCOMES
The Child/Parents
- State appropriate administration of medications, side effects, and when to contact physician concerning problems
- Utilize techniques to distract or decrease pain
- Keep appointment for follow-up care

The Child Requiring Play Therapy

Definition/Discussion

Play is the natural language of a child; it is the expression of a child's biopsychosocial being in relation to the environment. Therapeutic play is a supervised, semistructured play experience that is deliberately planned, observed, and evaluated in relation to its intended objectives.

Nursing Assessment

☐ **PERTINENT HISTORY**

Effective coping methods used by child in the past, prior experiences with stress/hospitalization, child's favorite play materials, changes/disruptions in routine or life-style

☐ **PHYSICAL FINDINGS**

Any physical limitations that would restrict child from certain activities

☐ **PSYCHOSOCIAL CONCERNS/ DEVELOPMENTAL FACTORS**

Developmental level of child, pattern of play at home

☐ **PATIENT AND FAMILY KNOWLEDGE**

Purpose, willingness to learn and participate in therapeutic play activities

Nursing Care

☐ **LONG-TERM GOAL**

The child will express ideas, feelings, and imagination through play; the child will adapt to the stress of illness/ hospitalization through play.

NURSING DIAGNOSIS #1
a. **Knowledge deficit** regarding hospitalization, treatments
b. **Ineffective individual coping** related to limited cognitive abilities, lack of available communication skills
c. **Diversional activity deficit** related to hospitalization, enforced activity restrictions

---

Rationale: During hospitalization, clinic visits, or illness experiences in the home, a child's emotional outlets may be restricted and fears intensified; and maladaptive behaviors may occur. The child may "act out" fear by aggression toward others, crying, denying the need for medical attention, or by withdrawing from interaction with others. Young children lack the cognitive/social/communication skills necessary to make sense out of the confusion they are experiencing. Play provides the child with a safe means of communicating thoughts, fears, concerns, and stressors. Health professionals may use therapeutic or goal-directed play to assist the child to relate to the environment and cope with injury, illness, hospitalization, discomfort, and separation from loved ones.

☐ **GOAL**

The child will communicate thoughts, feelings, concerns through play; will use play to decrease the stress of hospitalization; will cooperate with treatments and procedures.

☐ **IMPLEMENTATION**

• Refer to *Normal Growth and Development*, pages 231–245.
• Plan the specific purpose(s) of the play (e.g., to determine fears/concerns, relieve anxiety, express creativity, channel energy, distract from discomfort/pain, explain or teach a diagnostic or treatment procedure).
• Prepare a playroom for ambulatory children and a portable cart for children on bedrest; consult teachers, recreation specialists, parents, and children for suggested equipment and supplies; use your imagination; determine choice of equipment/ toys/supplies based on child's development and goal.
• Request consultative assistance and patient behavior information from coordinator/specialist.

- Be alert to behaviors/actions that reflect child's feelings.
- Validate impressions but do not restrict spontaneity; avoid interruptions.
- Be nonjudgmental; do not direct child or develop rules/guidelines that inhibit child's self-expression.
- Use up-coming special events as themes (e.g., "Tell a story about . . .").
- Encourage older children to write poems, stories, or plays; provide positive reinforcement for all accomplishments.
- Provide and encourage drawing, coloring, and water painting for self-expression; avoid use of "coloring books" and structured "art"; display if acceptable with child.
- Provide dolls, selected medical equipment so child can act out selected experiences (e.g., getting a shot, being anesthetized, removing sutures).
- Use age-appropriate books, drawings, models to demonstrate tests and procedures.
- Observe play; note failure to respond to age-appropriate toys and play materials; monitor types of play (e.g., solitary, parallel, interactional).
- Acknowledge feelings and encourage child to express them verbally; listen to what is and what is not revealed; share observations and findings with other health care professionals.
- Use community resource volunteers for entertainment (e.g., musicians, magicians, clowns, dancers, actors, puppeteers).
- Use tapes, records, books, and cartoon movies available on free loan from community libraries, schools, recreation centers; identify community resources.
- Ask parents to bring in child's favorite toys/activities if possible.
- Record pertinent observations regarding play experiences and responses, revealed fears, feelings, and indications of new insights.

☐ **EVALUATION CRITERIA/DESIRED OUTCOMES**

The Child
- Cooperates with treatment
- Shares fears/concerns
- Describes tests and procedures in own words

NURSING DIAGNOSIS #2

Knowledge deficit regarding value of play

Rationale: *Some parents are not aware of the benefits of play.*

☐ **GOAL**

Parents will understand usefulness of play in allowing child to explore feelings of fear, anxiety, pain, and happiness.

☐ **IMPLEMENTATION**

- Teach the relationship of play to ability to master developmental tasks and to cope with experiences in everyday life.
- Reinforce information about child's developmental level and cognitive abilities.
- Explain need for positive play experiences to promote child's self-esteem and sense of well-being.
- Role model appropriate activities/responses to facilitate optimal play.

☐ **EVALUATION CRITERIA/DESIRED OUTCOMES**

The Parents
- Verbalize an understanding of how play can assist child to resolve feelings of tension, bring life experiences into child's level of comprehension
- Assist child in creative play activities

The Child Experiencing Separation Anxiety

Definition/Discussion

Separation anxiety refers to the anticipation of danger or uncertainty that is generated by separating a child from significant others (usually parents). It occurs in older infants, toddlers, and in the early preschool years. The behaviors that accompany it can be divided into 3 recognizable stages or phases

- *protest*: begins with hospitalization or mother's absence and lasts from a few hours to 3 or 4 days; common protest behaviors (see Nursing Assessment) occur if another adult approaches child when the parents are absent
- *despair*: frequently called the mourning state or "settling in" stage, begins from 1 hour to several days following separation and lasts 1-2 days, or until discharge
- *detachment (or denial)*: period of seeming acceptance or adjustment as the child returns to normal patterns of behavior; has detached self from parents to cope with the emotional pain of wanting them, and easily goes from person to person forming superficial relationships

If the child has had an emergency admission or is placed in a pediatric intensive care unit (PICU), both child and family will encounter a varying combination of additional stressors that can potentiate the separation anxiety, such as

- nature and severity of child's illness
- restrictions and fright caused by necessary treatment (e.g., restraints, intrusive procedures, machines)
- sleep deprivation
- unfamiliar surroundings compounded by altered states of consciousness related to disease, fever, drugs
- imposed separation of family related to space limitations or unit policy
- the emotional impact of critically ill child on the parent (e.g., grief, shock, guilt)
- overwhelming sensory stimuli (e.g., noxious odors, noises)
- imposed bedrest
- threats to infant's/toddler's trust, security, and autonomy/initiative
- threats to older child's body image, integrity, control of functions, pain or fear of pain

Nursing Assessment

☐ **PERTINENT HISTORY**

Number of other siblings, birth order, experiences outside the home, other traumatic separations, previous reactions to separations

☐ **PHYSICAL FINDINGS**

Protest stage: puffy eyes, red face, restlessness and crying, crying out for and demanding presence of primary caretaker; listening for step and looking for approach of primary caretaker; intensified crying when parents leave and when demands are not met; refusal to go to sleep; refusal to cooperate with care or treatment procedures; fighting, struggling, resisting, or pushing caretakers away
Despair stage: regressive behavior (e.g., thumbsucking, holding blanket or toy, incontinence, whining, clinging, use of baby talk); apathy and withdrawal; sometimes hyperactive or overtly aggressive; no eye contact; staying in crib in a fetal position, pretending to be asleep; showing no pleasure when parents are present, crying when they appear, rejection of parents or clinging to them; demanding to be taken home; accepting nursing care passively; allowing staff to handle and touch him/her
Detachment stage: showing an interest in surroundings and others; accepting care and love from almost anyone; complacency; no acting-out behavior or frequent bursts of anger; playing well by self or with others; responding to parents no differently from anyone else

☐ **PSYCHOSOCIAL CONCERNS/ DEVELOPMENTAL FACTORS**

Rituals of child, time of awakening, feeding times and methods, naptimes and bedtime rituals; other significant behavioral patterns

☐ **PATIENT AND FAMILY KNOWLEDGE**

Understanding of behavior, developmental aspects of child care, concept of separation anxiety, level of knowledge, readiness and willingness to learn

Nursing Care

☐ LONG-TERM GOAL

The child will experience separation from caretaker during hospitalization with minimal traumatic/residual effects; the child will feel secure and trust others.

NURSING DIAGNOSIS #1

Ineffective individual coping related to separation, hospitalization

Rationale: *Learning to separate from parents is normally a gradual process achieved by the child as s/he comes to appreciate own separate individuality; it cannot be forced abruptly. The separation involved in hospitalization, coupled with the stress of illness, is usually beyond the normal adaptive capacity of a child aged 8 months to 6 years.*

☐ GOAL

The child will experience minimal effects of separation; will not injure self or others; will maintain a secure and trusting relationship with parents; will interact normally and effectively with peers and adults.

☐ IMPLEMENTATION

Protest stage
- Review *Normal Growth and Development*, pages 231–245, for age-appropriate needs.
- Provide one consistent care giver for child; have nurse meet child in presence of parent.
- Accept crying and anger; reassure child that parent will return.
- Use language appropriate for child's age and stage of development.
- Allow for safe areas like crib, playroom where no procedures are done.
- Delay intrusive procedures when possible if child is very upset or parents are absent.
- Stay visible but do not force contact with child; respond physically when child initiates contact, then cuddle and comfort as needed.
- Be warm, firm, and reassuring to child.
- Gently restrain if child attempts to escape or injure self or others; use crib nets or high-top cribs when necessary.
- Provide with familiar and cherished objects, if possible.
- Encourage one parent to room in if feasible.
- Encourage parents to visit often, participate in care whenever possible.
- Have parent leave something personal behind (e.g., purse or gloves) so child knows parent will return; have bedside pictures of family, pet, or best friend.
- Encourage visiting of siblings if hospital rules allow.
- Read to preschool child *Curious George Goes to the Hospital* or other appropriate books about hospitalization.
- Use puppets, comedy to attract child's attention and cooperation.
- Arrange for preschooler or older child to visit hospital (e.g., tour and preadmission party) if possible, to alleviate fears and reduce incidence of anxiety.
- Assess the actual effects of additional stressors and plan care according to individual needs of child/family; provide additional explanations, encouragement, touching/stroking, talking/soothing, environmental manipulation as indicated.
- Allow child to make some simple decisions, if able.

Despair stage
- Continue previous successful nursing actions.
- Allow, but do not foster or encourage regressive behavior.
- Provide for physical comfort and closeness; hold and rock child, establish trust.
- Attempt to maintain skills achieved at home (e.g., talking, toilet training); know that the last skill learned will be the first to disappear when child is stressed.
- Allow expression of anger through play with active toys (e.g., play clay, bang toys, balls) or dramatic play with puppets, dolls; refer to *The Child Requiring Play Therapy*, page 220.
- Use games like peek-a-boo or hide-and-seek to desensitize child (especially infant) to separation and to encourage the development of object permanence; tell stories in which people are reunited or brought together.
- Keep track of child's possessions and do not lose them; allow child to wear own clothes; have shoes at bedside so child can see that they are there when s/he needs them to go home.

Detachment stage
- Continue previous successful nursing actions.
- Talk about home, what the people are doing there now, about when child will be going home to room/school/brother/sister, and what s/he will do.
- Continue use of physical contact; explain to parents child's need to be held even if it appears that s/he rejects them.
- Help parents continue nurturing role (they may resent child's acceptance of the nurse and feel nurse is stealing child's love; if parents pull back from child, child may feel s/he is being abandoned).
- Allow child to have some control over own life and any procedures; encourage involvement with other children.

☐ EVALUATION CRITERIA/DESIRED OUTCOMES

The Child
- Is allowed to protest within limits
- Accepts care of nursing staff
- Accepts parents when they return
- Uses play activities to express fears
- Talks about home/family
- Interacts effectively with peers/adults
- Returns to previous level of social/interactive behavior

NURSING DIAGNOSIS #2

Knowledge deficit regarding child development, child-rearing practices

Rationale: If a knowledge deficit exists, parents can become overwhelmed by child's behavior and fear the child is acting abnormally or not responding appropriately.

☐ GOAL

The parents will verbalize an understanding of separation anxiety; will anticipate child's behavior and provide appropriate interventions.

☐ IMPLEMENTATION

- Explain the concept of separation anxiety and why the child is acting in certain ways.
- Encourage to verbalize feelings (e.g., confusion, sadness, anxiety).
- Encourage to visit even if child cries more at their appearance; explain this is child's way of coping and is a positive behavior.
- Discourage from "sneaking" away from child; encourage them always to say goodbye.
- Support in efforts at intervention; provide parents with general ideas for interventions but allow them to make the major decisions.

☐ EVALUATION CRITERIA/DESIRED OUTCOMES

The Parents
- Describe separation anxiety
- Express feelings toward child having separation anxiety
- Provide interventions for child to prevent separation anxiety

The Adolescent who Attempts Suicide

Definition/Discussion

Adolescence is a time of mood swings, depression, loneliness, anger, and other negative feelings balanced by positive new independence, sensations, experiences and relationships, achievements, and pleasures. These rapid changes may elicit a sense of loss of control over one's life—a sense of desperation that may lead to a functional fixedness through which the teen sees no other alternative but to end life. Feelings/motives that precipitate/precede a suicide attempt may include acting out (cry for help), impulsive acts, true death wish, desire to punish others or self, release from despair, or avoiding risk of rejection. An ongoing depressive process is usually present prior to suicide.

Nursing Assessment

☐ PERTINENT HISTORY

Precipitating factors, losses, past patterns of managing stress, chronic or terminal illness, school functioning, physical/sexual abuse, peer/family relations, alcohol/chemical abuse, promiscuity

☐ PHYSICAL FINDINGS

Hygiene, eating, sleeping, and elimination patterns; change in usual motor activity, nervous habits; scratches, bite marks, bruises, lacerations, or burns; orientation to person, time, place

☐ PSYCHOSOCIAL CONCERNS/ DEVELOPMENTAL FACTORS

Developmental level; interactional patterns; expression of affect; self-destructive behavior, rebellion, withdrawal, running away, social isolation, change in behavior, giving away possessions, irritability, low frustration level, restlessness, anger; sexuality, peer relationships, independence, school functioning; unusual sensations or thoughts; feelings of sadness, worthlessness, apprehension, fear of harm from others, inability to cope, difficulty concentrating; problem-solving skills

☐ PATIENT AND FAMILY KNOWLEDGE

Self-evaluation, parental perception of adolescent's behavior, patient and family's awareness of existence of a problem and willingness to work toward resolving issues; level of knowledge, readiness and willingness to learn

Nursing Care

☐ LONG-TERM GOAL

The adolescent will realize that life's frustrations and challenges do have possible solutions and will not attempt to end life; the adolescent will learn effective methods of communicating needs and feelings (e.g., loss, anger, guilt, failure, inadequacy, loneliness).

NURSING DIAGNOSIS #1

Potential for injury related to suicidal gestures/attempts

Rationale: Depending on the plan, the adolescent is at risk from self-harm. The more definitive the plan, the greater the risk. Suicidal gestures/attempts may include accidents as well as self-inflicted injuries.

☐ GOAL

The adolescent will not injure self.

☐ IMPLEMENTATION

- Take any comment or mention of death and suicide seriously.
- Do not promise to keep suicidal gesture a secret from individuals who can help.
- Discuss the suicidal ideation with the teen; assess lethality of comment (e.g., Does teen have a plan?, What is it?, Is it feasible?, Does teen have access to methodology?, What is the time frame?).
- Stay with adolescent at all times if lethality is moderate or high (e.g., plans to give overdose of

insulin, is diabetic, has access to materials needed—insulin, syringes).
- Remove potentially lethal objects from the environment.
- Place on one-to-one observation; make statements that indicate caring (e.g., "Staff care and are here to protect you and keep you safe until you are able to do that yourself.").
- Report findings to health care provider/mental health professional.
- Express "I care . . ." statements; articulate your concern for teen's safety and that you will protect him/her from harming self, even if that means informing others.
- Remain calm; be accepting and supportive; do not act shocked, make judgments, or instill guilt.

☐ **EVALUATION CRITERIA/DESIRED OUTCOMES**

The Adolescent
- Does not injure self
- Recognizes that someone cares enough to prevent the lethal behavior
- Participates in therapy

NURSING DIAGNOSIS #2

Potential for violence: self-directed related to anxiety, fear, dysfunctional grieving

Rationale: As teens progress through adolescence, they experience a variety of biopsychosocial changes. These may be perceived as threats to self-concept and create anxiety for the teen. Many events may precipitate fear in the adolescent (e.g., peer pressure, diagnosis of chronic illness, loss of a significant other, parental divorce, school failure, sexual development/activity, lack of knowledge about the biopsychosocial changes). The move to adolescence produces actual losses (e.g., childhood, identity, role) that must be grieved. In addition, the usual developmental changes of adolescence and the resulting confusion may cause the teen to experience an otherwise innocuous loss with increased intensity, or to experience disproportional and prolonged grief with a truly significant loss.

☐ **GOAL**

The adolescent will recognize own anxiety and coping patterns; will experience an increase in psychologic comfort; will develop/utilize effective coping skills.

☐ **IMPLEMENTATION**
- Encourage expression of feelings; refer to *Strategies for Counseling Adolescents*, page 252.

- Assess physical and psychologic symptoms that may accompany fear/anxiety/grief.
- Determine actual/perceived stressors/losses; define the significance; assist adolescent to define precipitating factor(s), real or imagined.
- Discuss past and present coping mechanisms; assist to identify effective and ineffective coping mechanisms.
- Assist to identify alternatives to suicide rather than merely postponing it; help find reason to live, something to look forward to.
- Assist to recognize behaviors indicating increased anxiety (e.g., increased restlessness, mood swings, apathy, poor concentration) and to develop mechanisms to manage behaviors (e.g., engage in physical activity, practice relaxation techniques, identify factors that can be controlled, make decisions when realistic, seek professional counseling); refer to *The Child/Family Experiencing Anxiety*, page 177.
- Instruct in use of relaxation techniques (e.g., deep breathing, meditation).
- Role play adaptive coping skills with teen; support and reinforce use.

☐ **EVALUATION CRITERIA/DESIRED OUTCOMES**

The Adolescent
- Expresses feelings
- Identifies stressors/losses
- Develops successful coping mechanisms
- Role plays new skills

NURSING DIAGNOSIS #3

Disturbance in self-concept related to distorted body image, decreased self-esteem

Rationale: One of the main developmental tasks of adolescence is to maintain a sameness with one's peers—not to be different. The suicidal adolescent often has a distorted view of self in relation to physical/social/emotional environment. Comparison of the self with a distorted environment can result in an altered sense of self and subsequent decreased self-esteem.

☐ **GOAL**

The adolescent will develop a realistic body image; will increase self-esteem.

☐ **IMPLEMENTATION**
- Note manner of dress and state of hygiene and grooming (e.g., disheveled, unkempt appearance).
- Engage in dialogue regarding feelings/opinions about self and personal appearance (e.g., likes/ dislikes, strengths/weaknesses).

- Explore feelings surrounding changes in body with onset of puberty.
- Encourage and reinforce any positive self statements; discuss ways to highlight good feelings about self (e.g., improving grooming/hygiene).
- Assist with hygiene and grooming as needed; reinforce any attempts toward improvement in hygiene/grooming.

☐ EVALUATION CRITERIA/DESIRED OUTCOMES

The Adolescent
- Participates in grooming and hygiene
- Makes positive statements about self

NURSING DIAGNOSIS #4

Alteration in family process related to suicidal ideation, gestures

Rationale: The normal supportive environment of the family is altered when an adolescent contemplates/attempts suicide. Members may become overly protective or ignore/deny the issue out of discomfort with the topic.

☐ GOAL

The family will achieve a productive functional state; will be supportive of the adolescent.

☐ IMPLEMENTATION

- Determine level of disruption in family functions and interactions.
- Provide opportunities for members to verbalize feelings (e.g., anger, disbelief) to nurse and one another.
- Assist adolescent/family to listen, hear, and acknowledge one another.
- Be accepting; both the adolescent and the family are feeling very vulnerable.
- Assist the family to identify and use supportive behaviors with one another through role play.
- Collaborate with the family to establish/facilitate goals and treatments.
- Encourage family to seek professional therapy; provide a list of community resources (e.g., men-

tal health clinics, Survivors of Suicide support group, clergy).

☐ EVALUATION CRITERIA/DESIRED OUTCOMES

The Family
- Participates in goal-setting and treatment
- Supports one another
- Participates in family/individual counseling

NURSING DIAGNOSIS #5

Knowledge deficit regarding adolescent suicide, early symptoms of suicidal behavior

Rationale: Many teens are unaware that many other "normal" teenagers also think about suicide; the adolescent is not different from the peer group in this respect. Teens who recognize problems, utilize coping skills and support systems are less likely to feel so hopeless. Parents often deny or ignore warning signs.

☐ GOAL

The adolescent/parents will recognize the scope of adolescent suicide; will know warning signs; will seek professional help if these signs appear.

☐ IMPLEMENTATION

- Discuss warning signs (e.g., behavior changes, mood swings, change in peer group or loss of peer group, school failure or absorption, decreased communication, expressing bad feelings about self, verbalizing suicidal ideation, making suicidal gestures/attempts).
- Give resource list of therapists proficient in adolescent and family therapy.
- Educate regarding the scope and seriousness of adolescent suicide.
- Identify community resources with counseling/information available to those contemplating suicide and their families (e.g., Suicide Hotline).

☐ EVALUATION CRITERIA/DESIRED OUTCOMES

The Adolescent/Parents
- Identify warning signs of suicide
- Verbalize the scope of the problem
- List community resources available

APPENDIX I
Nursing Diagnoses: Accepted List

Activity intolerance
Impaired *adjustment*
Ineffective *airway* clearance
Anxiety: mild, moderate, severe, panic
Alteration in *body* temperature: potential
Alteration in *bowel elimination*: constipation
Alteration in *bowel elimination*: diarrhea
Alteration in *bowel elimination*: incontinence
Ineffective *breathing pattern*
Alteration in *cardiac output*: decreased
Alteration in *comfort*: pain
Alteration in *comfort*: chronic pain
Impaired *communication*: verbal
Family *coping*: potential for growth
Ineffective family *coping*: compromised
Ineffective family *coping*: disabling
Ineffective individual *coping*
Diversional activity deficit
Alteration in *family process*
Fear
Alteration in *fluid volume*: excess
Fluid volume deficit
Impaired *gas exchange*
Anticipatory *grieving*
Dysfunctional *grieving*
Altered *growth and development*
Alteration in *health maintenance*
Impaired *home maintenance management*
Hopelessness
Hyperthermia
Hypothermia
Functional *incontinence*
Reflex *incontinence*
Stress *incontinence*
Total *incontinence*
Urge *incontinence*

Potential for *infection*
Potential for *injury*: poisoning, potential for; suffocation, potential for; trauma, potential for
Knowledge deficit (specify)
Impaired physical *mobility*
Noncompliance (specify)
Alteration in *nutrition*: less than body requirements
Alteration in *nutrition*: more than body requirements
Alteration in *oral mucous membrane*
Alteration in *parenting*
Post trauma response
Powerlessness
Rape trauma syndrome
Self-care deficit: feeding, bathing/hygiene, dressing/grooming, toileting
Disturbance in *self-concept*: body image, self-esteem, role performance, personal identity
Sensory-perceptual alteration: visual, auditory, kinesthetic, gustatory, tactile, olfactory
Sexual dysfunction
Altered *sexuality* patterns
Impairment of *skin* integrity
Sleep pattern disturbance
Impaired *social* interaction
Social isolation
Spiritual distress (distress of the human spirit)
Impaired *swallowing*
Ineffective *thermoregulation*
Alteration in *thought* processes
Impaired *tissue integrity*
Alteration in *tissue perfusion*: cerebral, cardiopulmonary, renal, gastrointestinal, peripheral
Unilateral neglect
Alteration in patterns of *urinary elimination*
Urinary retention
Potential for *violence*: self-directed or directed at others

APPENDIX II
Guidelines for Teaching Patients and Families

The 3 most important basic learning conditions for teaching skills or procedures are

- *Contiguity:* The individual steps of the procedure must be taught in continuous order or sequence. Teaching may begin with the first step and work to the last one, or start with the last step and work backwards; it does not matter as long as the steps are in sequence.
- *Practice:* This permits the patient to rehearse the sequence until each step is learned satisfactorily. Practice will be most effective when the patient distributes it over a period of time (e.g., several times a day for several days) rather than trying to perfect the entire sequence all at once.
- *Feedback:* This provides the patient knowledge of progress. It is the most important variable in learning, and is highly motivating to the patient. A return demonstration of learning can be critiqued and corrected.

Individuals learn, accept, and cope with things at different rates. Thus, the *time* a patient requires for each step, or the entire procedure, may vary widely. Some patients will require more practice, and more explanation, than others. Be patient, and caution your patient to be likewise. The *learning/comprehension level* will vary from patient to patient, and you will need to adjust the level of your presentation accordingly. Ensure that you use terms, words, etc., that the patient understands. Some patients may benefit from *reading* about the procedure. If possible, supply reading materials, such as booklets or pamphlets.

☐ ASSESSMENT

Age, relevance of proposed teaching methods; sex; attention span; memory; coordination (eye-hand, posture, balance); vision (color, focus, acuity); hearing; reading and writing ability; educational/cognitive level; ability to use telephone and to seek, accept, and effectively use help; cultural, ethnic, sexual, or racial influences; beliefs and attitudes regarding health, illness, medical treatment; availability of a family member or friend who wants/needs to learn about patient's care; emotional acceptance of condition, psychologic adjustment, and willingness to talk about this in personal terms; motivation and desire to learn, willingness and ability to modify life-style as indicated by disease/disability management or rehabilitation

☐ SPECIFIC TEACHING TECHNIQUES

- Consult sources of educational materials available for care of a given condition; try to obtain both materials suitable for giving to patient and those recommended for teaching yourself.
- Use or develop an assessment form to guide your interview of patient/family, to assist in developing a relevant, individualized teaching plan, and to serve as a permanent record along with patient/family education record of learning attained.
- Prepare an individualized, detailed lesson plan and assemble audiovisual teaching aids.
- Arrange list of specific, measurable, *realistic* objectives (expected outcomes) in sequential steps, from simple to complex, considering also the patient's most pressing needs/problems/concerns.
- Involve the family and friends (as well as the patient) in the planning, implementation, and evaluation of the teaching program.
- Consider a written or verbal contract, identifying what specific changes in life-style and behavior are needed, desired, and agreed to by the patient in order to maintain the desired level of health and disease control.
- Whenever possible, assign only 1 person to teach in order to minimize confusion, contradiction, and incompleteness; whenever possible, have that person present when supplementary teaching is done by a consultant specialist (e.g., dietician, volunteer expatient, pharmacist); reinforce information as needed.
- Schedule teaching sessions according to patient's receptivity (e.g., fatigue, distractibility, interest, readiness, comfort); let patient set pace and choose topics of most interest.
- Provide a quiet, well-ventilated, distraction-free setting for learning.
- Provide information using visual aids.
- Obtain feedback by asking questions; do not say, ''Do

you understand?" but rather, "Tell me how you can do this yourself," or, "How can you use this information in your care at home?" or, "Tell me what your situation is," to help reveal patient's feelings, perceptions, misconceptions, and need for reiteration of facts; correct gaps in knowledge or errors in thinking and repeat information.
- Maintain optimism and patience; compliment patient for effort and for each increment of learning.
- Provide a means for patient to learn more (or reinforce what was taught); consider supplying leaflets, written instructions, referrals to health and education service agencies, the name and number of a community health nurse or of a successfully rehabilitated expatient who is willing to help; attach a copy of the teaching record to the referral form.
- Administer tests to patient to determine learning; use oral or written quizzes, or return demonstrations.
- Keep a written record of what has been learned, not just what was taught and by whom; share this with nurse, family member, or friend who will care for patient at home; provide a means for the patient to evaluate own learning and to sign record; save to reactivate, update, and review teaching plan if patient is readmitted.
- Consider sending patient a letter following discharge to evaluate patient compliance and your teaching effectiveness.

☐ EVALUATION OF TEACHING

A variety of techniques can be used to evaluate the effectiveness of patient teaching
- Return demonstration
- Verbal description of content in own words
- Verbal list of pertinent content
- Achievement of the goal for which teaching was instituted (e.g., weight loss achieved/maintained; blood pressure controlled within stated limits; remaining free from hypoglycemic/hyperglycemic episodes)
- Selection of appropriate menu

APPENDIX III
Normal Growth and Development: Infant

Definition/Discussion

Infancy is the initial period of an individual baby's life cycle, generally spanning from 4 weeks to 18 months.

- Childhood is sequentially divided into stages or critical periods to denote a specific span of time that is maximally favorable for the accomplishment of a new developmental process or task.
- Developmental task (Erikson's central problem) to be resolved in infancy is the development of a sense of *trust* versus *mistrust*.
- Overall nursing responsibilities during infancy include meeting the infant's needs for nutrition, warmth, sucking, comfort, sensory stimulation, security, and love; supporting and guiding the parents to a responsible, nurturing, and understanding relationship with their child; observing, assessing, and recording normal and abnormal patterns of infant growth and development.
- The common parameters of physical development and behaviors for the infant are outlined below; corresponding nursing implications and parental teaching or guidance suggestions follow in *italics*.

☐ AGE 1 TO 6 MONTHS

Weight: gains 5–8 oz/week (14–22 gm); average American baby now doubles birth weight by 4⅔ months.
- *Review with parents the accuracy of their knowledge on formula or breast-feeding techniques. Reinforce that baby does not need solid foods until 4–6 months.*
Height: grows approximately 1 in/month (2.5 cm).
- *Teach normal growth, development, and safety needs to parents, repeating as necessary.*
Posterior fontanel: closes by about 2 months.
- *Show parents how to handle head gently while fontanels remain open, but not to be afraid to wash scalp.*
Skin: diaper rashes common; infantile acne on face at about 4–5 weeks is common; lasts 4–6 weeks, disappears without treatment; is thought to be associated with disappearance of mother's hormones and the activation of baby's oil and sweat glands.
- *Wash baby clothes prior to use in mild detergent (not soap as it decreases flame retardancy) and rinse well.*
- *Remind parents to keep diaper area clean, dry, and aerated; change diapers frequently washing area with warm water, mild soap after bowel movements; avoid perfumed soaps, bubble bath products, and overuse of commercial diaper wipes (contain alcohol, fragrance, and other additives); protect skin with a thin layer of water-barrier ointment (e.g., zinc oxide, Desitin, A&D), not petroleum jelly, which predisposes to yeast infections; lay infant on pad without diaper and leave area open to air for short periods; teach that using powder is not necessary but if parents insist, then to apply small amount to their hand away from baby's face and then put on baby; do not let baby play with powder container.*

Immunity: passive immunity received from mother is lost unless infant is breast-feeding; then immunity to some diseases remains through breast-feeding period.
- *Encourage parents to seek health care at recommended intervals, usually 2 weeks, 2, 4, 6, 9, 12, 15, and 18 months. Ascertain that parents have a health care provider who is available, accessible, and within transportation and financial means.*
- *Remind parents of need to have immunizations at recommended visits; inform of risks/benefits of immunizations so they can make an informed choice.*
- *Review common signs of illness and importance of early medical attention.*

Teething: begins at approximately 5–6 months; salivation increases at 3 months when salivary glands mature; drooling, which occurs as infant has not yet learned to swallow saliva effectively, is not a sign of teething though may become more evident when teething begins.
- *Suggest a bib to absorb saliva. Teach that prior to eruption, baby's gums are swollen and tender, baby is irritable and restless, may have slight fever or change in bowel habits. Rubbing gums with finger, a cold spoon, or chilled teething rings may ease discomfort. Sometimes the dentist will prescribe a medication to numb the gums. Symptoms subside when teeth erupt.*
- *Teach parents that high fever, diarrhea, or upper respiratory symptoms are not teething symptoms; these illnesses should be reported promptly to health care provider.*

Reflexes: sucks reflexively in response to touch; quiets in response to sucking.
- Strong palmar grasp reflex; reaches to mouth; "mouths" objects and fist at 2 months; chews at 4–6 months.
  - *Encourage parents to allow baby to satisfy sucking needs (other than during feeding) by permitting baby to suck fingers or thumb, or by using a pacifier.*
  - *Warn parents to be sure that all objects within baby's reach are too large to be swallowed; provide washable, safe toys.*
- Moro (startle) reflex present from birth to 4 months.
  - *Try to avoid loud noises or startling moves around baby.*

- Tonic neck reflex response reaches peak about 3 months, then gradually disappears.
  - *Tell parents to turn baby's head periodically to prevent unsightly flattening and balding of head from sleeping too much with head turned to preferred side since baby exhibits a definite preference for turning head to one side.*
  - Suggest reversing crib's position in room or hanging bright objects on the neglected side of the crib to stimulate interest.

COMMON BEHAVIORS
2 Months
Movement: can move in crib; holds head erect in mid position for a few seconds, but still wobbly.
  - *Be certain crib slats are no greater than 2 3/8 in (6 cm) apart; mattress should fit snugly. Secure infant seat so it cannot tip over with baby's movement. Restrain infant when in seat (a 3-point restraint is more effective than a lap belt only).*
  - *Reinforce and emphasize car seat safety; use only approved car seats that meet Federal safety standards; always use car seat and buckle baby in correctly; start early and be consistent and firm in use to make compliance expected and to foster appropriate "car behavior." The safest place in the car is the back seat, optimally the middle. Car seats should be rear facing until the infant can sit and hold head erect (about 6 months), then may be forward facing.*

Play: likes bright, colorful, large toys of varied shapes, configurations, and textures; spongy, squeeze toys that make sounds.
  - *Turn feeding, dressing, bathing, and diapering into pleasurable play.*
  - *Provide washable, durable toys without sharp edges or small, loose pieces; avoid fuzzy toys (present an inhalation danger).*
  - *Use crib gyms with stable items for grabbing (infants get frustrated by items that always swing out of reach when they grab for them); rotate toys in crib or playpen to provide various stimuli.*
  - *Use infant seats and swings for awake baby but caution against excessive use. Sometimes place baby in prone position and surround with toys; other times, use back or chest carrier to keep baby close to mother.*
  - *Hold baby and dance to music while humming or singing along.*

Crying: becomes differentiated as to cause (e.g., pain, cold, offensive odors, loud noises).
Smiling: an open-eyed, alert smile involving whole face, eyes crinkling; responds to another's smile.
Vision: can follow a bright, moving object from outer corner of eye to midline; stares indefinitely at surroundings, fixating on 1 or 2 objects (especially moving objects); prefers person to object; begins to coordinate senses (e.g., sucking at sight of bottle, anticipating or looking for sound of objects); attempts to bat or grab objects; begins to hold objects for a few moments.
  - *Teach parents that there is no really "average" baby; each is unique with its own pattern of eating, sleeping, crying, temperament, and activity.*
  - *Encourage to ward off a deluge of unsolicited advice and to take questions and concerns to someone they trust (e.g., health care provider).*
  - *Urge to interview and train at least 2 or 3 mature, reliable baby sitters, or to use licensed child care persons. Try to have sitter spend time with baby while parent is there. Have parent fully explain and demonstrate details of baby's routine, as well as special likes and dislikes.*
  - *Encourage to employ, when possible, healthy nonsmokers;*

children who are exposed to a lot of second-hand smoke have been shown to have a higher incidence of upper respiratory infections and a possibly higher risk of developing cancer.

Sleep: 18–20 hours/day; may sleep 7 hours at night after a late night feeding; shows a definite preference for sleep position; stays awake longer with social interaction.
Feeding: needs approximately 115 cal/kg/day; eats approximately every 4 hours and anticipates feedings. Breast-feeders may eat more frequently.
  - *Hold baby for feedings, looking down and talking to baby, thus providing both stimulation and positive interactions for both baby and care giver.*

Bathing: enjoys bath, kicking, and splashing; exhibits delight and excitement.
  - *Encourage water play during bath time. Pick up baby's legs and move them in circles while singing a song or saying a rhyme. Baby may like being nude, being stroked, massaged, and tickled slightly.*

3 Months
Movement: moves arms and legs vigorously; begins purposeful movements; when on stomach, raises head and chest, supported by forearms; holds hands in front and stares at them, wiggling fingers; reaches for objects, bringing hands together in front; puts hands and objects in mouth. Coordinates looking/grasping/sucking movements.
Play: similar to that of a 2-month-old.
Crying: less.
Smiling: more spontaneous.
Vocalization: babbles and coos in response to sounds. Begins to localize sounds, voluntarily turning toward them; distinguishes speech sounds from other sounds and responds.
  - *Keep diaper pins and other small, loose objects out of baby's reach.*
  - *Move baby from bassinette to a full-sized crib and from mother's bedroom to another room if this has not yet been done. Establish satisfactory sleep patterns by using crib only for sleep, by avoiding stimulation just before bedtime, by setting a consistent habit of presleep activities, and by putting baby in preferred sleep position.*
  - *Rock, cuddle, hum, or play soft music, but avoid practice of putting baby to bed with a propped bottle, as this will foster dental caries, ear infections, and promote association of feeding with bedtime. "Nursing bottle" decay occurs when naptime or bedtime bottles of sweetened liquids are given; the decay process begins during the sleeping hours.*

Sleep: 16–20 hours/day; may sleep 10 hours at night, although may awaken and fret; will fall back to sleep if left undisturbed.
  - *Babies who sleep on their stomach "nest" down, appearing to burrow into mattress; therefore be sure mattress is firm with no loose plastic sheets or pillows to cause smothering.*

4 Months
Appearance: birth hair is gradually replaced by permanent hair. Eye changes to permanent color (although some babies will retain blue eyes up to 2 years before changing color).
Movement: holds head steady and erect for a short time; lifts head and shoulders off surface at 90° angle when prone; supports body with hands. Rolls from back to abdomen and from stomach to side, gradually able to go from stomach to back. Begins "swimming" motions preliminary to creeping and crawling. Picks up objects with whole hand, or may take small objects between index and second fingers.
  - *Never leave infant alone on bed, table, or sofa; use playpen (those with mesh sides must always have them up; children can roll into the mesh and be smothered), crib with rails up, or an infant seat that is securely anchored.*

Play: likes brightly colored rings, large plastic or wooden beads, spoons, keys, noisemakers. Shows preference for certain toys or blankets.

- *Hold toys within baby's vision so s/he can reach for them, but do not put on string that can strangle a neck or wrist.*
- *Toys should be safe for chewing but not able to be swallowed.*

Smell: distinguishes between and shows interest in different smells.

- *Provide opportunities for baby to smell different foods, fragrances, etc.*

Vision: eyes can focus at different lengths and follow different objects for 180°. Stares at place from which an object drops; discriminates between familiar and strange faces, responding with more pleasure to familiar, smiling faces than strangers.

- *Give brightly colored toys to hold; put brightly colored pictures with simple designs in line of vision; put in front of mirror.*

Socialization: likes attention, having people around to handle, play, and talk to him/her; becomes fussy, demanding, or bored if ignored. Enjoys sitting up and being part of a busy environment. Listens, recognizes voices, turns head toward sounds; is quiet and attentive to music.

- *Keep infant in close proximity to others; smile at/talk to frequently while doing chores, encourage siblings to interact with infant while playing nearby, play various types of music (avoid loud noises that may damage hearing).*

Vocalization: expresses moods of enjoyment or protest; makes sounds, laughs, gurgles, or shrieks; laughs in response to light tickling.

- *Repeat sounds baby makes; call by name; laugh with baby; talk to baby about environment, things that are occurring.*

Sleep: sleeps through nights for up to 10 or 11 hours (although some babies will continue to wake at night and demand a feeding for as long as a year).

Feeding: needs approximately 110 cal/kg/day; learning to eat from a spoon may be possible now.

- *Encourage mother to breast-feed infant as long as desired; formula feeding should continue through the first year. Avoid overfeeding or excessive calories.*
- *Introduce solid foods at 4–6 months depending on health care provider's recommendation, care giver's desire, and baby's readiness. Introduce solid foods, one at a time, each week, watching carefully for allergies or intolerances (e.g., rashes, vomiting, diarrhea). Begin with single-grain enriched cereals: rice, barley, oatmeal (delay offering wheat, corn cereals, or mixed grain cereals for several weeks).*
- *Do not force feed, keep mealtime pleasant, happy; let baby play with spoon, get used to smell and taste of new food as well as feel in mouth.*
- *Give vitamin supplements as directed; fluoride supplements may be needed if water supply for homemade formula is not fluoridated. Breast-fed infants need fluoride supplements.*
- *Encourage parents to let baby meet sucking needs (e.g., bottle of water, fingers, pacifiers); if using pacifier, NEVER put it on a string around baby's neck or attached to gown.*

5 and 6 Months

Movement: sits momentarily without support in forward-leaning position, gradually extending time able to sit. Hitches (moves backward in a sitting position). Begins creeping (moves along with abdomen on floor). Gradually able to roll completely over, from stomach to back to stomach. Touches knees, brings feet to mouth; can be pulled up to standing position easily. Tonic neck reflex disappears. Likes to sit in high chair to watch family activity. Enjoys outings in carriage or stroller.

- *Be sure to strap in seat safely; use harness in carriage or food shopping cart.*
- *Keep floor clear of small and dangerous objects; keep cords out of reach; cap all unused electrical outlets.*
- *Close off open stairwells; block off unsafe step-downs.*

Play: enjoys unrestricted movement, to exercise limbs and to observe environment. Likes to look at self in mirror. Enjoys bath and noisy water toys. Likes large soft balls and musical balls. Has longer attention span; can roll, play with toys for an hour or so. Shows interest in books, pictures, paper; likes being read nursery rhymes. Loves social games.

- *Provide opportunities for baby to have unrestricted movement (e.g., carpeted floor, large playpen); let creep around in front of large mirror; limit walker use. Play social games (e.g., peek-a-boo, pat-a-cake, piggy-went-to-market).*

Socialization: distressed around strangers.

- *Give baby an opportunity to be around strangers before they hold/care for baby.*

Vocalization: utters syllables such as "ma," "ba," "da," adding new ones each week; crows, squeals, grunts, purrs, clicks, coughs, babbles.

Feeding: begins to finger-feed, hold bottle and spoon.

- *Limit formula amounts to approximately 20–24 oz daily, while increasing solids to meet development and weight needs.*
- *Add vegetables and fruits, 1 new each week, checking for food allergies and intolerances.*
- *Neither approve nor scold the spitting back or blowing of food; be persistent and encouraging, patiently spooning food off face, chin, or bib back into mouth.*
- *Realize that amounts and portions of foods vary depending on the baby's size, activity, health status, and appetite, as well as the number of other foods taken and amount of formula given. Offer bottle after eating solids.*
- *Allow baby to be part of family at mealtime; provide with finger food.*

☐ AGE 7 TO 12 MONTHS

Weight: gain after 6 months slows to approximately 4–5 oz/week (11.4–14 gm).

- *Evaluate child's growth status in terms of self; comparisons with charts or siblings may be inappropriate.*

Height: approximately 26–28 in (65–70 cm) at 6 months; grows ½ in/month (1.25 cm).

- *Arrange for 6-month check-up.*
- *Because of baby's rejection of strangers at this time, try to do as much of the exam as possible while baby is sitting in mother's lap. Proceed with the less distressing tasks first, giving baby something to interest and distract.*
- *Remember to smile and talk to baby while conducting examination.*

Teeth: begin to erupt around 6 months; 2 central lower incisors first, then 2 central upper incisors, then upper and lower lateral incisors.

- *Show mother how to clean newly erupted teeth of placque by using a clean washcloth. "Baby" teeth or primary teeth are important for chewing, for appearance, for proper development of jaws and mouth, and for reserving space for permanent teeth. Placque and decay need prompt care to control.*

COMMON BEHAVIORS
7 to 9 Months

Movement: toe sucking common. Sits alone well by 9 months. Raises self to sitting position. Tries various ways to move body; some may crawl (on all 4 limbs with abdomen up off floor). May start pulling self to a stand, learning later how to return to floor. Bounces and bears some weight in standing position.

- *Hand things to baby directly in front of eyes and chest; don't try to change way baby tries to grasp them.*
- *Never leave alone in bathtub; keep electrical appliances (e.g., can openers, hair dryers) out of reach.*
- *Keep wastebaskets hidden and out of reach; avoid pinching baby's fingers when closing doors, cupboards, drawers.*
- *Strap baby safely into strollers, carriages, grocery carts, high chairs. Close off stairs or teach baby how to crawl down them, feet and legs first.*

Play: likes large plastic and wooden blocks, nesting boxes or cups, stacking rings, water toys, paper to crumple, plastic keys, measuring cups and bowls.

- *Use play pen, cushioned furniture to practice standing and improve muscle tone. Play "hide-a-toy" with baby. Continue social games; give toy telephone; play music of many kinds, provide simple rhythm instruments (e.g., drum, bells, xylophone); read rhymes, poems, sing-song stories with repetitive sounds (Dr. Seuss-type) and ABC rhyme books with pictures.*

Socialization: wriggles and giggles in anticipation of play; learns meaning of "no" by voice tone; pats mirror image; resists doing what s/he doesn't want to do. Wants to play in presence of family; perform for audience. Shows open and fond affection for family members; exhibits comfort around children; fear of strangers reaches peak, then starts to lessen. Begins to understand disappearance concept, may look to floor for object dropped in front of him/her. Imitates adult movements such as clapping, swaying, making sounds and noises.

- *Because of stranger anxiety, cost of sitters, and baby's comfort around children, it is tempting and convenient to involve older siblings in a large amount of baby care while mother is otherwise busy; safety of baby and maturity of older child must be prime considerations, as well as possibility of sibling rivalry and the need of older child to have usual routines of afterschool activities.*

Vocalization: loves to imitate; coughs, clicks, buzzes; says syllables like "ma," "da," "ga."

Sleep: 14–16 hours/day, including 1–2 daytime naps.

Feeding: eats 3 meals/day; holds spoon, drinks from a cup, enjoys finger foods, tastes everything; may or may not show readiness for weaning; still has strong sucking needs and the emotional need to be held even though willing to hold own bottle.

- *Allow longer time for feeding so child can practice new skills.*
- *Show excitement at baby's achievements.*
- *Gradually decrease amount and frequency of formula or breast-feedings, while increasing foods of various kinds and textures; include meat, soft pieces of fruit, cheese, toast.*
- *When eating 3 meals/day, milk intake should be approximately 24 oz/day.*
- *Avoid foods that can cause choking (e.g., raw carrots, nuts, popcorn). Start good nutritional habits by avoiding too many sweet cookies and salty crackers. Do not introduce candy or ice cream.*

10 to 12 Months

Movement: crawls and creeps well; climbs up and down from furniture; climbs up stairs, but needs to be taught how to crawl down backwards. Pulls self to feet; by 12 months, can stand alone for a few minutes and pivot body 90°. "Cruises" or sidesteps along furniture (average 11 months). Begins walking (average 12 months). Stoops, squats, bends, leans, reaches, opens drawers, lifts lids. Begins to help dressing self. Can pick up objects now and can voluntarily release them. Can hold 2 or more objects in hand; can

"store" object in mouth or under arm while grabbing another one. Likes to handle, shake, bang, roll, fill, empty, push, spin, drop, and otherwise manipulate all objects.

- *Allow freedom to creep and walk in safe, baby-proof areas; never leave alone in bathtub.*
- *For babies who can climb out of crib, use a net or put crib side down, placing crib next to a bed to cushion descent.*
- *Baby-proof bedroom and be sure baby cannot open door. Close off stairways or teach baby how to crawl down backwards, safely.*
- *Use only toy hampers without lids to prevent pinched fingers.*
- *Assure parents of a "quiet" baby (or one that is "late" developing motor skills) that when baby is ready, learning and practice time is often shorter than for those babies who started to crawl, climb, or walk earlier; some babies show interest in movement, others in vocalization, still others in passive study and observation.*
- *Whether babies should learn to walk in bare feet or soft-or hard-soled shoes is controversial. Consult health care provider and consider own needs and environment. When purchasing shoes, buy them only ½ in longer and ¼ in wider than baby's foot to allow natural spread and growth. Too-large shoes are clumsy, cause blisters, and force unnatural foot position to develop. Too-small shoes also cause problems, so check size and fit at least monthly.*
- *Minor toeing-in is normal for the new walker and can correct itself when baby's balance is better.*
- *Teach baby meaning of "hot" and "don't touch." Set firm, consistent limits. Try to be patient and persevering. Join a parent support group for mutual aid and help.*
- *Show love openly; touch, hold, rock, be active with child.*
- *Supervise older children "sitting" with or playing with baby, so they don't frighten or inadvertently hurt baby; help older children express frustrations at baby's behavior in socially acceptable and safe ways.*
- *Do things as a family, showing love and respect for older child's needs.*

Play: likes rocking horse and riding toys. Likes to play chase. Prefers push toys to pull toys. Likes to rock, sway, keep time and "dance" with someone to music. Actively searches for vanished objects.

- *Provide new and different toys that stimulate curiosity (e.g., milk cartons, fabric or cardboard boxes, containers to fill and spill, pots).*
- *Do not pretend to be something fearful or jump out at baby with loud noises.*
- *Play music in baby's bedroom or playroom.*
- *Play "hide-a-toy"; let baby see the object covered, then search for it.*

Socialization: may begin temper tantrums. Seeks approval but is not always cooperative. Shaking head "no" is easier than nodding "yes." Shows moods.

- *Walk away from baby having a temper tantrum, or place in own room. Reward verbally for cooperative behavior.*

Verbalization: responds to own name. Identifies (by pointing to) objects such as sky, airplane, familiar animals, and people. May be able to say 3 or 4 words (e.g., "ma-ma," "no," "hi," "hot").

- *Be alert to detect early hearing losses. See a pediatric audiologist if baby does not respond to own name, cannot imitate simple sounds, or cannot point to familiar objects.*

Sleeping: some active babies sleep only 11–12 hours at night with 1-hour daytime nap. Some babies still wake at night to stand, to be rocked, to have a bottle.

Feeding: will eat less solid food if formula or breast-feeding not correspondingly reduced; gains less weight as movement increases.

- *Do not force baby to eat more than s/he wants or force foods that baby dislikes. Allow longer mealtime if baby is feeding self. Allow baby to use fingers and do not force spoon usage at all times. Give baby a spillproof plastic cup; a plastic sheet or newspapers on floor during mealtimes will ease cleanup of spills.*

☐ AGE 12 TO 18 MONTHS

Weight: average 20–24 lb (9–11 kg), triples birth weight by 12 months, gaining 2–6 lb in next 6 months.
- *Recommend 1-year physical check-up, with Hgb, Hct, urinalysis, Tb skin test.*

Height: approximately 29 in growing to approximately 33 in by 18 months.

Size: head and chest circumference are about equal at 12 months.

Pulse: 100–140/minute. Respirations: 20–40/minute.
- *Measure vital signs at rest.*

Reflexes: Babinski sign disappears.

Anterior fontanel: closes (average 10–24 months).
- *Evaluate fontanel and cranial configurations.*

Abdomen: protrudes.

Teething: continues with 10–14 primary teeth by 18 months, including lower and upper molars and cuspids. Good chewing, sucking, and swallowing movements.
- *Urge dental hygiene (e.g., brushing, fluoridated drops, encourage weaning from bottle, no candy/raisins).*

COMMON BEHAVIORS

Movement: able to walk alone with a widebased gait. Climbs upstairs, holding onto hand or rail, 1 step at a time. Throws, turns pages in a book, builds a tower of 3 objects/blocks. Helps in dressing self with hat, shoes, lifting arms or legs appropriately.
- *Protect child from kitchen accidents (e.g., hot liquids, overhanging handles, cords on appliances, long table cloths).*
- *Reinforce importance of earlier safety teaching. If not done earlier, lock up all medicines, poisons, gasoline, fertilizers, cleaning agents.*
- *Check all houseplants, keeping them out of reach; discard poisonous varieties.*
- *Keep matches out of reach.*
- *Put safety plugs in electrical outlets.*
- *Supervise yard play.*
- *Never leave alone in bath water, wading or other pools.*

- *Always use seat belts and approved car seats.*
- *Use safety devices on cabinet drawers and all doors.*

Play: Likes large cars and trucks, dolls, mops, brooms, kitchen utensils, stuffed animals, 2- to 10-piece puzzles, balls, picture books. Loves to throw and retrieve objects. Delights in pushing, pulling, or riding toys; climbing up, down, and through indoor gym/slide combinations. Enjoys solitary play or watching others.

Socialization: explores everything with rapid attention shifts. Curious; trial and error behavior teaches s/he can control some things around self; enjoys new skills; shows pride in achievements. Imitates and mimics household chores. Security is focused on one object (e.g., doll, blanket, stuffed animal, thumb, diaper).
- *Know that the parents' reaction to child's failure or accomplishment affects the child's self-concept. Showing anxiety over minor injuries, anger at childish carelessness, or ignoring accomplishments can have an unhealthful effect on child's self-esteem. Try to treat minor injuries, failures, with casual acceptance.*
- *Show pleasure at new social or physical skills. Set firm, safe limits.*

Verbalization: can point to parts of body when asked; can say 3 to 12 meaningful single words (e.g., "ma-ma," "da-da," "no," "hi," "hot," "bye-bye," "go," "baby," "wa-wa" [water]). Begins to follow a few simple commands (e.g., "Give it to me," "Show me the _____ ").

Elimination: may be able to control bowel movements or void at will on potty chair, but usually not interested.
- *Delay bowel/bladder training until baby's readiness is evident (e.g., shows interest and cooperation, able to express needs, walk to bathroom).*

Feeding: feeds self with spoon and drinks from cup by 18 months; appetite decreases with decreasing growth rate. Needs 100 cal/kg or approximately 1,300 cal/day (range: 900–1,800 cal).
- *Do not force feed, coax, wheedle, bribe, threaten, or punish poor appetite or feeding if growth rate is proceeding normally.*
- *Give regular table foods in a 3-meal-a-day pattern with nutritious between-meal or bedtime snacks. Give very small helpings. Keep child at table only as long as interested in eating. Do not give snacks as an alternative to mealtime eating.*
- *Do not appease a fussy or crying baby with a cookie or sweets. Do not use food as a reward, as a comfort for small hurts, or as a substitute for love and attention.*

Normal Growth and Development: Toddler/Preschooler

Definition/Discussion

Toddlerhood is the developmental period in a child's life between 18 months and 3 years. Preschool covers from 3 to 6 years of age.
- Rate of growth and development as well as task mastery varies with each individual child. Parental and environmental influences may stimulate and nurture or retard development, but innate differences and individual readiness will strongly affect level and rate of achievement.
- Developmental task (Erikson's central problem) to be resolved during toddlerhood is *autonomy or independence* ver-

sus *shame or doubt*, and during the preschool period it is *initiative* versus *guilt*. Successfully achieved, the youngster develops pride, high self-esteem, and good will to self and others.
- Special fears of toddlers and preschoolers are of abandonment and separation from parents. Learning to separate from parents and to cope effectively is an important task of the young child. Success can be achieved when the child experiences positive periods of short separation and feels trust and security with those who care for him. Coping skills begin to include modes of self-expression and elementary self-

reliance. Familiar surroundings and care giver's presence are no longer always necessary for the child to feel secure.

- Cognitive abilities develop rapidly in the preschool years and the child learns many things. The toddler has a concept of time limited to the present experience, focuses on only one aspect of objects, problem solves through trial and error, imitates language heard, and perceives through senses. Piaget calls this the "sensorimotor" stage of cognitive development. The preschooler's thinking, termed "preoperational," is literal, concrete, and absolute (e.g., good/bad, right/wrong, hurt/doesn't hurt). S/he views the world and people's actions in terms of own self and consequences to self, refusing others' viewpoints. The preschooler asks "why" and "how" frequently, extends concept of time to include past as well as present, and has a longer memory span than toddlers.
- Imagination is heightened in the preschooler; fantasy and reality are often interchangeable. Imaginary companions people this fantasy world, are often blamed for the youngster's own misbehavior, and serve as coping mechanisms for controlling situations, especially stressful ones.
- Play in the toddler period is active, informal, spontaneous, and often centered around motor activity. Characteristically, toddler play is singular and referred to as "parallel play" (when 2 children play alongside but not with each other). When the child learns to give in order to receive, s/he makes the transition into the preschool type of play known as cooperative or associative play.
- Ritualism is a common behavioral pattern of these 2 periods; activities of daily living are best scheduled and performed precisely and regularly in order to provide security and stability for the child in a rapidly changing period of growth and development.
- Negativism and the consistent use of the word "no" for everything is characteristic of this period. It is the toddlers' way of controlling people and events, acting on their own terms, doing things by themselves ("Me do it myself!"); the negative response becomes quite an automatic one.
- Temper tantrums are the young child's way of expressing frustration and releasing anger at people, things, and self in an effort to gain control. An angry, kicking toddler in the midst of a tantrum cannot be effectively dealt with by threats or reasoning for s/he is oblivious to reality. Walk away from a child having a tantrum; do not be a sympathetic or angry bystander; reward verbally for cooperative, socially acceptable behavior.
- The common parameters of physical development and behaviors for the toddler and preschool child are outlined below; corresponding nursing implications and parental teaching or guidance suggestions follow in *italics*.

☐ **AGE 18 MONTHS TO 3 YEARS (Toddler)**

Weight: average 28–30 lb (13 kg) (birth weight quadruples by 2½ years).

Height: average 33–37 in (82.5–92.5 cm) (approximately 50% of eventual adult height at 2 years).

- *Caution parents that appetite and weight gain level off during this period; thus child can eat less and still maintain activity levels. Recommended daily dietary intake is about 41–45 cal/lb (90–100 cal/kg).*
- *Provide appropriate counseling for children above 95th percentile or below 5th percentile for height or weight. Any child whose pattern has changed markedly (e.g., from 50th to 10th percentile or vice versa) also should be further evaluated.*
- *Check all measurements and ascertain that they are accurate. Norms are based on children being weighed with no clothing except light undergarments.*

Pulse: 90–120/minute; respirations: 20–35/minute.
- *Count for 1 full minute.*

Teeth: 16 at 2 years, acquiring a full set of 20 primary teeth by 3 years.
- *Establish nutritious, noncariogenic dietary and snacking habits for proper tooth formation and bone development. Offer pretzels, fruits, fruit juice, and raw vegetables. Avoid carrot sticks, popcorn, and nuts because of possible choking. Keep candy, cookies, raisins, pastries, sweetened soft drinks and gum to a minimum.*
- *Encourage parents to take child for first dental visit by age 2 or before all 20 primary teeth have erupted. Take to dentist immediately for any cavities noticed or for injuries to teeth. Make first dental visit a pleasant, friendly one, preparing child with a positive, matter-of-fact explanation. Read child a book about visiting the dentist. Remember that parental attitudes and examples can mold a child's feelings about dental care for many years.*
- *Teach, demonstrate, and supervise cleaning (brushing and flossing) of teeth.*
- *Apply topical fluoridation treatments for additional decay protection. Continue fluoride supplements for children who do not live in community with fluoridated water supply.*

Vision: visual acuity is approximately 20/70 in the 2-year-old. Depth perception remains poor (cerebral rather than visual developmental function); increasing development of the neurovisual pathways leaves most 3-year-olds with good ability to assess size and location of objects.
- *Recommend a complete eye exam by a specialist for every child between 1 and 3 years of age.*
- *Provide address for free brochure on children's vision (The Children's Eyesight Society, 7420 Westlake Terrace, Suite 1509, Bethesda, MD 20034).*

Body proportions: changing, with abdomen protruding, arms and legs lengthening rapidly, and trunk and head growing slowly. Falls and stumbling may increase during this period due to changing body proportions and rapidly increasing motor skills. In addition, toddlers assert autonomy and overestimate physical capabilities.
- *Supervise constantly and initiate precautions necessary to minimize accidents.*
- *Install stairway rails, sturdy high fences; remove loose throw rugs, tables with sharp edges, glass objects that can topple over.*

Immunization: current CDC guidelines suggest that *H. influenzae* type B (HIB) vaccine be given to all children 24 months and older. Toddlers 18–24 months old in daycare centers should also receive the vaccine but need to be revaccinated when they reach 24 months.
- *Reinforce need for well child check-ups at 18 and 24 months.*

COMMON BEHAVIORS
2-Year-Old

Movement: gait is steady; walks, runs, jumps with both feet. Climbs stairs one at a time with both feet on each step, holding rail. Can open doors and turn knobs. Can kick a ball without falling, even when running. By 2½ can ride a "kiddy" car and tricycle. Can throw objects overhead, string large beads, and begin to use scissors. Can scribble and copy vertical and straight lines. Assists with dressing and undressing self. Washes and dries hands. Uses toothbrush, but not skillfully.
- *Supervise carefully all outdoor and indoor play.*
- *Teach child street and traffic safety.*
- *Use fire-retardant night clothes.*
- *Lock up all dangerous products.*
- *Lock doors or put plastic holders over doorknobs to prevent toddler usage.*

- *Use car seats for every car ride.*
- *Post a poison chart with poison control center phone number.*

Play: has short attention span; needs combination of motor activities with quiet play. Enjoys stories, music, TV, sandbox with toys, Play-Doh, clay, mud, and finger paints. Likes construction toys, cars, trucks, pull toys, wagons, doll buggies, and riding toys like fire engines, tricycles, kiddy cars. Enjoys climbing and swinging playground apparatus, puzzles with large pieces, drawing paper, musical and rhythm instruments, dolls, stuffed animals, and toy household items for imitative play (e.g., brooms, lawnmowers). Parallel play predominates.

- *Supervise water play constantly.*
- *Encourage swim lessons to begin if pool is present and accessible, even if only occasionally.*
- *Make sure riding toys are in good working order.*
- *Provide opportunities to practice and develop skills.*

Socialization: is egocentric, the center of own world, viewing all in relationship to self. Treats other children almost as if they were objects. May bite in anger or frustration or just to use teeth. Other frequently observed behaviors include self-stimulation (e.g., rocking, masturbation), thumbsucking, ritualism, and negativism.

- *Do not expect child to do more than s/he is able to do. Child has a need for peer companionship, even if unable to share.*
- *Teach parents that biting back, slapping, shouting, or putting something unpleasant in mouth (e.g., soap or hot sauce) usually do not work. Verbal disapproval, removal of child from stressor, or addressing cause (e.g., sibling rivalry) may have some positive effect.*
- *Accept the normalcy of behavior for this stage. Remain consistent in discipline; provide periods of special quiet time alone with child, reading stories, playing music, cuddling, and providing individual attention.*
- *Give choices when possible. Do not offer choices where none are present.*

Verbalization: has vocabulary of about 200 words, understands more. Begins using phrases of two to four words (e.g., "go bye-bye," "more cookie," "where daddy," "me do it"). Most popular words: "no," "me," "my," "mine."

- *Include child in conversations; have child use words to express wants; use concrete examples of words (let child handle object and identify the name for it; look at books, magazines, and identify objects).*

Elimination: may gradually become toilet trained at least during daytime.

- *Introduce toilet training if child shows signs of readiness (ability to stand and walk well, hold urine for 2 hours at a time, regular schedule of bowel movements, willingness to please care giver, ability to indicate need to eliminate).*
- *Stress to not start toilet training during stressful periods (birth of a sibling, weaning, moving, family separations, illness).*
- *Make teaching positive, pleasant, nonpunitive, nonpressured, and geared to the particular child.*
- *Expect accidents when child is tired, excited, preoccupied, busy with play, or otherwise in a stressful situation. React casually and noncommittally.*
- *Keep potty chair accessible or a step stool near a standard toilet fitted with a smaller seat adaptation.*
- *Be consistent in reinforcements (rewards); use praise, not sweets. Use correct terminology for body parts. Begin foundation for health/sex education; refrain from negative responses for normal curiosity. Child may want to see elimination products or not want them flushed away immediately; postpone it temporarily.*
- *Recommend loose-fitting, easily removed outer clothing and training pants that child can manage without help.*

Sleeping: 10–14 hours/day, including an afternoon nap. Does not go to sleep immediately, prolongs process of going to bed.

- *Monitor TV programs; avoid violent programs.*
- *Reinforce bedtime ritual; have quiet time at consistent hour; play soothing music, read stories.*
- *Teach parents not to use going to bed as punishment; use familiar stuffed animal, nightlight if afraid of dark.*

Feeding: drinks/feeds self without spilling, plays with food.

- *Keep portions small; choose foods from basic 4 food groups; limit milk to 2–3 glasses/day to avoid excessive calories and leave room for nutrients provided by other foods; do not rush child.*

☐ **AGE 3 YEARS TO 6 YEARS (Preschool)**

Weight: approximately 44 lb; 4- to 6-year-olds require approximately 36–41 cal/lb (80–90 cal/kg).

Height: approximately 44 in (100 cm) (about double birth length at 4 years). Height and weight are about even at age 5.

Pulse: 80–120/minute; respirations: 20–30/minute.

- *Count for 1 full minute.*

Blood pressure: 85–90/60 mm Hg.

- *Use child-size blood pressure cuff. Let child handle equipment and listen to own heart beat.*

Teeth: begins to lose primary teeth at approximately 5–7 years.

Immunizations: per schedule

Vision: visual acuity is approximately 20/40 in 3-year-old, 20/30 in 4-year-old, and normal 20/20 by age 6. Depth perception is developing and color vision fully established.

- *Evaluate physical condition, immunization, vision, hearing, and kindergarten readiness skills before starting school; provide appropriate corrections and assistance.*

Body proportions: loses much of baby fat and protruding abdomen; waist not discernible; legs continue to grow rapidly equaling approximately 44% of total length.

COMMON BEHAVIORS
3-Year-Old

Movement: climbs stairs, alternating feet, but still holding rail. Tries to draw a picture, a mass of lines and circles. Can hit a pegboard with a hammer with more accuracy than before, ride a tricycle. Dresses self with help on grippers, zippers, buttons, and shoe tying. Can help with minor tasks such as drying dishes, emptying waste baskets, getting or putting away items such as cleaning utensils or groceries.

- *Continue supervision and safety precautions, even though child shows signs of using more caution and responsibility.*
- *Teach child what to do if lost while shopping or in new situation. Encourage ID bracelet. Teach child name, age, and phone number, including area code.*
- *Give small errands or jobs to do around house. Watch and wait before offering help or suggestions.*

Play: uses blackboard and chalk, activity related dolls (e.g., can feed, dress, take for stroller rides), housekeeping toys, windup musical toys, child's typewriter, record player, tape player, mechanical games, increasing numbers and varieties of books, puzzles, trucks, building toys.

- *Assist parents to expand child's world with same age group play experiences (e.g., babysitting co-ops or playgroups, nursery or Sunday schools, trips to zoo, playgrounds, story hours).*
- *Encourage development of cooperative, sharing, or associative play skills.*

Socialization: tolerates short periods of separation, especially if child is in a happy, play-type situation with competent adults.

- *Encourage child to express feelings verbally and accept*

feelings, while redirecting unacceptable behavior to more acceptable behavior.

Verbalization: has mastered most vowels, half the consonants; speaks in 3-or-more-word sentences that become more complex. Has a rapidly expanding speaking vocabulary of about 1,000 words. Frequently repeats words and syllables as a means of learning them. 90% of 3-year-olds should be readily understood by others. Knows first and last name, age, and sex. May stutter as attempting to learn complex pronunciation skills. Questions with "what?" "when?" "why?" and "how?" Understands simple explanations of cause and effect.

- *Teach parents to help develop child's language skills by talking aloud about what they are doing, thinking, and feeling; also by "parallel" talk describing what someone else may be doing, thinking, feeling while it happens. Ignore stuttering.*
- *Provide simple but honest explanations, patiently, upon request. Show and describe how things work and why something is dangerous or unwise to handle.*

Elimination: Goes to bathroom with minimal help.

- *Remind child to go before going outside or when playing busily.*

Sleeping and feeding: similar to 2-year-old.

4-Year-Old

Movement: walks with a freeswinging, adultlike stride; walks backwards; can walk upstairs without grasping rail. Can stand on 1 foot for 5 seconds. Runs well. Hops 2 or more times. Throws ball overhead with control and increasing accuracy to someone. Uses scissors to cut out pictures, following outline with increasing accuracy. Can draw a picture of a person with head, eyes, and 2 other parts.

- *Check play areas to remove unsafe hazards. Clear trash heaps; cover holes, ditches, tunnels; lock empty refrigerators or remove doors; properly discard faulty appliances, paint cans, plastic bags, aerosol cans.*

Play: is cooperative; dramatic, imitative play predominates. May have an imaginary companion. Likes jumpropes; play tools; paste and various scraps (e.g., cloth, leaves, paper) to arrange in collage; easels with paints; tires and very large boxes to climb around in; gym sets.

- *Provide dressup clothing for imitative play (e.g., cowboy hats, guns, holster, purses, jewelry, adult clothes).*
- *Take to children's plays, musical performances, puppet shows.*
- *Enroll in dance classes, swim lessons, exercise classes, and other learning opportunities.*

Socialization: brags, shows off, looks for praise, criticizes others, tattles. Developing a conscience that influences behavior. Develops romantic fantasies about parents of opposite sex. Common age for nightmares, castration fears, fears of scary objects and animals. As nightmares are common at this age, child may want to sleep with parent.

- *Invite friends over for parties, play activities, group games.*
- *Start child in own bed, perhaps with light on and relaxing music.*
- *Stress that temporary cuddling in parents' bed for nightmares can be condoned, but when child falls asleep, return to own bed. Patience and persistence, along with growing out of this stage will return the child to a regular, secure sleeping routine.*

Verbalization: has a speaking vocabulary of 1,500 words, expanding approximately 600 words/year depending on stimulation by adults and older siblings. Understands prepositions and opposites. Talks/questions incessantly; knows phone number, and some know

address. Begins use of socially unacceptable words for their shock effect. Knows primary colors, some numbers and alphabet letters.

- *Reinforce new knowledge with toys, games, books about numbers, colors, and letters.*

Sleeping: 11–12 hours/day, napping only occasionally when very tired or ill.

Feeding: rarely needs assistance, interested in setting table, pours well from pitcher.

- *Have rules concerning table manners; encourage setting table, serving self; make mealtime a pleasant experience (give everyone a chance to talk about their day).*

5-Year-Old

Movement: can run and play games at same time; hops and skips well; some may attempt to ride a 2-wheel bicycle without training wheels. May be able to swim standard swim strokes a distance of 25 yards. Begins to use fork and knife. May be able to print first name, sometimes a short last name. Some may be able to tie shoelaces, but many are unable to do this until 6–8 years. Draws a recognizable person with body, head, arms, legs, and 4 other parts. Counts to 20 and may recognize coinage of a penny, nickel, dime. Washes self without wetting clothes. Brushes teeth correctly with reminders and some supervision.

- *Teach safe use of toys and riding or moving equipment (e.g., bikes, skates, skateboards).*
- *Teach safe street crossing, obeying traffic lights and crosswalk lines.*
- *Teach how to phone for help (e.g., fire, police, paramedics, emergency 911).*
- *Reinforce how to recite name, age, phone number, and address.*

Play: can use rollerskates, iceskates, sleds, scooters, skateboards, riding toys. Likes building sets, toy soldiers, plastic people, toy animals, doll houses.

- *Add more books, games, puzzles, involving increasing manipulative and cognitive skills. Do not pressure to achieve but let child enjoy the activity.*

Socialization: takes some responsibility for actions, following directions and rules. Increased respect for truth. Growth of modesty and wish for privacy. Able to sit quietly for 10–15 minutes to hear a story or lesson. Interested in meaning of family relationships (e.g., aunts, uncles, cousins, grandparents).

- *Teach personal safety habits (e.g., always tell care giver where they will be, walk with other children in well travelled areas, never talk to strangers or go near strange cars, yell "This isn't my daddy," scream, kick, bite if someone grabs them; don't let anyone do things to their body they shouldn't do; "say no to drugs").*
- *Keep behavior rules simple, enforce consistently; avoid prolonged arguments.*
- *Keep in close touch with kindergarten teacher to learn more about child's progress, abilities, needs, and to get suggestions for helping and guiding child. Help to build child's self-confidence by praising new skills, positive attitudes, and acceptable behavior.*

Verbalization: has a vocabulary of 2,000+ words. Can explain to others how and why of games or activities. Begins sentences with "I" instead of "me," "he" instead of "him." Although child may mispronounce some sounds and make some grammatical errors, most of the time language should closely match that of the family and neighborhood. Stuttering is inappropriate past the sixth birthday.

- *Get further evaluation from health care provider for suspected problems.*

Normal Growth and Development: School-Age Child

Definition/Discussion

The school years are the developmental period in an child's life between 6 and 11 years of age.

- Developmental task (Erikson's central problem) to be resolved during this period is *industry* versus *inferiority*. The child moves out into many different social groups and, while the family remains the chief socializing agent, s/he learns new and important skills and attitudes from peers: (1) the art of compromise, cooperation, and persuasion; (2) fair play through competition; (3) increased autonomy from the home; (4) reinforcement of appropriate sex-role behaviors; and (5) an ongoing development of self-concept.
- Cognitive development: time is now well understood and the child can plan ahead. There is a mature concept of causality. Formal logical thinking is present, which is based on perceptually concrete events, not abstractions. Conservation, the ability to see changing states of matter as unchanging, develops during this period. The child expands knowledge rapidly through formal and informal educational means. The child begins to combine others' viewpoints with his own. S/he is capable of prolonged interest and attention span. The memory is good for concrete sequences of numbers and letters and for 2 meaningful and related ideas.
- Special fears of this period are those of bodily injury, concern about death, fear of parental loss, school phobia/failure, fear of the dark, and fear of embarrassment from criticism or ridicule.
- Play is centered around groups of same sex after 6 or 7 years of age; "gang" activities predominate in both school and recreational interests (e.g., clubs, teams, scouts, parties, enrichment classes, neighborhood play groups). Peer-group influence becomes important and peer criticism begins for deviation from sex roles, intellectual or physical skill differences, sociocultural differences, and noncomformity in language, dress, social behaviors. Quarrels are frequent but usually short lived. The school-age child has now learned to share and take turns and can participate in organized games requiring coordinated efforts.
- The common parameters of physical development and behaviors for the school-age child are outlined below; corresponding nursing implications and parental teaching or guidance suggestions follow in *italics*.

☐ AGE 6 TO 11 YEARS

Weight: 45 lb (20 kg) at 6 years, child gains 5–7 lb/year on average; 62 lb (28 kg) at 7–10 years.

Height: 46 in (117 cm) at 6 years; growth occurs in spurts; overall height increases average approximately 3 in (7 cm)/year to approximately 52 in (132 cm) at 7–10 years.

Pulse: 80–100/minute at 6 years; approximates adult norm at 10–11 years.

- *Refer to growth charts as guidelines, but do not use as rigid criteria.*

Respirations: 18–20/minute at 6 years; approximates adult norms at 10–11 years.

- *Encourage annual well-child check-ups.*

Blood pressure: 95–108/60–68; approximates adult norms at 10–11 years.

- *Immunization: verify compliance with state requirements.*

Vision: 20/20 by 7 years.

- *Promote vision testing every 2 years.*
- *Encourage children to sit no closer than 4 ft to TV.*

Nutrition: calorie requirements for 7 to 10-year-old are 32–36 cal/lb (70–80 cal/kg).

- *Assess nutritional status and further evaluate children in the upper or lower percentiles of weight. Have parent keep food diary for 1 week (with child's help). Reinforce basic nutrition ideas and stress healthful eating habits.*

Teeth: first permanent molars come in at 6–7 years; primary teeth are lost in order of eruption; has 10–11 permanent teeth by 10–11 years.

- *Remind parents to schedule twice-yearly dental check-ups and to continue supervision of correct brushing and flossing techniques.*

Sex characteristics: early development may begin in girls as soon as 8 years, and in boys as soon as 10 years. Early developers are often subject to ridicule and embarrassment. Adolescent growth spurt often begins by 10–11 years but may not occur until nearly 14.

- *Provide education and counseling to assist children to understand and accept the changes in their bodies.*
- *Help parents increase their effectiveness in providing sex education for their children.*

COMMON BEHAVIORS
6-Year-Old

Movement: large muscle ability exceeds fine motor coordination. Girls are ahead of boys in fine motor skills, physical development, and achievement. High energy levels; very active, impulsive, and constantly in motion. Balance and rhythm are good. Can hop, skip, run, jump, gallop, and climb. Can kick, throw, and catch a ball well. Can ride a 2-wheel bicycle without training wheels. Able to draw a recognizable human figure, house, flowers. Dresses self with almost no help; can master buttons, grippers, zippers, and shoelaces.

- *Reinforce traffic safety, provide adult supervision of play.*
- *Teach child to avoid strangers, never get in an unknown car, never take candy, food, or pills from strangers.*
- *Provide for a balance of rest and activity.*
- *Teach cold prevention (e.g., separate drinking cups) and good health practices, including reinforcement of dangers of drug abuse and taking medicines or pills not prescribed by a physician.*

Play: plays well alone, but enjoys groups of both sexes in small groups. Likes simple games with basic rules. Likes to make things (starts many, but finishes few). Likes imaginary, dramatic play with real costumes, running games of tag, hide-and-seek, rollerskating, kickball, soccer, jumprope games, hopscotch, iceskating, skiing, and skateboarding. Plays house; builds with plastic blocks. Still plays with dolls, airplanes, cars, and trucks. Enjoys electronic and musical games, puzzles, and books with words as well as pictures. Likes to draw, color, paint, paste, and cut.

- *Give some responsibility for household duties within ability and maturity level.*

Socialization: boisterous, verbally aggressive, assertive, bossy, opinionated, outgoing, active, argumentative, sometimes whiny, and know-it-all. Expresses sense of humor in riddles, practical jokes, and nonsense. Moods and feelings (fear, joy, affection, anger, shyness, jealousy, sadness) expressed in extremes. Can use a telephone. Has a strong need for teacher approval, affection, and acceptance. Very aware of teacher's social attitudes and values as communicated by behavior. Learns concepts of coinage, right and left, morning and afternoon, days of week, months of year, beginning reading and printing. Peer-group influence also becoming important.

- *Assure parents that aggressiveness is normal for age; suggest sidestepping power struggles; offer choices when possible.*
- *Frequently reassure the child of his/her competence, basic worth and lovability.*
- *Encourage parents to visit school, talk with teacher and resolve problems. Successful school experience is critical at this age to establish positive attitudes to learning and later educational experiences.*

Verbalization: has a vocabulary of 2,000–3,000 words. Communicates to share thoughts and ideas with others. Understanding of language greater than ability to use it. Can verbalize similarities.

- *Note any speaking or language difficulties; seek further evaluation and necessary remediation. Confer with school authorities first.*

Nutrition: needs approximately 2,000 cal/day. Eats 3 meals/day plus several snacks.

- *Provide snacks like fruit, raw vegetables, cheese, milk, and juice; have a snack shelf in refrigerator for child to help self.*

7-Year-Old

Movement: motor control has improved, but it is not as important at this age. Capable of fine motor hand movements.

- *Continue to reinforce safety guides.*
- *Assist parents to tolerate "quiet" days and periods of shyness as part of growing up. May be subjected to various fears and nightmares; do not permit child to sleep with parent; reassure, comfort, but do not oversympathize or give undue attention and importance to these unless they increase in severity and frequency (then see counselor).*
- *Stress the importance of teaching and setting examples regarding harmful use of drugs, alcohol, smoking.*

Play: begins to prefer to play with own sex. The importance of the peer group becomes central now. Enjoys games that develop physical and mental skill. Wants more realism in play. Collects things for quantity, not quality (rocks, bottle caps, baseball cards, shells). Enjoys illusion and magic tricks. Likes table and card games, dominoes, checkers. Likes books to read by self; also radio, records, TV; skateboards and bicycles. Girls this age often ready also for lessons in dancing, piano, or gymnastics.

Socialization: is less impulsive and boisterous in activities; quiet and reflective. Begins to deal with the complex organization of concrete concepts; can count by 2s, 5s, and 10s; can add and subtract; can tell time, days, months, and seasons; anticipates things like Christmas, birthdays, holidays. Thinks before acting; thought is more flexible now. Begins to classify and group objects on a general level. Nervous habits are common. Mutilation, body image, and castration fears develop. Wants to be like friends; competition is important. Likes school, considers ideas of teacher important.

- *Help parents form realistic expectations of child's school achievement, development, and behavior. Parents need affirmation that child's unpredictable and changing behavior is normal and expected.*

8-Year-Old

Movement: returns to an active, vigorous phase with fine motor coordination acquired. Movements are more graceful.

- *Teach safety around autos including using seat belts, knowing rules of bike safety.*

Play: enjoys making detailed drawings. Reads comic books, cartoons and books (often adventure stories). Likes board games, electronic games, craft kits, sports of all types.

Socialization: again gregarious, becomes a self-assured and pragmatic character on home ground. Eager to absorb the world around and render opinions on all matters. Curiosity is boundless; able to collect and classify objects in a qualitative manner now. Increasingly modest about own body. Strongly prefers the company of own sex; is selective in choice of company; likes group projects, clubs, and outings. Uses language as a tool; likes riddles, jokes, and word games; has a sense of humor. Art work begins to show new perception of subjects.

- *Reinforce the need to be considered important by adults and given small responsibilities.*
- *Provide simple explanations, honest answers to questions regarding sex.*
- *Avoid negative reinforcement of teasing, nailbiting, enuresis, whining, poor manners, swearing.*

Nutrition: needs approximately 2,100 cal/day.

- *Plan meal and snack times, as child is often too busy to take time for eating proper amounts with good eating habits.*

9-Year-Old

Movement: active, constantly on the go; plays and works hard, often to the point of fatigue. Large group skills and activities predominate (swimming, other sports, dancing). Uses tools fairly well. Uses both hands independently.

- *Have parents teach safety with firearms including storing them away from the bullets, handling them carefully, never referring to them as a toy.*
- *Assess health knowledge and spend time with child discussing health habits.*

Play: peer activities dominate with strong sex differences in play choices; hopscotch, jacks, jumprope, and crafts for girls; war games, fort building, tag, and football for boys. Both sexes like soccer, kickball, and softball. Board games, electronic games, afterschool hobbies, music and dancing lessons popular. Reading still enjoyed by many, but school-age children now thought to watch more than 20 hours TV/week.

Socialization: rules become a guiding force in all aspects of life. Overly concerned with peer-imposed rules. Interested in family life, activities, and vacations, but parents are excluded from a major portion of child's life. Shows a consuming interest in how things are made; how and what makes weather, seasons; outer space, rockets, and science fiction. Much antagonism and rivalry between sexes and between siblings, leading to frequent quarrels and teasing. Lying and stealing to gain recognition or attention may become a problem.

- *Avoid harsh and severe punishment; try to restrict to room or home, cancel treats; try system of rewards with charts or lists of desired behavior. Understand and accept the child as s/he is.*
- *Stress importance of parents knowing playmates and their parents.*

10-Year-Old

Movement: very active with good coordination. Marked differences in motor skills between the sexes appear, with boys surpassing girls in strength, endurance, and agility while girls may exceed in flexibility and graceful movement; training and interests are determining variables.

- *Parental guidance and support are the strongest influence on school achievement.*
- *Competitiveness in school activities may lead to difficulties for the child in handling failure. Low self-esteem is often related to learning difficulties, below average physical skills, family and neighborhood problems.*
- *Assist to seek counseling and help if problems occur.*

Play: likes gangs and clubhouse with secret codes, rules and rituals; experiments in all areas. Enjoys crafts like weaving, jewelry and leather work; singing in choral groups. Likes mystery stories and TV. Interested in hobbies (e.g., collections of stamps, coins, rocks, shells, beer cans, bottle caps, license plates). Parental involvement and commitment are needed to encourage participation of child in organized clubs, sports, and youth groups.

- *Stress importance of serving as "team parent" or helper as most of these activities are organized and conducted by volunteer, interested parents. Parents need to understand that while child needs time alone or with friends, there is still a need to supervise and protect child from harmful companions and influences (e.g., "R" rated movies and some TV programs [including cable TV]).*

Socialization: is happy, cooperative, casual, and relaxed; usually courteous and well-mannered with adults. Has a growing capacity for thought and conceptual organization; is able to discuss problems, see other person's point of view, think about social problems and prejudices. The peak of the gang age; companionship is more important than play activities. Needs occasional privacy; wants independence. Can understand transformations of state in size, shape, weight, and volume. Has the ability to plan ahead.

- *Provide list of organized community programs for "latchkey" children (youngsters under 12 who are on their own and unsupervised after school while both parents are working).*
- *Continue sex education and preparation for adolescent body changes. Since peers share sexual (mis)information, be sure children are given correct facts. Become involved with the health education program at child's school.*

Nutrition: needs approximately 2,400 cal/day.

11-Year-Old

Movement: differences between sexes may become more noticeable, as girls no longer compete on an equal basis with males in some areas of physical strength. Manipulative skills nearly equal to those of adults. May be the start of a stormy, active period of constant activity like finger-tapping, foot-drumming, or restless leg swinging while sitting.

Play: enjoys projects and working with hands in metal craft, ceramics, auto mechanics, bicycle repair, knitting and crocheting. Likes to do jobs and run errands that will earn money (e.g., gardening, babysitting). Very involved in sports, dancing, and talking on telephone. Likes participation in all aspects of drama (e.g., production, stage manager, makeup, props, publicity). May show an interest in golf, tennis, racquetball, jogging/running, water sports, and both street and ice hockey. Indoor games of choice may include arcade games, electronic games, Ping-Pong, pool, volleyball, and basketball. Enjoys listening to popular music; wants

records, tapes of favorite stars and to attend rock concerts or movies.

- *Encourage inactive preteens to engage in some organized, regular play or physical exercise. Establish life-long habits of regular exercise for physical and mental well-being.*

Socialization: rebels at routines, doing homework, or household chores. Has wide mood swings with rapid changes from moodiness to cheerfulness. May cry and lose temper if hair doesn't look "perfect" before going somewhere. Begins to take daily showers, shampoos without urging, especially as s/he begins to take notice of opposite sex. Peers are very significant; "put-downs" and taunting over physical attributes, clothing, or school skills are very common. Participates actively in community, team, and school affairs. Wants unreasonable amounts of freedom to do as s/he wishes. Wants to be trusted and given responsibility; wants to earn extra money over allowance (e.g., washing cars, mowing lawns, babysitting). Boys begin to tease girls to get attention. Hero worship is prevalent. Can be very critical of selves, own work or skills. Interested in whys of health measures; beginning to understand reproduction when accurately taught.

- *Set realistic limits that can be tolerated by both sides. Offer support and give democratic guidance as child works through feelings. Help channel energy in the right direction.*
- *Assist parents to set clear expectations and enforceable limits on preteen behavior.*
- *Help schools arrange for suitable educational materials on smoking and alcoholism by contacting local agencies of PTA and American Cancer Society. Use power of suggestion rather than dictating behavior; set good examples of moderation and moral values for children.*
- *Provide explanations of body changes and special understanding for child that surges ahead or lags behind. Recognize that they may have a need to rebel and deprecate others.*
- *Encourage parents and schools to address sex education (e.g., reproduction, venereal disease, taking responsibility for own actions, the right to say no, birth control) since the time of menarche continues to occur at earlier ages (it is not unusual to see menstruation occur at age 11, also some pregnancies).*
- *Encourage parents to discuss beliefs (e.g., religion and birth control).*

Sleep: needs approximately 8–10 hours/night.
Nutrition: boys need approximately 2,500 cal/day; girls approximately 2,250 cal/day.

- *Discourage excessive sugar snacks and junk foods. Reinforce basics of good nutrition.*

Normal Growth and Development: Adolescent

Definition/Discussion

Adolescence spans the developmental period terminating childhood, from 12 through 19 years of age.

- Developmental task (Erikson's central problem) to be re-solved in adolescence is *identity* versus *identity diffusion* (e.g., Who am I really? Who do I want to be? How am I

different from others?). During this period the adolescent continues to develop a self-concept and identity that is acceptable to him/her and to significant others. To this end s/he "tries on" many different roles in deciding what career, role, and personality characteristics are most desirable.

- Acceptance is a critical element in the adolescent's pursuit for a self-concept; conformity of dress, eating, activities, appearance, and beliefs are all efforts or attempts at acceptance by the peer group.

- The overriding importance of peers of the last period of the middle years of childhood takes on a different character during adolescence as peer groups are no longer restricted exclusively to one sex; the individual has significant peer relationships in groups of both sexes serving different needs.
- The all-consuming importance of rules for the school-age child gives way to a severe criticism of authority and rule and a desire to change the world, making it a better place to live. To this end the adolescent joins activist groups and groups promoting civic change to make a contribution and effort at achieving his high goals for mankind.
- Stress-related disorders in adolescents (e.g., anxiety and phobic reactions, eating disorders, depression, alcohol and drug abuse, suicidal and delinquent behaviors) are more prevalent today than in previous generations due to increased social pressure and expectations of peers versus parents. Teenagers often need help to learn that everyone has problems, conflicts, tensions; that help is available from caring others, that s/he can successfully face own feelings and understand and accept self; and that by developing stress management skills, s/he will be able to cope effectively with own problems.
- More than 12 million teenagers are sexually active (Guttmacher Institute Report, 1982). While use of contraception is increasing, more than 1 million teenage girls get pregnant each year. About 75% of these pregnancies are unintended. Studies show teenagers to be seriously misinformed on basic sex education facts. More than two-thirds never practice contraception, or do so inconsistently. Nearly 50% of the sexually active teenage females think they can't get pregnant, yet 20% of teenage pregnancies occur within the first month after start of intercourse; half the pregnancies occur within the first 6 months. Studies show that peers and the media (movies, TV) are the primary source of adolescent sex education. Less than 25% of teenage students receive a significant amount of school-based sex education. A heightened awareness and concern among the public, along with a strong commitment, may help correct this growing problem.
- Adolescence is a special period of childhood where the individual undergoes numerous physical and emotional changes to develop into the unique individual s/he has been maturing into throughout childhood. Due to the uniqueness of each individual, it becomes difficult to set rigid standards for patterns of development, yet there is a sequential progression of behaviors during this period.
- The common parameters of physical development and the broad changes in behaviors for the adolescent are outlined below; corresponding nursing implications and parental teaching or guidance suggestions follow in *italics*.

☐ AGE 12 THROUGH 19 YEARS

Weight and height
- girls
  11–14 years: 101 lb (46 kg); 62 in (157 cm)
  15–19 years: 120 lb (55 kg); 64 in (163 cm)
- boys
  11–14 years: 99 lb (45 kg); 62 in (157 cm)
  15–18 years: 145 lb (66 kg); 69 in (176 cm)
  19 years: 147 lb (67 kg); 70 in (178 cm)
- *Provide information regarding weight gain, growth spurts, and episodes of fatigue that accompany adolescent physiologic changes.*
- *Counsel in a patient, supportive manner to bolster self-confidence.*

- *Encourage sound dietary practices and hygiene.*
- *Provide a wide degree of variability based on individual differences.*
- *Screen for scoliosis and refer as needed.*
Pulse: 50–100/minute.
Respirations: 15–24 minute.
Blood pressure: 110–118/65–74.
Teeth: Wisdom teeth usually come in, if at all, by 18–20 years. Caries common during this period.
- *Arrange at least twice yearly dental check-ups; screen for orthodontic problems.*
Female Sex Characteristics
- *primary:* increase in size of internal and external genitalia; changes in endometrial lining and vaginal secretions; ovulation and menarche (average age of onset 12–13 years)
- *secondary:* increase in breast size, bone growth, basal metabolic rate; changes in shape of pelvis, pubic and axillary hair patterns; increased fat deposits in breasts, buttocks, and thighs; increasingly smooth and soft skin
Male Sex Characteristics
- *primary:* growth and development of testes, scrotum, and penis; production of mature sperm
- *secondary:* changes in body hair distribution; increase in size of vocal cords; increased thickness of skin, sebaceous secretions, basal metabolic rate, and bone growth with broadening of shoulders
- *Answer questions regarding the physical changes in their systems in an honest and direct manner to prevent misconceptions and to foster a positive self-image. Listen sympathetically to expression of feelings (e.g., worries, fears) regarding changes; initiate conversation on points the adolescent may be reluctant to discuss (e.g., unequal breast size).*
- *Provide information on antiprostaglandin preparations (Motrin, Ponstel, Anaprox) to help with dysmenorrhea. They should be taken at the onset of menstrual period and stopped as the flow subsides. They are also useful for decreasing heavy bleeding, but not shortening the period. They should be taken with milk or food, but not with aspirin or any other medication. Caution teenagers not to take each others' prescriptions. Each girl should be examined by a competent physician to evaluate whether cause of the dysmenorrhea is primary or secondary to some organic problem, infection, or tumor.*
- *Teach girls to use sanitary pads or tampons (regular-size only), and to change them at least every 4 hours. Caution against use of tampons used when girl is being treated for any pelvic inflammatory disease or vaginal infections.*
- *Have an open discussion about menstruation to encourage sharing of questions, beliefs, and feelings. If girls have been raised in families comfortable with occasional discussions of growth and sex, the beginning of menstruation will be accepted naturally with little embarrassment or tension. Simply dropping a book on the subject in the girl's hands is unwise, unless requested or read together by mother and daughter. The action of giving the child something to read can be interpreted as lack of caring, unwillingness, or inability on the part of the mother to discuss such private subjects.*
- *Provide clear, concise, accurate information about menstruation in a matter-of-fact way to enable the girl to reject inaccurate information shared among her friends.*
- *Assure girls that they can continue with normal activities, that discomfort is often only temporary, and that their periods may be very irregular for a year or more.*
- *Teach youth to cleanse face thoroughly (washing gently, not scrubbing) with a mild, unscented soap; rinse; apply a 5% or*

10% benzyl peroxide gel 1–2 times daily for pimple prevention as well as treatment.

COMMON BEHAVIORS

12 to 15 Years

Movement: often awkward and uncoordinated, as the adolescent adjusts to physical changes in height and size. Frequently displays poor posture. Physically active, but tires easily.

- *Provide reassurance and help in accepting changing body; parents need to reinforce positive qualities, seek professional help for health problems (e.g., skin eruptions, vaginal discharge, dental caries, drug use).*
- *Set realistic but firm limits that can be mutually agreed upon for security reasons; avoid threats.*
- *Exercise authority with tact.*

Leisure/play: enjoys activities centered around peer group (usually same sex, gradually mixing at social and sporting events). Enjoys school-related events (e.g., sports, dances, concerts, rallies, parties, plays, and various competitions). Likes shopping, talking on telephone, listening to music, spending time on grooming, sun bathing, watching soap operas and other TV, movies, cooking, sewing, reading popular magazines, and baby sitting, watching or participating in sports activities, working on bikes, cars, motorscooters, or other mechanical interests, watching/playing arcade/electronic games. Wants free time, unsupervised by adults, to "do my own thing." Shows interest in getting part-time jobs for extra spending money over regular allowances.

- *Provide opportunities for child to earn money and have some financial independence.*
- *Encourage independence and allow person to be an individual, to feel s/he has some control over what happens to him/her; however, be available and allow child to utilize parent, as s/he needs to do so.*
- *Provide honest answers to questions; repeat explanations as needed.*
- *Arrange for driver education prior to 16th birthday.*

Socialization: has an increasing interest in the opposite sex. "Going around" (liking each other but not really dating yet) progresses to group dates, then couple dating alone. Peer-group acceptance is strongest in early adolescence and the pressure to conform to group norms is nearly overwhelming to many teens. Strong friendship bonds are formed with 1 or 2 close peers. Age varies on dating, as some do not date a single person until late adolescence. Shows increasing hostility and alienation towards parents or authority figures. Expresses strong opinions and beliefs contrary to those of parents and school staff. Verbal conflicts over restrictions are common. Concerned with morality, ethics, religion, and social customs; is in the process of developing own values and standards, but peer group beliefs are strong influences. Idealism is prevalent. Reasoning is mature; thinking now includes abstract ideas. Wide variations in academic abilities and interests. Day-dreaming and sexual fantasies are common. Girls are more socially adept than boys; will take initiative to telephone boys and plan parties or other group activities. In early adolescence (age 12), girls have more interest than boys in physical appearance, physical development and attractiveness. By age 14, both sexes worry and fret over hair, skin, size of body parts, clothing, and physical details. As interest in opposite sex grows, so does the frequency of showers, shampoos, teeth brushing, and grooming habits.

- *Assist parents to provide gentle encouragement and guidance regarding dating; avoid strong pressures of either extreme.*
- *Continue to provide teenagers a warm, affectionate, loving, parental relationship (e.g., tell children you love them; tell them they are attractive, interesting, worthwhile, and special; encourage positive mental attitude; show them respect by*

helping to build their self-confidence and self-esteem; praise often, criticize less).
- *Explain that feelings do not have to be denied; that it is normal to have varied and changing moods and feelings (e.g., anger, irritability, tenderness, sensitivity, romantic longings, jealousy, guilt, anxiety, fear, embarrassment). Help adolescents to get in touch with feelings by talking about it with a trusted other, family member, or good friend. Parents need to understand child's conflicts as s/he attempts to deal with social, moral, political, and intellectual issues.*
- *Let the adolescent know it is OK to masturbate to avoid increasing the level of guilt and anxiety about it.*
- *Provide information and counseling regarding venereal disease, professional birth control resources.*
- *Encourage open discussion of problems, concerns, and questions.*
- *Assist to seek family counseling for coping with an adolescent who has problems of drug abuse, pregnancy, depression, learning handicaps, or other difficulties.*
- *Consider a parent support group to cope with parental feelings of guilt, fear, anger, and hopelessness.*

Sleep: approximately 7–9 hours/night.

Eating: prefers easy-to-obtain junk foods such as candy, carbonated drinks, potato chips. Concern over appearance may lead to crash diets, poor eating patterns, or serious eating disorders. Girls need approximately 1,500–3000 calories/day (average 2,200 cal/day). Boys need approximately 2,000–3,700 calories/day (average 2,700 cal/day)

- *Vitamin and iron supplements are often recommended.*

16 through 19 Years

Movement: has increased energy as growth spurt tapers. Muscular ability and coordination increase.

Leisure/play: enjoys working for altruistic causes. Sports activities (as both participant and observer) are well-attended. Likes beach and recreational activities like surfing, skiing, sailing, tennis, volleyball, hiking. Reading, TV, music, radio, and telephone are all still important. Likes challenging games (e.g., chess, bridge, poker, crossword puzzles). May explore new interests via volunteer work, summer jobs, high school occupational programs, part-time employment, and vacation trips. Dancing is popular; also enjoys attending concerts, plays, etc. Enjoys high-risk, competitive sports such as car racing.

- *Assist to set goals with adolescents and help them develop independence and competence in such things as grocery shopping, preparing nutritionally balanced meals, checkbook management, home and yard maintenance, first aid, health and safety measures.*

Socialization: continues to refine language, reasoning, thinking, and communicating skills. Begins to realize that inadequacies in these areas adversely affect job opportunities and limit career choices. Has achieved a more mature, interdependent relationship with parents. At 15 or 16, confides more in friends than in parents; at 18 or 19, parental advice and support is sought and the transition to adulthood is made. Dating in pairs and groups is common; romantic love affairs develop. Some look for permanence in a relationship; others decide to postpone permanent relationships until completion of college or establishment of job security. Has an increased ability to balance responsibility with pleasure. Develops an identity for self and an image of the kind of person s/he will become. Tries to develop characteristics thought to be desirable in a mate. Learns through satisfactions and frustrations of the problems living full time with peers, either in college or apartment settings. Peer group affiliation is not as rigid. Despite continuing peer influence, independent judgment emerges. Constantly seeks satisfactory part-time jobs to pay for car, dating, and other personal expenses. Effort is directed to become independent and self-supportive. Summers are spent working or getting extra course work for college. Plans more realistically for career. Assumes major responsibility for deciding on post-high school plans. More women are now seeking educational majors and careers that were formerly dominated by men (e.g., engineering, business, medicine).

- *Encourage parents to provide assistance as needed and desired (e.g., selecting a college, obtaining a scholarship and financial assistance, getting a job, planning a wedding,*

buying a car, getting insurance or a loan, using an acceptable, appropriate birth control method, resolving a health problem).
- *Assist parents to adjust to the loss of their dependent child.*

Sleep: 6–8 hours/night.

Nutrition: Girls need approximately 1,200–3,000 cal/day (average 2,100 cal/day); boys need approximately 2,100–3,900 cal/day (average 2,800 cal/day).

- *Continue vitamin and iron supplements as recommended.*

APPENDIX IV
Mental Status Exam

Definition/Discussion

A mental status exam is an assessment of observable aspects of the patient's/client's psychological functioning.

☐ General Considerations

- The mental status assessment is a *method* of organizing clinical observations that provides a baseline for the patient's psychologic state; it also provides specific information to assist in establishing diagnoses, planning goals, interventions, and subsequent evaluation.
- In the practice of psychiatric nursing, the mental status is an integral part of the initial assessment. The complete psychiatric examination includes a physical and neurologic study by the physician, as well as a psychiatric history, that includes the statement of the problem, a careful identification of the present episode with the reason why the patient came in at this particular time, a personal history, and a family history.
- The mental status exam is a useful assessment tool in all areas of nursing practice. Additions to the initial assessment are made by daily observations in inpatient and day treatment facilities, as well as other community settings.
- The nurse may be the first to pick up symptoms of organic brain disease, alcohol or drug use, suicidal ideation, and inappropriate speech activity or behaviors; the patient can then be referred for a thorough medical and psychiatric examination by a physician.
- The mental status examination usually includes areas of
  - appearance and behavior
  - consciousness
  - speech activity
  - thought process, content, and perceptions.

Components of Assessment	Examples of Abnormalities
Appearance and Behavior	
• Observe for dress, grooming, and personal hygiene; colors, makeup, condition of clothes; skin color and condition.	Inappropriate to age or place; condition of clothes unusual; unkempt appearance, unshaven, body odor; pediculosis or other unusual skin condition.
• Describe posture: erect, seated, horizontal.	Stooped, slumped; note open or closed posture.
• Describe gait.	Shuffles, limps, fast, slow, akathisia. Signs of anxiety: moist hands, restlessness or retarded movement, dilated pupils, carotid pulses visibly noticeable or bounding, pacing.
• Describe motor behavior: ability to relax, level and pattern of activity, relationship to topics of discussion or activities and people around area.	
• Describe affect (facial expression and mobility): sad, serious, smiling, immobile, flat (no expression).	Grimacing, tremors, parkinsonism, and bizarre movements of head and neck in phenothiazine reactions.
• Examine for scars and other marks.	Birthmarks, operative scars, needle marks, wounds, trauma on wrist, etc.
• Note prostheses: eyeglasses, contact lenses, cane, dentures, etc.	
• Note culture, growth, and development tasks.	Inappropriate behaviors for culture, stage of growth and development.

Components of Assessment	Examples of Abnormalities

Consciousness

- Determine orientation to time, place, and person by asking questions about the time of day, date, year, duration of hospitalization. Use direct questioning if appropriate: "What day is today?" or "How long have you been here?"

Disoriented to time, place, or person; stuporous, confused, clouded, unconscious.

- Note sensorium: if patient is aware of his surroundings, his sensorium is said to be clear.

Unaware of surroundings.

Speech Activity

- Describe quality: loudness, clarity, pitch, tone, inflection.
- Note quantity: pace volume.
- Assess organization: coherence, relevance, circumstantiality.

Slow, monotonous, flight of ideas; incoherent, circumstantial speech with neologisms (self-coined words); slurred speech, speech defect.

Thought Processes and Content, Perceptions

- Assess feelings by verbal questioning such as: "How are your spirits? How are you managing? Do you get pretty depressed (discouraged, blue)? How do you feel about that? How low do you feel? How do you feel right now? What do you see for yourself in the future?"

Important to assess for depression and suicidal risk; refer to *The Patient Experiencing Depression*, page 57; *The Patient with Manic-Depressive (Bipolar) Psychosis*, page 89; and *The Patient who is Suicidal*, page 144.

Note evasiveness, hostility, anger, elation, tearfulness, distrustfulness, resentment, apathy, lack of openness and approachability.

- Observe the way patient describes own history, symptoms, feelings; follow leads provided by patient's own words.

Incoherent, disorganized thoughts; blocking, irrelevance, loose associations, talkative, silent, aphasic.

- Ask appropriate questions such as: "What do you think about at times like this?" "Sometimes when people get upset, things seem unreal. Is this happening now to you?"

Note indications of compulsions (repetitive acts that patient feels driven to do), obsessions (recurrent, uncontrollable thoughts), doubting and indecision, phobias (irrational fears), free-floating anxieties (feelings of dread or impending doom; ill-defined dread).

- Inquire about feelings of unreality, depersonalization (a sense that one's self is different, changed, unreal, has lost identity), feelings of persecution (a sense that patient is disliked, persecuted, being plotted against), feelings of influence (a sense that others are controlling or manipulating patient), feelings of reference (a sense that outside events such as TV or radio are related to patient, communicating to patient or about patient).

Feelings of unreality, depersonalization, persecution, influence, reference, delusions (false, fixed beliefs), illusions (misinterpretation of sensory stimuli), hallucinations (subjective sensory perceptions); assumes listening or watchful posture; attitude may indicate hallucinations.

- Assess for memory of recent events by asking about events in recent past; assess for retention and recall by reciting several consecutive numbers and asking patient to repeat them. Ask patient to give chronologic account of his/her life to assess past memory; ask about birthdays, anniversaries.

Poor recent memory in organic brain disease or high anxiety state. Poor retention and recall.

Components of Assessment	Examples of Abnormalities

Thought Processes and Content, Perceptions *(cont'd)*

- Assess for attention and concentration: say you want to test patient's ability to concentrate. Read a series of digits, starting with shortest set and enunciating each number clearly at a rate of 1/second; ask patient to repeat them back to you. If patient makes a mistake, give a second try with a different series (e.g., 8-5-6-3, 3-5-6-8-2, or 9-7-6-6-3-2). Ask patient to repeat digits backwards. Ask patient to count backwards from 100 by 5s. Note effort required, speed, and accuracy of responses.

Poor performance of digit span is characteristic of organic brain disease; performance is also limited by mental retardation.

Unable to repeat at least 5 to 8 digits forward, or 4 to 6 backwards (the usual number).

- Assess judgment: ask about patient's daily life; note ability to compare thoughts, events, relationships, and draw solid conclusions. Ask "What should you do if you are stopped for a traffic/speeding ticket?" "What should you do if you miss the bus?"

Unable to make comparisons of thought and events, understand the relationships, draw valid conclusions.

- Assess abstract thinking: ask the patient to interpret simple proverbs such as "A rolling stone gathers no moss," or "Don't cross your bridges until you come to them."

Concrete responses may indicate organic brain disorder, schizophrenia, low intelligence.

- Assess insight: as assessment interview progresses, does patient show understanding of his/her present situation? How does s/he describe his/her problems or the cause of present state?

Unaware of current problems or present situation; unaware of mental illness or abnormal behaviors; unable to link cause and effect (these are associated with neurotic disorders).

APPENDIX V
Problem Solving

Definition/Discussion

Problem solving is a systematic method of reasoning or organizing data in order to find useful and effective alternative ways to cope with a situation, need, or concern that constitutes a problem. Effective problem solving is essential to mental health and is a learned behavior; with practice, the learner can improve problem-solving ability. Components of problem solving are: awareness of problem area, problem definition, data collection and analysis, formulation of alternative solutions, discussion of possible consequences, selection of best alternative, implementation of trial run, evaluation, and summary.

Nursing Assessment

Behaviors that may indicate a need for problem solving include:

- physical discomfort
- powerlessness
- shame or stigma
- passivity
- incompetence in coping with ADL (activites of daily living)

- Conflict
- emotional threat
- hopelessness
- increased stress
- non-assertion
- distorted reality

- anxiety
- low self-esteem
- frustration
- guilt
- immaturity
- aggression

Nursing Care

☐ **Long-Term Goal**

The patient/client/staff member will learn and demonstrate the steps and methods of problem solving; the patient/client/staff member will demonstrate increased ability to solve problem.

☐ **SPECIFIC CONSIDERATION #1**

Awareness of the Problem Area

☐ **GOAL**

The patient/client/staff member will see, hear, feel, or experience awareness of specific situation or problem area.

☐ **IMPLEMENTATION**

- Focus on situation, need or concern; ask person to recall and describe details, including feelings and issues, what was seen and heard, who was involved, when and how event occurred.
- Know that awareness is the first step of change; listen and explore without giving advice or jumping to conclusions.

☐ **SPECIFIC CONSIDERATION #2**

Problem Definition

☐ **GOAL**

The problem(s) will be identified and defined; goals/objectives/expected outcomes will be specified.

☐ **IMPLEMENTATION**

- Define needs and goals/objectives/expected outcomes; set priorities in terms of most pressing problems.
- Identify issues and different aspects involved; separate complex problems into subgroups.
- Determine what creates the problem by asking: "Why is it a problem? Who is affected by this? Who else is involved? Who else could be involved in problem solving? Why am I motivated to change the situation?"
- Identify who, what, when, where and which; ask open-ended questions (e.g., "How do you manage _____ ?" "What is it about this situation that concerns you?").

☐ **SPECIFIC CONSIDERATION #3**

Data Collection and Analysis

☐ **GOAL**

Data will be collected, organized, and analyzed in an appropriate way

☐ IMPLEMENTATION

• Decide on a method to collect data relevant to the situation (e.g., literature search; create data collection tool to be used to interview in person, by mail, or by telephone survey); problem solving group may be created to bring together individuals with similar problem to share information and offer group support, encouragement.
• Organize and classify data, using outline or numbering method; large file cards or computer system may be helpful.
• Validate findings with other persons; clarify issues; identify gaps or discrepancies in information.
• Analyze data by discussion, comparing and contrasting issues and information.
• Interpret data by making a relationship between facts; use the process of induction or deduction to form a conclusion; identify causes of problem and influencing factors.

☐ SPECIFIC CONSIDERATION #4

Alternative Solutions

☐ GOAL

Alternative solutions will be formulated and discussed with consideration of possible consequences.

☐ IMPLEMENTATION

• Formulate tentative alternative solutions, using data analysis and conclusions; consider all possible courses of action; list each as a possible solution.
• Discuss each alternative and identify its possible consequences, including pros and cons, strengths and weaknesses; role play alternatives, paying attention to feelings and physiologic responses.
• Be aware of person's attitudes, values, and feelings that influence determination of pros and cons.
• Assess for lack of knowledge or experience to initiate alternative; teach as needed in assertiveness, communication skills, interpersonal relationship skills.

☐ SPECIFIC CONSIDERATION #5

Trial Run and Evaluation

☐ GOAL

An alternative solution will be chosen and a trial run will be implemented and evaluated:

☐ IMPLEMENTATION

• Choose one possible solution that seems most appropriate; plan and initiate trial run; complex plans should be broken down into small steps.
• Identify specific actions to be taken; estimate time needed and anticipate factors that may facilitate or hinder the action.
• Know that trial runs usually have to be modified or revised; continue collecting data to revise or modify as needed.
• Be flexible and open-minded; if the alternative is not satisfactory, try another one. *There are always other alternatives!* You may find that you need to start back at the first or second step with awareness and redefinition of the problem.
• Evaluate effectiveness of alternative solution in relation to the previously set goals and objectives.

☐ SPECIFIC CONSIDERATION #6

Summary

☐ GOAL

The problem-solving method will be summarized, including problem-solving process and content; anticipatory guidance will be offered to cope with next problem.

☐ IMPLEMENTATION

• Summarize the problem-solving process, using the problem-solving components and the specific content; this may be done verbally or with charts, graphs, audio visuals, or written reports may be created to share the conclusion or results with others.
• Identify future situations that may be potential problem areas and use anticipatory guidance to apply conclusions, alternative solutions, or problem-solving methods to these situations; give positive reinforcement for ability to apply new knowledge to potential problem situations.
• Recognize and give verbal and nonverbal positive reinforcement for willingness to learn and use problem-solving methods and for demonstrations of increased ability to problem solve.

APPENDIX VI
Behavior Modification

Behavior modification is a teaching technique for dealing with observable and measurable behavior problems. It is designed to assist individuals to modify behavior that stands in the way of health and well-being. The basic tenet of behavioral theory is: behavior that is reinforced tends to be repeated. Behavioral theory indicates that both positive and negative behaviors are learned and can be modified. Initially positive or negative reinforcement should be given each time the problem behavior occurs; after the desired behavior or change is established, intermittent reinforcement (e.g., every 2-3 times) is more desirable. *Terminal behaviors* are the desired new behaviors to be learned. *Positive reinforcement* means a desired response or behavior is followed by a positive or desired consequence; reinforcement works best when applied immediately. *Aversive consequences* are undesirable consequences that can be used to decrease occurrence of behavior. *Generalization* is the transfer of an already learned response to another situation.

☐ Assessment

- Identify problem behavior needing intervention; behavior should be observable and measurable (target behavior).
- Determine how this behavior interferes with care, health, and the patient's well-being (e.g., patient is 50 lb overweight, has erratic diet habits, and wants to lose weight as part of treatment plan to decrease blood pressure).
- Instruct patient to keep a diary for 1 week and write down information needed to gather baseline date (e.g., how many times does the behavior occur in a specific time period).
- Observe sequence and pattern of behavior (e.g., patient's weight is 190 lb; daily diet diary indicates no breakfast, a high-calorie 10 A.M. snack, a sandwich and malt for lunch, peanuts and wine at 5 P.M. and a large dinner with dessert at 8 P.M.
- Assess for events that precede and follow behavior; pay attention to feelings as well as to who, what, when, how, and why.
- Involve the patient/family in this analysis; encourage the patient to count and keep track of behavior and feelings that accompany it by keeping a journal, diary, or chart.

- Assess for deficits in behavioral repertoire (e.g., skills and abilities the patient has not learned or is not currently using). Example: Patient eats to give self treat; does not know how to nurture self in other ways. Gets up too late for breakfast and eats lunch out because there is nothing in the house to take for lunch. Eats dinner late to eat with husband. Snacks to cope with anxiety and depression. Willing to work on anxiety and depression by learning new ways to cope.

☐ PLAN/IMPLEMENTATION

- Set and write out behavioral objectives to modify the target behavior to the desired terminal behavior; include the setting or conditions under which the desired behavior is expected to occur, the specific desired behavior that can be observed and measured, and the criteria for how and when the behavior will be performed.
- Include the patient in setting goals and planning program; such as selecting appropriate positive reinforcers and suitable aversive consequences.
- Nursing behaviors for positive reinforcement should include spending time with patient, verbal praise and encouragement, smiling, showing interest in discussion of specific subjects, providing opportunity for patient to have special experiences or treats.
- Aversive consequences could include discontinuing special experiences or treats, participating in chores that are disliked by patient, or nursing behaviors of lack of interest, frowning, turning face away, or spending less time with patient.
- Teach patient that all behavior has consequences and that each individual can choose among many alternative actions and resulting consequences.
- Set a specific time for trial run of program and agree to evaluate effectiveness at that time. Example: Patient will reduce diet intake to ingest 1,200 calories/day, to include 3 meals plus 2 snacks in a well-balanced diet. Patient will weigh in once a week and will be able to plan and have a nonfood treat (e.g., flowers, music, new clothes, perfume) each time s/he loses 5 lb. Patient will swim or walk 15 minutes daily. If no weight lost or if weight gained, patient agrees to clean out garage or wash down walls for neighbor.
- Offer specific plan to practice modified behavior; en-

courage attitude of positive and matter-of-fact expectance that modified behavior will occur. Example: Plan acceptable diet and snacks with some unusual low-calorie treats; plan shopping to include items for breakfast and lunch.

- Break behavior into small steps in a sequence pattern; plan practice of small steps.
- Include some known desired behaviors that cannot be done simultaneously with target behavior. Example: Play guitar or flute instead of snacking; chew gum while cooking dinner instead of tasting food; folk dance or swim instead of drinking alcohol.
- Begin with known steps and then attempt unknown or new steps; choose simple, unthreatening situations and then gradually include more complex and difficult ones.
- Instruct patient to keep diary or journal of practice, including log of new steps and modified behavior, plus feelings and concerns. Steps might include: buy low-calorie acceptable food, prepare lunch the night before, get up early to eat breakfast, take guitar/flute lessons, prepare and eat low-calorie, well-balanced meals, keep a journal of all food ingested plus feelings and concerns.
- Reinforce small, discrete steps in adaptive direction (shaping).
- Provide information of behavior change to patient, verbally and with charts.
- Reinforce progress, using plan of positive reinforcement; ensure that each step taken toward the terminal/expected behavior is reinforced.

- Involve family and friends in giving feedback and encouragement for steps in adaptive direction. Appreciation is not only much valued at this point, but also helps shape the desired behavior.
- Involve patient in keeping own record or chart of desired terminal behavior, thus increasing awareness of own behavior and allowing for increased intrinsic motivation. Example: Patient can keep own weight chart and could negotiate with husband, friend, or co-worker to give verbal encouragement. Nurse can give praise and encouragement plus listen attentively to concerns, read patient's journal, and discuss patterns.
- Assist patient to transfer modified behavior to other similar situations and environments by role playing and using problem-solving method.
- Explore and anticipate with patient the natural positive reinforcement that could be expected or planned for with modified behavior. Example: Anticipate and role play dining-out situations in which patient asks for fresh fruit or vegetable substitute for high-calorie item. Anticipate camping trip or vacationing with 1,200-calorie diet. Encourage patient to imagine self buying smaller-sized vacation clothes and having more energy and lower blood pressure.

☐ EVALUATION

The Patient
- Demonstrates willingness to participate in program
- Demonstrates desired change in behavior

APPENDIX VII
Strategies for Counseling Adolescents

Long-Term Goal

Through this period of rapid change and turmoil, the adolescent will develop necessary skills to solve problems of daily living and to adapt to puberty and independent adult life; the adolescent will demonstrate an appreciation of, and security in, his/her own uniqueness, abilities, limits, values, feelings; will demonstrate responsibility for own behavior.

☐ General Considerations

Adolescence spans the developmental period from puberty to adulthood, usually from 12 through 19 years of age. Refer to *Normal Growth and Development: Adolescent*, page 241, for information on development, nursing implications, and suggestions for guidance.

Adolescents need adults to trust in them as they learn to cope with the changes of puberty and the challenges of independent adult life. As problems and issues emerge, adolescents experience conflict between dependent and independent roles. They need adult role models to offer hope that they are able to learn problem-solving and coping skills, and to impart positive feelings about the growth process.

Behavior cues that may indicate a need for counseling include conflicts with parents, problems in school (e.g., acting out, getting poor grades, dropping out), running away, substance abuse (e.g., drugs, alcohol), nutritional problems (e.g., obesity, anorexia, bulimia, inadequate nutrition for growth), depression, suicidal behavior, sexual problems (e.g., lack of knowledge, pregnancy, venereal disease, prostitution, sexual abuse, incest, rape), acting out or antisocial acts (e.g., stealing, aggression, violence), and lack of skills necessary for independent adult life.

- Assessment
  - degree of mastery of developmental tasks
    * identity: knows values and beliefs, can describe self in realistic way, has direction for future
    * peer relationships: establishes friendships at school and home

* independence from family, relationships with family
* performance at school or work
* sexuality: accepts body changes with maturation; has knowledge of body function, birth control, sexual relationships
* plans for present and future goals
  - level of self-esteem: realistic perception and acceptance of self
  - perception of environment: home, school, hospital, or clinic (realistic versus unrealistic)
  - behavior problems
  - physical problems
  - strengths and abilities, weaknesses and learning needs
  - response to counseling and treatment plan
  - parents: response to adolescent (quality of parent-adolescent interactions), perceptions, attitudes, expectations, level of knowledge, coping patterns, communication patterns, quality of parent-parent interactions/relationship, strengths and weaknesses of family unit, response to counseling and treatment plan.

☐ Strategies for Counseling Adolescents

1. Create a comfortable environment: use posters, pictures, bulletin boards, magazines, and books that appeal to the teenager; use plants, light, and color to help create an informal and welcoming atmosphere. Set aside a special time for teens (after school or on Saturdays in outpatient setting, or specific hours in an inpatient setting). Keep appointments fairly short and allow for choices of appointment time. Provide privacy in interviewing and examination rooms.
2. Contract for confidentiality: state that information shared with you will not be discussed with parents or anyone else unless teen gives permission to do so. Explain that the only exception would be if the teen indicates plan to harm self or others; then protective action would be taken, including talking with parent and others. Make the same contract with parents.

3. Provide an initial interview with teen and parents or group: everyone can be introduced to hospital/clinic program and verbalize requests for services; family or group interactions can be observed during the initial interview and appointments for further sessions can be made.

4. Approach the adolescent with respect: avoid authoritarian attitude; let the adolescent be the expert about him/herself; use open-ended questions and be nonjudgmental. Do not try to be "hip" or use adolescent jargon (it changes almost daily; only teens can keep up with it and adults who try to be one-of-the-gang create distance and distrust). If teen uses jargon or is unclear about situations or events, ask for clarification; do not act as if you understand when you don't.

   Listen for and explore issues; observe for nonverbal cues that may be symptoms of increased anxiety, stress, or unexpressed feelings (e.g., looking down or away from interviewer; stuttering, pausing; flushing; wringing hands; looking bored, frustrated, upset). Avoid the use of "why" questions; the answer to "why" is always "because," and it evokes defensiveness and intellectualization rather than increased awareness and exploration. Avoid giving advice; instead, teach and assist the teen to use a problem-solving approach.

5. Outline what the clinic/hospital/staff can offer, the purpose of the sessions, appropriate/expected behavior, and the limits of the situation/staff. Teens need to test limits as part of their learning about themselves and acceptable behavior in different situations; firm limits tend to promote trust and to prevent acting-out and disorganized behavior. Allow some things to be negotiable, but state what is and is not (learning to accept reasonable limits is a necessary skill for adult life).

6. Provide the option of individual or group sessions: ask the adolescent for a preference about who is to be present during counseling (best friend, parent, both parents, sibling(s), group of same sex or with same problem, or mixed group of teens, etc.) and negotiate for an arrangement that is appropriate to teen, setting, and nurse. Group work offers certain advantages to teens (e.g., some may feel more comfortable sharing ideas and feelings with a supportive friend, peer, or family member). Discussion and practice sessions can be continued on the group's own time; there is an opportunity for increased insight and understanding of self and others, and for group support. Groups are usually cost effective.

7. Assist the adolescent to clarify values (the process of developing own values with self-awareness so that beliefs, values, and behavior can be congruent): adolescence is a time to develop one's own value system by questioning, learning, and trying out alternative value systems. When beliefs, values, and behaviors are incongruent, the individual experiences conflict, confusion, and ambivalence. The adolescent is often unaware of these sources of confusion and ambivalence.

Provide opportunities to examine beliefs and values and compare own with others, noting differences and commonalities. Devise exercises to increase awareness of feelings, thoughts, and ideas concerning adolescent issues (i.e., relationships with peers, parents, body image, sexuality), e.g., "I strongly agree/strongly disagree." (See articles by Adams, Reighley in Recommended References.) As the adolescent becomes more aware of own values and beliefs, the next step is to learn to articulate values, to problem solve with awareness, to choose from alternatives, to consider consequences, and to take actions.

8. Offer opportunities to explore feelings and to develop adaptive strategies to cope with feelings: the unpredictable emotional state of the adolescent is characterized by extreme highs and lows, related to hormonal activity and adjusting to puberty and adult life. The adolescent may lose control of self in an emotional outburst, which releases accumulated anxiety, and then becomes overwhelmed by feelings of embarrassment, guilt, and fear over the loss of self-control. When staff provides support, the adolescent can withdraw, plan adaptive coping methods, and try the situation again. Examples of support: accepting expression of feelings; acknowledging human commonalities (e.g., "This is upsetting for you; it would be for most people your age"), providing hope that the adolescent will learn to cope. Teaching can include saying, "It's OK to cry," or "What else about that made you mad?"

9. Teach assertive communication skills: help adolescent complete "I" statements (e.g., "I feel;" "I want;" "I don't want;" "I like;" "I don't like;" "I am willing to;" etc.). Avoid "you" statements (e.g., "You make me mad. You are sloppy;" instead, say "I'm mad at you. I'm upset with the way this room is messed up." "You" statements tend to evoke defensive reactions and block communication.). By using assertive communication skills, the adolescent is able to negotiate a workable compromise.

   Role play assertive communication by using simple, nonthreatening situations, with characters (participants) from the individual's or group's everyday life. This is a way to rehearse new behaviors for future use. After simple and nonthreatening situations are mastered, each individual can design more difficult practice situations, and use group members or nurse for feedback as s/he learns to cope adaptively with difficult situations and threatening people. Ask the adolescent to keep a journal of daily life situations in which s/he notes behaviors of assertion, aggression, and nonassertion; instruct teen to include feelings and body sensations. The journal can be shared or kept private as preferred. See Recommended References for books on assertion.

10. Teach stress-management skills: assess learning needs and teach alternative ways to relax such as progressive relaxation, autogenic training exercises, diaphragmatic breathing, hobbies, exercise, use of imagery and positive affirmations.

11. Offer opportunities to learn risk taking with support of nurse (going from childhood to adolescence and adulthood involves living with change and taking risks): common risks during adolescence include separating from family to form a peer group, developing relationships with the opposite sex, learning to drive a car, daring to be different from peer group and expressing unique values and behaviors, and leaving home; all the while wanting emotional and financial support while craving independence and freedom.

Use role playing and problem solving with guided imagery to explore new behaviors, possible choices, and consequences of behaviors. Use positive affirmations and values clarification to increase adaptive risk taking.

BIBLIOGRAPHY

Acquired Immune Deficiency Syndrome

Acquired immune deficiency syndrome (AIDS): Precautions for health care workers and allied health professionals. (1983). *Public Health Letter*, November.

Acquired immunodeficiency syndrome (AIDS) update—United States. (1983). *Morbidity & Mortality Weekly Review, 32*, 450-451.

Allen, J., & Mellin, G. (1982). The new epidemic. *American Journal of Nursing, 82*, 1718-1722.

Bennett, J. (1985). AIDS epidemiology update. *American Journal of Nursing, 85*, 968-972.

Bennett, J. (1985). The HTLV-III/AIDS link. *American Journal of Nursing, 85*, 1086-1089.

Irish, A. (1983). Straight talks about gay patients. *American Journal of Nursing, 83*, 1169-1170.

Kennedy, M. (1987). AIDS: Coping with the fear. *Nursing87, 17*(4), 44-46.

Koop, C. (1987). *Surgeon General's Report on Acquired Immune Deficiency Syndrome.* U. S. Department of Health & Human Services.

Lillard, J., Lotsperch, P., Gurich, J., & Jesse, J. (1984). Acquired immunodeficiency syndrome (AIDS) in home care—maximizing helpfulness and minimizing hysteria. *Home Healthcare Nurse, 2*(6), 11-16.

Peabody, B. (1986). Living with AIDS: A mother's perspective. *American Journal of Nursing, 86*, 45-46.

Popkin, J., et al. (1983). Caring for the AIDS patient. *Nursing83, 13*(9), 50-55.

Questions and answers on acquired immune deficiency syndrome (AIDS). (1982). *California Morbidity Supplement, 12*(10), 48.

Turner, J., et al. (1986). AIDS: a challenge for contemporary nursing. *Focus on Critical Care, 13*(3) 53-61.

Aggression

Boettcher, E. (1983). Preventing violent behavior: An integrated theoretical model for nursing. *Perspectives in Psychiatric Care, 21*(2), 54-58.

Fernandez, T. (1986). Classic: How to deal with overt aggression. *Issues in Mental Health Nursing, 8*(1), 79-83.

Moran, J. (1984). Aggression management: Response and responsibility. *Nursing Times, 80*(5), 28-31.

Schultz, J., & Dark, S. (1982). *Manual of psychiatric nursing care plans.* Boston: Little, Brown.

Alcoholism

"Alcoholism" (and other publications). National Council on Alcoholism, Inc., 2 Park Avenue, New York, NY 10016.

Eells, M. (1986). Interventions with alcoholics and their families. *Nursing Clinics of North America, 21*, 493-504.

Fisk, N. (1986). Alcoholism: Ineffective family coping. *American Journal of Nursing, 86*, 586-587.

Anger

Green, C. (1986). How to recognize hostility and what to do about it. *American Journal of Nursing, 86*, 1230-1234.

Rambo, B. (1984). Coping problems of the self-concept. *Adaptation Nursing*, Philadelphia: Saunders, 277-298.

Anorexia Nervosa

Carino, C., & Chmelko, P. (1983). Disorders of eating in adolescence: Anorexia nervosa and bulimia. *Nursing Clinics of North America, 18*, 343-352.

Claggett, M. (1980). Anorexia nervosa: A behavioral approach. *American Journal of Nursing, 80*, 1471-1472.

Edmands, M. (1986). Overcoming eating disorders: A group experience. *Journal of Psychosocial Nursing, 24,*(8), 19-25.

Forsyth, D. (1982). Binge-vomit disorder may follow anorexia cure. *RN, 45*, 115.

Kiecolt-Glasser, J., & Dixon, K. (1984). Postadolescent onset male anorexia. *Journal of Psychosocial Nursing, 22*(1), 10-20.

Richardson, T. (1980). An overview. *American Journal of Nursing, 80*, 1470.

Sanger, E., et al. (1984). Eating disorders: Avoiding the power struggle. *American Journal of Nursing, 84*, 10-20.

Twiss, J. (1986). The plight of the female adolescent: Anorexia or bulimia. *Issues in Comprehensive Pediatric Nursing, 9*(5), 289-298.

Antisocial Personality Disorder

Frosch, J. (1983). The treatment of antisocial and borderline personality disorders. *Hospital and Community Psychiatry, 34*(3), 243-248.

McMorrow, M. (1981). The manipulative patient. *American Journal of Nursing, 81*, 1188-90.

Anxiety/Stress Management

Jaffee, D. (1980). *Healing from within.* New York: Knopf.

Muller, P. (1987). Avoiding burnout through prevention. *Journal of Post-Anesthesia Nursing, 2*(1), 53-58.

Segal, J. (1981). *Feeling great: Images to health and well being.* Santa Cruz: Unity.

Seyle, H. (1976). *The stress of life,* (revised ed.). New York: McGraw-Hill.

Smitherman, C. (1981). Your patient's anxious: What should you do? *Nursing81, 11*(2), 72-73.

Trygstad, L. (1986). Stress and coping in psychiatric nursing. *Journal of Psychosocial Nursing, 24*(10) 23-27.

Vogelsang, J. (1987). Nursing interventions to reduce patient anxiety. *Journal of Post-Anesthesia Nursing, 2*(1), 25-31.

Autism

Baker, B. (1982). The use of music with autistic children. *Journal of Psychosocial Nursing, 20*(4), 31-34.

Dudziak, D. (1982). Parenting the autistic child. *Journal of Psychosocial Nursing, 20*(1), 11-16.

Verzemnieks, I. (1984). Developmental stimulation for infants and toddlers. *American Journal of Nursing, 84*, 749-752.

Zoltak, B. (1986). Autism: Recognition and management. *Pediatric Nursing, 12*(2), 90-94.

Behavior Modification

Elder, J. (1986). Behavioral management training for families of emotionally handicapped and/or developmentally delayed children. *Issues in Mental Health Nursing, 8*(1), 37-49.

Montgomery, C. (1987). How to set limits when a patient demands too much. *American Journal of Nursing, 87*, 365-366.
Roberts, M., et al. (1980). Behavior modification with a mentally retarded child. *American Journal of Nursing, 80*, 679-680.
Steckel, S. (1980). Anorexia nervosa: Patient behavioral approach. *American Journal of Nursing, 80*, 1471-1472.
Steckel, S. (1980). Contracting with patient-selected reinforcers. *American Journal of Nursing, 80*. 1596-1599.

Borderline Personality Disorders

Egan, J. (1986). Etiology and treatment of borderline personality in adolescents. *Hospital and Community Psychiatry, 37*, 613-618.
Gallop, R. (1985). The patient is splitting. *Journal of Psychosocial Nursing, 23*(4), 6-10.
Hickey, B. (1985). The borderline experience: Subjective impressions. *Journal of Psychosocial Nursing, 23*(4), 24-29.
Kaplan, C. (1986). The challenge of working with patients diagnosed as having a borderline personality disorder. *Nursing Clinics of North America, 21*, 429-438.
Kerr, N. (1987). Patterns of interaction with borderline clients. *Comprehensive psychiatric nursing.* New York: McGraw Hill, 585-600.
McEnany, G., & Tescher, B. (1985). Contracting for care—One nursing approach to the hospitalized patient. *Journal of Psychosocial Nursing, 23*(4), 11-18.
O'Brien, P., Caldwell, C., & Transeau, G. (1985). Destroyers—Written treatment contracts can help cure self-destructive behaviors of the borderline patient. *Journal of Psychosocial Nursing, 23*(4), 19-23.
Platt-Koch, L. (1983). Borderline personality disorder. *American Journal of Nursing, 83*, 1666-1671.

Bulimia

Carino, C., & Chmelko, P. (1983). Disorders of eating in adolescence: Anorexia nervosa and bulimia. *Nursing Clinics of North America, 18*, 343-352.
Kelter, N. (1984). Bulimia: Controlling compulsive eating. *Journal of Psychosocial Nursing, 22*(8), 24-29.
Moore, J., & Coulman, M. (1981). Anorexia nervosa—Patient, family and key family therapy interventions. *Journal of Psychiatric Nursing, 19*(5), 9-14.
Sanger, E., et al. (1984). Eating disorders: Avoiding the power struggle. *American Journal of Nursing, 84*, 30-33.
Twiss, J. (1986). The plight of the female adolescent: anorexia or bulimia. *Issues in Comprehensive Pediatric Nursing, 9*(5), 289-298.
White, J. (1984). Bulimia—Utilizing individual and family therapy. *Journal of Psychosocial Nursing, 22*(4), 22-28.

Chronic Illness

Kodalek, S. (1985). Working with the chronically ill. *Nurse Practitioner, 10*(3), 45-48.
Knafl, K., & Deatrick, J. (1986). How families manage chronic conditions: An analysis of the concept of normalization. *Research in Nursing and Health, 9*(3), 215-222.
Reich, N., & Otten, P. (1987). What to wear: A challenge for disabled elderly. *American Journal of Nursing, 87*, 207-210.
Sexton, D., & Munro, B. (1985). Impact of a husband's chronic illness on the spouse's life. *Research in Nursing and Health, 8*(1), 83-90.
Schmidt, M. (1985). Meet the health care needs of older adults by using a chronic care model. *Journal of Gerontological Nursing, 11*(9), 30-34.

Chronic Organic Brain Syndrome (OBS)

Charatan, F. (1980). Therapeutic supports for the patient with OBS. *Geriatrics*, September, 100-102.
Coyle, M. (1987). Organic illness mimicking psychiatric episodes. *Journal of Gerontologic Nursing, 13*(1), 31-35.
Richardson, K. (1982). Hope and flexibility—Your keys to helping OBS patient. *Nursing 82, 12*(6), 65-69.

Confusion

Campbell, E., Williams, M., & Mlynarczyk, S. (1986). After the fall—Confusion. *American Journal of Nursing, 86*, 151-154.

Hays, A., & Borger, F. (1985). A test in time. *American Journal of Nursing, 85*, 1107-1111.
Langland, R., & Panicucci, C. (1982). Effect of touch on communicating with elderly, confused clients. *Journal of Gerontological Nursing, 8*(3), 152-155.
Montgomery, C. (1987). What you can do for the confused elderly. *Nursing87, 17*(4), 54-56.

Crisis Intervention

Baird, S. (1987). Helping the family through a crisis. *Nursing87, 17*(6), 66-68.

Denial

Elliott, S. (1980). Denial as an effective mechanism to allay anxiety following a stressful event. *Journal of Psychiatric and Mental Health Services, 18*(10), 11-15.
Hagerty, B. (1980). Denial isn't all bad. *Nursing80, 10*(2), 58-60.
Smitherman, C. (1981). Dealing with the patient's denial: What should you do? *Nursing81, 11*(12), 70-71.

Dependent Personality Disorder

Davister, K. (1985). The demanding patient. *Nursing Life, 5*(1), 41.
King, J. (1984). Your health in your hands. *Nursing Times, 80*(44), 51-52.
King, J. (1984). A question of attitude. *Nursing Times, 80*(45), 51-52.

Depression

Field, W. (1985). Physical causes of depression. *Journal of Psychosocial Nursing, 23*(10), 6-11.
Mellencamp, A. (1981). Adolescent depression: A review of the literature with implications for nursing care. *Journal of Psychosocial Nursing and Mental Health Services, 19*(9), 15-20.
Minot, S. (1986). Depression: What does it mean? *American Journal of Nursing, 86*, 283-291.

Depression: Severe

Gordon, V., & Ledray, L. (1985). Depression in women. *Journal of Psychosocial Nursing, 23*(1), 26-34.
Holden, C. (1986). Depression research advances, treatment lags. *Science, 233*(4765), 723-726.
Miller, J. (1985). Inspiring hope. *American Journal of Nursing, 85*, 22-25.
Vogel, C. (1982). Anxiety and depression among the elderly. *Journal of Gerontological Nursing, 8*(4), 213-216.
Author. (1986). Depression (Parts I-IV). *American Journal of Nursing, 86*, 284-288, 288-291, 292-294, 294-297.

Developmental Disability

Bullard, I., and Dohnal, J. (1984). The community deals with the child who has a handicap. *The Nursing Clinics of North America, 19*(2), 309-108.
Elder, J. (1986). Behavioral management training for families of emotionally handicapped and/or developmentally delayed children. *Issues in Mental Health Nursing, 8*(1), 37-49.

Drug Abuse

Anderson, M. (1982). Personalized nursing: A unique approach to drug dependent women. *Journal of Emergency Medicine, 14*, 225-231.
Gary, N., et al. (1983). Barbiturates and a potpourri of other sedatives, hypnotics and tranquilizers—clinical aspects of drug intoxication. *Heart and Lung, 12*, 122-127.
Halpern, J. (1983). Street speed. *Journal of Emergency Nursing, 9*(4), 224-227.
Pallikkathayil, L., & Tweed, S. (1983). Substance abuse: Alcohol and drugs during adolescence. *Nursing Clinics of North America, 18*, 313-322.

Dying/Terminal

Barry, P. (1984). *Psychosocial nursing assessment and intervention.* Philadelphia: Lippincott.
Bourne, E. (1987). What a dying patient needs from you. *RN, 50*(6).
Carpenito, L. (1983). *Nursing diagnosis.* Philadelphia: Lippincott.

Dealing with death and dying. In *New Nursing Skill Book* (2nd ed.). (1984). Springhouse, PA: Nursing84 Books, Springhouse.

Eggerman, S., & Dustin, D. (1985-6). Death orientation and communicating with the terminally ill. *Omega, 16*(3), 255-265.

Gonka, T., & Ruark, J. (1984). *Dying dignified—The health professionals guide to care.* Menlo Park, CA: Addison Wesley.

Henderson, M. (1985). Assessing the elderly: Altered presentations. *American Journal of Nursing, 85,* 1103-1106.

Hover, M. (1985). What Rosie taught us about dying. *RN, 48*(ll), 17-18.

Kubler-Ross, E. (1969). *On death and dying.* New York: Macmillan.

Martocchio, B. (1982). *Living while dying.* Bowie, MD: R. Brady.

Papowitz, L. (1986). Life—Death—Life. *American Journal of Nursing, 86,* 416-418.

Pasquali, E., et al. (1985). *Mental health nursing* (2nd ed.). St. Louis: Mosby.

Pflaum, M., & Kelley, P. (1986). Understanding the final messages of the dying. *Nursing86, 16*(6), 26-29.

Scott, F., & Brewer, R. (1971). *Confrontations of death.* Oregon Center of Gerontology, Eugene, OR. Portland: Continuing Education Publications.

Slaby, A., & Glicksman, A. (1985). *Adapting to life-threatening illnesses.* New York & Philadelphia: Praeger Special Studies, Praeger Scientific.

Snyder, C. (1986). *Oncology nursing.* Boston: Little, Brown.

Stedeford, A. (1984). *Facing death—Patients, family and professionals.* Portsmouth, NH: Wm. Heinemann Medical Books Ltd.

Stuart, G., & Sundeen, S. (1983). *Principles and practice of psychiatric nursing* (2nd ed.). St. Louis: Mosby.

Trent, C. (1985). Your patient is dying. *Nursing Life, 5*(6), 18-21.

Grief

Cowles, K. (1984). Life, death, and personhood. *Nursing Outlook, 32*(3), 168-172.

Jillings, C. (1985). Loss and grief: Unravelling two complex phenomena. *Critical Care Nurse, 5*(5), 7-9.

Williams, M. (1984). Use of a concluding process to assist grieving families. *Journal of Emergency Nursing, 10*(5), 254-258.

Guilt

Johnson, S. (1984). Counseling families experiencing guilt. *Dimensions of Critical Care Nursing, 3*(4), 238-244.

Knowles, R. (1981). Managing guilt. *American Journal of Nursing, 81,* 1850.

Knowles, R. (1981). Worry journal and guilty time. *American Journal of Nursing, 81,* 2035.

Manic Behavior

Brenners, D., Harris, B., & Weston, P. (1987). Managing manic behavior. *American Journal of Nursing, 87,* 620-623.

Manipulation

Chitty, K., & Maynard, C. (1986). Managing manipulation. *Journal of Psychosocial Nursing, 24*(6), 9-13.

Mental Status Exam

Harris, E. (1981). Mental status assessment . . . Programmed instruction. *American Journal of Nursing, 81,* 1493-1518.

Noncompliance

Magnani, L. (1985). The man who wrote too much. *American Journal of Nursing, 85,* 867-877.

Obsessive-Compulsive Disorder

Runck, B. (1983). Research is changing views on obsessive-compulsive disorder. *Hospital and Community Psychiatry, 34,* 597-598.

Pain

Dolan, M. (1982). Controlling pain in a personal way. *Nursing82, 12*(1), 144.

Heidrich, G., Perry, S. (1982). Helping the patient in pain. *American Journal of Nursing, 82,* 1828-1833.

McGuire, L., & Dizard, S. (1982). Managing pain in the young patient. *Nursing82, 12*(2), 52-55.

Meinhart, N., & McCaffery, M. (1983). *Pain: A nursing approach to assessment and analysis.* Norwalk, CT: Appleton-Century-Crofts.

Olsson, G., & Parker, G. (1987). A model approach to pain assessment. *Nursing87, 17*(5), 52-57.

Panayotoff, K. (1982). Managing pain in the elderly patient. *Nursing82, 12*(2), 53-57.

Snyder, C. (1986). *Oncology nursing.* Boston: Little, Brown.

Willoughby, S. (1985). Pain. In J. McNally, J. Stair, & E. Somerville (Eds.), *Guidelines for cancer nursing practice.* Orlando: Grune & Stratton.

Phobic Disorder

Davis, J. (1982). Treatment of a medical phobia including desensitization administered by a significant other. *Journal of Psychosocial Nursing, 20*(8), 6-8.

Post-Traumatic Stress Disorder

Allen, I. (1986). Post-traumatic stress among black Vietnam veterans. *Hospital and Community Psychiatry, 37*(1), 55-61.

Burgess, A. (1985). *Psychiatric nursing in the hospital and the community.* Englewood Cliffs, NJ: Prentice-Hall.

Christenson, R., Walker, J., Ross, D., & Maltbie, A. (1981). Reactivation of traumatic conflicts. *American Journal of Psychiatry, 138*(7), 984-985.

Davidson, P., & Jackson, C. (1985). The nurse as a survivor—Delayed post-traumatic stress reaction and cumulative trauma in nursing. *International Journal of Nursing Studies, 22*(1), 1-13.

Frye, J. (Ed.), & Stockton, R. (1982). Discriminant analysis of post-traumatic stress disorder among a group of Vietnam veterans. *American Journal of Psychiatry, 139*(1), 52-56.

Horowitz, M. (1986). Stress-response syndromes: A review of post-traumatic and adjustment disorders. *Hospital and Community Psychiatry, 37*(3), 241-249.

Laufer, R., Brett, E., Gallops, M., & Phil, M. (1985). Symptom patterns associated with post-traumatic stress disorder among Viet Nam veterans exposed to war trauma. *American Journal of Psychiatry, 142*(11), 1304-1311.

McFarland, G., & Wasli, E. (1986). *Nursing diagnosis and process in psychiatric mental health nursing.* Philadelphia: Lippincott.

Mullis, M. (1984). Vietnam—The human fallout. *Journal of Psychosocial Nursing, 22*(2), 27-31.

Resing, M. (1982). Mental health problems of Vietnam veterans. *Journal of Psychosocial Nursing, 20*(9), 40-43.

Schottenfeld, R., & Cullen, M. (1985). Occupation induced post-traumatic stress disorder. *American Journal of Psychiatry, 142*(2), 198-202.

Schwartz, H. (Ed.). (1984). *Psychotherapy of the combat veteran.* New York: Spectrum Publications Medical and Scientific Books.

Powerlessness

Kritek, P. (1981). Patient power and powerlessness. *Supervisor Nurse, 12*(6), 26-31.

Lambert, V., & Lambert, C. (1981). Role theory and concept of powerlessness. *Journal of Psychosocial Nursing, 19*(9), 11-14.

Psychotropic Medications

Cohen, M., et al. (1981). Medication group for psychiatric patients. *American Journal of Nursing, 81,* 343-345.

DeGennaro, M., et al. (1981). Antidepressant drug threapy. *American Journal of Nursing, 81,* 1304-1310.

Divson, D. (1981). Manic-depression: An overview. *Journal of Psychiatric Nursing, 19*(6), 28-31.

Harris, E. (1981). Antipsychotic medications. *American Journal of Nursing, 81,* 1316-1319.

Harris, E. (1981). Extrapyramidal side effects of antipsychotic therapy. *American Journal of Nursing, 81,* 1324-1328.

Harris, E. (1981). Lithium. *American Journal of Nursing, 81,* 1310-1315.

Harris, E. (1981). Sedative-hypnotic drugs. *American Journal of Nursing, 81,* 1329-1334.

Preventing excessive weight gain from psychotropic drugs. (1981). *Nurses Drug Alert, 5*(1), 5.

Preventing psychotropic-induced seizures. (1981). *Nurses Drug Alert, 5*(3), 23.

Selander, J., & Miller, W. (1985). Prolixin group: Can nursing intervention groups lower recidivism rates? *Journal of Psychosocial nursing, 23*(11), 16-20.

Rape Trauma Syndrome

DiNitto, D., Martin, P., Norton, D., & Maxwell, M. (1986). After rape: Who should examine rape survivors? *American Journal of Nursing, 86,* 538-540.

DiVasto, P. (1985). Measuring the aftermath of rape. *Journal of Psychosocial Nursing, 23*(2), 33-35.

Leach, A. (1982). Threat to the nurse's sexual identity. In *Comprehensive psychiatric nursing* (2nd ed.). New York: McGraw-Hill.

Moynihan, B., et al. (1981). Symposium on emergency nursing. The role of the nurse in the care of sexual assault victims. *Nursing Clinics of North America, 16* 95-100.

Tolbert, S., et al. (1980). Improving emergency department care of the sexual assault victim. *Annals of Emergency Medicine*, June, 293-297.

Reality Orientation

King, K. (1982). Reminiscing psychotherapy with aging people. *Journal of Psychosocial Nursing, 20*(2), 21-25.

Langston, N. (1981). Reality orientation and effective reinforcement. *Journal of Gerontological Nursing, 7,* 224-227.

Remotivation/Resocialization

Carter, C., & Galliano, D. (1981). Fear of loss and attachment. *Journal of Gerontological Nursing, 7,* 342-349.

Ryden, M. (1981). Nursing intervention in support of reminiscence. *Journal of Gerontological Nursing, 7,* 461-463.

Schizophrenia

Field, W. (1985). Hearing Voices. *Journal of Psychosocial Nursing, 23*(1), 8-14.

Kahn, E. (1984). Psychotherapy with chronic schizophrenics. *Journal of Psychosocial Nursing, 22*(7), 20-25.

Seymour, R., & Dawson, N. (1986). The schizophrenic at home. *Journal of Psychosocial Nursing, 24*(1), 28-30.

Tousley, M. (1984). The paranoid fortress of David J. *Journal of Psychosocial Nursing, 22*(2), 8-16.

Strategies for Counseling Adolescents

Adams, B. (1983). Adolescent health care: Needs, priorities and services. *Nursing Clinics of North America, 18,* 237-248.

Moss, N. (1984). Child therapy groups in the real world. *Journal of Psychosocial Nursing, 22*(3), 43-48.

Numerof, R. (1980). Assertiveness training. *American Journal of Nursing, 80,* 1796-1799.

Reighley, J. (1982). Going with the risk. In *Nurses in Business*, M. Neal, Ed. Pacific Palisades, CA: Nurseco.

Rice, M. (1983). Review: Identifying the adolescent substance abuser. *MCN: The American Journal of Maternal-Child Nursing, 8,* 139-142.

Smith, M. (1975). *When I say no I feel guilty.* New York: Dial.

Suicide

Assay, J. (1985). The suicide prevention contract. *Perspectives in Psychiatric Care, 23*(3), 99-103.

Moore, I. (1986). Ending it all. *Nursing Times, 82*(7), 48-49.

Pallikkathayil, L., & McBride, A. (1986). Suicide attempts: The search for meaning. *Journal of Psychosocial Nursing, 24*(8), 13-18.

Valente, S. (1985). The suicidal teenager. *Nursing85, 15*(12), 47-49.

Violent Behavior

Jones, M. (1985). Patient violence: Report of 200 incidents. *Journal of Psychosocial Nursing, 23*(6), 12-17.

Oertz, B. (1980). Training for prevention of assaultive behavior in psychiatric setting. *Hospital and Community Psychiatry, 31,* 628-632.

Roper, J., Coutts, A., Sather, J., & Taylor, R. (1985). Restraint and seclusion: A standard and standard care plan. *Journal of Psychosocial Nursing, 23*(6), 18-23.

INDEX

259

physical/mental deficit, 198
regressed behaviors, 155, 158
ritualistic behavior, 101
Self-concept, disturbance in: body image,
    self-esteem, role performance,
    personal identity related to
altered body structure or function, 27,
    184
chronic illness, 39
decreased self-esteem, 226
distorted perceptions of body size, body
    image, 36, 195, 226
feelings of inadequacy, 91
feelings of unworthiness and lack of
    trust, 95
guilt associated with traumatic
    experience, 111
illness, hospitalization, 70, 135
impact of specific illness characteristics,
    188
inability to master autonomy, 32
inability to trust, 122
ineffective coping, 91
lack of appreciation for own value and
    abilities, 55, 58
lack of confidence in ability to
    accomplish what is desired, 55
life changes, 172
maladaptive situational, maturational,
    or physiologic factors, 146
misperceptions of body size, 17
parental abuse, 215
perceived loss of control, function, or
    propriety, resulting in feeling of
    humiliation, 132
real or threatened losses, 64
threat to self-esteem, 128
weak ego formation, 32
withdrawal from contact with others,
    122
Sensory-perceptual alteration: visual,
    auditory, kinesthetic, gustatory,
    tactile, olfactory related to
aging, 165
amount and meaningfulness of
    environmental stimuli, 129
distortion, 167
monotony, 167
overload, 167

Sexuality patterns, altered, related to
    physiologic limitations and life-style
    changes imposed by disease process,
    7
Skin integrity, impaired/impairment of,
    related to
decreased nutritional intake, 209
immunosuppression, 4
Sleep pattern disturbance related to
anxiety caused by stressful event(s),
    113, 178, 195
fears, 195
hyperactivity, 90
inability to fall asleep within 20 minutes
    of bedtime, 130
inactivity, 195
physiologic disturbances caused by
    anxiety, 23
sleeping during day and staying awake
    at night, 130, 195
Social interaction, impaired, related to
alteration in thought processes, 124
dysfunctional behavior, 180
fear, 172
grieving over diagnosis, 6
isolation precautions, 6
lack of experience with group process,
    172
shyness, 172
Social isolation related to
alterations in life-style, 171
confusion, 44
depression, 112
fear of being unable to obtain warmth
    and companionship from others, 162
feelings of alienation, 112
impaired interpersonal relationships,
    20
instability of social and interpersonal
    relationships, 31
lack of meaningful relationships, 171
limitations in outside contacts and
    activities imposed by chronic illness,
    40
limited verbal communication, 63
parents' gradual withdrawal from
    friends and community resources
    after diagnosis of chronic illness in
    their child, 189

separation from familiy, friends, and
    confinement to hospital environment,
    75, 204
societal nonacceptance of disease, 6
withdrawal, 44, 63, 112
Spiritual distress related to
disturbance in belief system, 76
hopelessness, 76
inability to participate in services, 76
loss of life and suffering, 87
Swallowing, impaired, related to
esophagitis, 5

Thought processes, alteration in, related
    to
anger, 101
anxiety, 91, 101
apathy, 168
cerebral pathology, 7, 159
cognitive, mental deterioration, 165
confusion, 156
disinterest, 168
forgetfulness, 156
inability to cope with feelings, 91
inability to evaluate reality, 123
inability to perceive realistically or
    interact appropriately with others,
    156
metabolic disturbances, 43
misinterpretations of reality, 64
neurologic trauma or dysfunction, 43
short attention span, 168

Violence, potential for, related to
feelings of anger, hostility, 62
impulsive, acting-out behaviors, 20, 30
inability to control anger, 30
intense feelings of anger, betrayal, or
    fear, 112
physically destructive behavior, 10
sensory-perceptual alteration, 151
suicidal ideation, 62
Violence, potential for: self-directed,
    related to
anxiety, 226
dysfunctional grieving, 226
fear, 226
inability to control behavior, 149
suicidal ideation, 145